T0213355

RADIOBIOLOGY
SELF-ASSESSMENT GUIDE

RADIOBIOLOGY SELF-ASSESSMENT GUIDE

Edited by

Jennifer S. Yu, MD, PhD
Associate Staff Physician
Departments of Radiation Oncology and Stem Cell Biology and Regenerative Medicine
Taussig Cancer Institute and Lerner Research Institute
Cleveland Clinic
Cleveland, Ohio

Mohamed E. Abazeed, MD, PhD
Associate Staff Physician
Departments of Radiation Oncology and Translational Hematologic and
Oncologic Research
Taussig Cancer Institute and Lerner Research Institute
Cleveland Clinic
Cleveland, Ohio

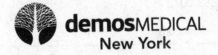

demosMEDICAL
New York

Visit our website at www.demosmedical.com

ISBN: 9781620701140
e-book ISBN: 9781617052910

Acquisitions Editor: David D'Addona
Compositor: diacriTech

Medicine is an ever-changing science. Research and clinical experience are continually expanding our knowledge, in particular our understanding of proper treatment and drug therapy. The authors, editors, and publisher have made every effort to ensure that all information in this book is in accordance with the state of knowledge at the time of production of the book. Nevertheless, the authors, editors, and publisher are not responsible for errors or omissions or for any consequences from application of the information in this book and make no warranty, expressed or implied, with respect to the contents of the publication. Every reader should examine carefully the package inserts accompanying each drug and should carefully check whether the dosage schedules mentioned therein or the contraindications stated by the manufacturer differ from the statements made in this book. Such examination is particularly important with drugs that are either rarely used or have been newly released on the market.

Library of Congress Cataloging-in-Publication Data

Names: Yu, Jennifer (Jennifer S.), editor. | Abazeed, Mohamed E., editor.
Title: Radiobiology self-assessment guide / editors, Jennifer Yu, Mohamed Abazeed.
Description: New York: Demos Medical, 2016. | Includes bibliographical references and index.
Identifiers: LCCN 2016028793 | ISBN 9781620701140 | ISBN 9781617052910 (e-book)
Subjects: | MESH: Radiologic Health | Radiobiology | Examination Questions
Classification: LCC QH652.A1 | NLM WN 18.2 | DDC 612/.01448—dc23 LC record available at https://lccn.loc.gov/2016028793

Special discounts on bulk quantities of Demos Medical Publishing books are available to corporations, professional associations, pharmaceutical companies, health care organizations, and other qualifying groups. For details, please contact:

Special Sales Department
Demos Medical Publishing
11 West 42nd Street, 15th Floor,
New York, NY 10036
Phone: 800-532-8663 or 212-683-0072
Fax: 212-941-7842
E-mail: specialsales@demosmedical.com

Printed in the United States of America by McNaughton & Gunn.
16 17 18 19 20 / 5 4 3 2 1

To my dearest Yoon and Daniel, our parents, David and Min and their families, for their love, compassion, and inspiration.

–Jennifer S. Yu

Nanos gigantum humeris insidentes.

–Mohamed E. Abazeed

CONTENTS

Contents

Mohamed E. Abazeed, MD, PhD
Associate Staff Physician
Departments of Radiation Oncology and
  Translational Hematologic and Oncologic
  Research
Taussig Cancer Institute and Lerner Research
  Institute
Cleveland Clinic
Cleveland, Ohio

Alex Almasan, PhD
Staff
Department of Cancer Biology
Cleveland Clinic
Cleveland, Ohio

Sudha Amarnath, MD
Assistant Professor
Department of Radiation Oncology
Cleveland Clinic
Cleveland, Ohio

Marc Apple, MD
Staff
Department of Radiation Oncology
Cleveland Clinic Florida
Weston, Florida

Ehsan H. Balagamwala, MD
Resident Physician
Department of Radiation Oncology
Cleveland Clinic
Cleveland, Ohio

Salim Balik, PhD
Medical Physicist
Department of Radiation Oncology
Cleveland Clinic;
Assistant Professor
Department of Medicine
Lerner College of Medicine of
  Case Western Reserve University
Cleveland, Ohio

Eli Bar, PhD
Assistant Professor
Department of Neurological Surgery
Case Western Reserve University School of
  Medicine and Case Comprehensive Cancer
  Center
Cleveland, Ohio

Camille Berriochoa, MD
Resident Physician
Department of Radiation Oncology
Cleveland Clinic
Cleveland, Ohio

HyeonJoo Cheon, PhD
Project Staff
Department of Cancer Biology
Lerner Research Institute
Cleveland Clinic;
Assistant Professor
Department of Molecular Medicine
Cleveland Clinic Lerner College of Medicine
Cleveland, Ohio

Taoran Cui, PhD
Medical Physics Resident
Department of Radiation Oncology
Cleveland Clinic
Cleveland, Ohio

Sharvari, Dharmaiah, BA
Graduate Student/Research Assistant
Department of Stem Cell Biology and
    Regenerative Medicine
Lerner Research Institute
Cleveland Clinic
Cleveland, Ohio

Frank Dong, PhD
Medical Physicist
Department of Diagnostic Radiology
Cleveland Clinic;
Associate Professor
Lerner College of Medicine of
    Case Western Reserve University
Cleveland, Ohio

Andrew Godley, PhD
Assistant Professor
Department of Radiation Oncology
Cleveland Clinic
Cleveland, Ohio

John F. Greskovich, Jr., MD, MBA
Medical Director
Department of Radiation Oncology
Cleveland Clinic Florida
Weston, Florida

Haidong Huang, PhD
Postdoctoral Fellow
Department of Stem Cell Biology and
    Regenerative Medicine
Lerner Research Institute
Cleveland Clinic
Cleveland, Ohio

Nikhil Joshi, MD
Associate Staff/Assistant Professor
Department of Radiation Oncology
Cleveland Clinic
Cleveland, Ohio

Aditya Juloori, MD
Resident Physician
Department of Radiation Oncology
Cleveland Clinic
Cleveland, Ohio

Jeffrey A. Kittel, MD
Former Resident
Department of Radiation Oncology
Cleveland Clinic
Cleveland, Ohio

Susan Kost, PhD
Medical Physics Resident
Department of Radiation Oncology
Cleveland Clinic
Cleveland, Ohio

Daesung Lee, MD
Staff Physician
Department of Radiation Oncology
Cleveland Clinic
Cleveland, Ohio

C. Marc Leyrer, MD
Resident Physician
Department of Radiation Oncology
Cleveland Clinic
Cleveland, Ohio

Bindu V. Manyam, MD
Resident Physician
Department of Radiation Oncology
Cleveland Clinic
Cleveland, Ohio

Anthony Mastroianni, JD, MBA, MD
Staff Physician
Department of Radiation Oncology
Cleveland Clinic
Cleveland, Ohio

Mihir Naik, DO
Staff
Department of Radiation Oncology
Cleveland Clinic Florida
Weston, Florida

Steven Oh, MD
Former Resident
Department of Radiation Oncology
Cleveland Clinic
Cleveland, Ohio

Yvonne Pham, MD
Resident Physician
Department of Radiation Oncology
Cleveland Clinic
Cleveland, Ohio

Peng Qi, PhD
Medical Physicist
Department of Radiation Oncology
Cleveland Clinic
Cleveland, Ohio

Vinay Rao
Research Assistant
Department of Stem Cell Biology and
    Regenerative Medicine;
Research Technician
Department of Cellular and Molecular Medicine
Lerner Research Institute
Cleveland Clinic
Cleveland, Ohio

Richard Blake Ross
Medical Student
School of Medicine
Case Western Reserve University
Cleveland, Ohio

Chirag Shah, MD
Associate Staff
Department of Radiation Oncology
Cleveland Clinic
Cleveland, Ohio

Matthew C. Ward, MD
Resident Physician
Department of Radiation Oncology
Cleveland Clinic
Cleveland, Ohio

Michael A. Weller, MD
Associate Staff
Department of Radiation Oncology
Cleveland Clinic
Cleveland, Ohio

Neil Woody, MD
Associate Staff
Department of Radiation Oncology
Cleveland Clinic
Cleveland, Ohio

Kevin Wunderle, MSc
Medical Physicist
Department of Diagnostic Radiology
Cleveland Clinic
Cleveland, Ohio

Choamei Xiang, PhD
Former Postdoctoral Fellow
Department of Stem Cell Biology and
    Regenerative Medicine
Lerner Research Institute
Cleveland Clinic
Cleveland, Ohio

Kailin Yang, PhD
Medical Student
Lerner Research Institute
Cleveland Clinic
Cleveland, Ohio

Brian D. Yard, PhD
Postdoctoral Fellow
Department of Translational
    Hematologic and Oncologic Research
Cleveland Clinic
Cleveland, Ohio

Jennifer S. Yu, MD, PhD
Associate Staff Physician
Departments of Radiation Oncology and
    Stem Cell Biology and Regenerative
    Medicine
Taussig Cancer Institute and Lerner Research
    Institute
Cleveland Clinic
Cleveland, Ohio

Xingjiang Yu, PhD
Postdoctoral Fellow
Department of Stem Cell Biology and
    Regenerative Medicine
Lerner Research Institute
Cleveland Clinic
Cleveland, Ohio

PREFACE

We are pleased to introduce the inaugural edition of *Radiobiology Self-Assessment Guide*. This guide provides up-to-date comprehensive concepts in classical radiation biology and contemporary research on stem cell biology, tumor immunology and immunotherapy, and radiogenomics.
It succinctly covers topics that are germane to the understanding of radiobiology and related disciplines in oncology. It uses more than 700 questions in a flash-card question-and-answer format to stimulate active learning and reinforce key concepts. Schematics and figures are used to clarify important ideas and references are included with each answer to facilitate independent in-depth learning.

This guide complements *Radiation Oncology Self-Assessment Guide* and *Physics in Radiation Oncology Self-Assessment Guide*. Together, these guides provide a thorough review of the clinical management of cancer, medical physics, and radiation biology.

We are indebted to the many experts from the Cleveland Clinic and Case Comprehensive Cancer Center who contributed to this book. We hope that this guide will prove an invaluable and high-yield resource for anyone interested in classical and contemporary radiation biology.

Jennifer S. Yu
Mohamed E. Abazeed

1

INTERACTION OF RADIATION WITH MATTER

JOHN F. GRESKOVICH, JR., MIHIR NAIK, AND MARC APPLE

Question 1
What type of decay does Radium-226 undergo, and what particles are produced in the decay?

Question 2
What are the names of the types of photons within the electromagnetic spectrum from lowest and highest energy?

Question 3
What is the relationship between photon energy, wavelength, and frequency?

Question 4
What is a photon?

Turn page to see the answers.   3

Question 1 *What type of decay does Radium-226 undergo, and what particles are produced in the decay?*

Answer 1

Radium-226 decays by α-decay, creating radon gas (Rn-222) and an alpha particle plus 4.87 MeV of released energy. An alpha particle is a helium nucleus consisting of two protons and two neutrons. The emission of an alpha particle decreases the atomic number by two and the mass number by four.

Hall EJ, Giaccia AJ. Physics and chemistry of radiation absorption. In: Hall EJ, Giaccia AJ, eds. *Radiobiology for the Radiologist*. 7th ed. Philadelphia, PA: Lippincott Williams & Wilkins; 2012:3–11.

Question 2 *What are the names of the types of photons within the electromagnetic spectrum from lowest and highest energy?*

Answer 2

Photons travel as electromagnetic waves, described by the electromagnetic spectrum. This spectrum defines regions based on their energy (and hence wavelength or frequency). From lowest energy (and lowest frequency, highest wavelength) the spectrum starts with radio waves, then microwaves, infrared waves, visible waves, ultraviolet waves, x-rays, and gamma rays.

Hall EJ, Giaccia AJ. Physics and chemistry of radiation absorption. In: Hall EJ, Giaccia AJ, eds. *Radiobiology for the Radiologist*. 7th ed. Philadelphia, PA: Lippincott Williams & Wilkins; 2012:3–11.

Question 3 *What is the relationship between photon energy, wavelength, and frequency?*

Answer 3

The higher the photon energy, the higher the frequency and the smaller the wavelength. Therefore, photon energy is proportional to frequency and inversely proportional to wavelength. This is formalized in the relationship called Planck's equation: $E = h\nu$ where E is energy in Joules (J), h is Planck's constant, 4.13×10^{-18} keV-sec, and ν is the frequency in Hertz (Hz, sec^{-1}). Using the electromagnetic wave equation, $c = \lambda\nu$ we can arrive at the equation $E = hc/\lambda$ where c is the speed of light, 3.0×10^8 m/sec.

A useful equation is: Energy (keV) = $12.4/\lambda$(angstroms) where angstrom = 10^{-10} m.

Hall EJ, Giaccia AJ. Physics and chemistry of radiation absorption. In: Hall EJ, Giaccia AJ, eds. *Radiobiology for the Radiologist*. 7th ed. Philadelphia, PA: Lippincott Williams & Wilkins; 2012:3–11.

Question 4 *What is a photon?*

Answer 4

A photon is the fundamental particle of electromagnetic radiation, typically described dually as "packets" of energy (Quantum Theory) and as waves of electrical and magnetic energy (Wave Theory). A photon has no mass or charge.

Hall EJ, Giaccia AJ. Physics and chemistry of radiation absorption. In: Hall EJ, Giaccia AJ, eds. *Radiobiology for the Radiologist*. 7th ed. Philadelphia, PA: Lippincott Williams & Wilkins; 2012:3–11.

Question 5
What is the energy range for visible light? x-rays and γ-rays? Why doesn't visible light cause ionization in tissue?

Question 6
What is ionization? What is excitation? Which photons in the electromagnetic spectrum are ionizing and which are nonionizing?

Question 7
What is the difference between x-rays and γ-rays?

Question 8
Describe the Compton scatter photon interaction.

Question 5 *What is the energy range for visible light? x-rays and γ-rays? Why doesn't visible light cause ionization in tissue?*

Answer 5

Using the equation Energy (keV) = 12.4/ λ (angstroms), we can calculate the energy of visible light as 1 to 3 eV since the λ for visible light is 4,000 to 7,000 angstroms. The energy for x-rays and γ-rays are typically in the keV to MeV range since the λ for x-rays and γ-rays are in the 10^2 to 10^{-4} angstrom range. Visible light does not cause ionization in tissue since the average energy for an ionizing event is 34 eV, significantly higher than the 1 to 3 eV energy of visible light.

Hall EJ, Giaccia AJ. Physics and chemistry of radiation absorption. In: Hall EJ, Giaccia, AJ, eds. *Radiobiology for the Radiologist.* 7th ed. Philadelphia, PA: Lippincott Williams & Wilkins; 2012:3–11.

Question 6 *What is ionization? What is excitation? Which photons in the electromagnetic spectrum are ionizing and which are nonionizing?*

Answer 6

Ionization is when enough energy is delivered to eject an electron from an atom or molecule, leading to an electron–ion pair. The average energy dissipated after an ionizing event is 34 eV, enough energy to break a carbon=carbon bond (C=C binding energy is 4.9 eV). Ionizing radiation consists of photons in the ultraviolet, x-ray, and γ-ray range. Nonionizing radiation consists of radio waves, microwaves, infrared (heat) radiation, and visible light. Excitation is the raising of an electron to a higher energy shell without ejection of the electron from the shell.

Hall EJ, Giaccia AJ. Physics and chemistry of radiation absorption. In: Hall EJ, Giaccia AJ, eds. *Radiobiology for the Radiologist.* 7th ed. Philadelphia, PA: Lippincott Williams & Wilkins; 2012:3–11.

Question 7 *What is the difference between x-rays and γ-rays?*

Answer 7

X-rays and γ-rays are two forms of high-energy electromagnetic radiation. They are not different in their physical properties, but their designation reflects the different ways that they are produced. X-rays are produced extranuclearly and γ-rays are produced intranuclearly. For example, x-rays are produced in an electrical device that is used to accelerate electrons and stop them abruptly in a target made of a metal like tungsten or gold (i.e., linear accelerator). However, γ-rays are emitted by radioactive isotopes and represent excess energy that is given off as an unstable nucleus breaks up and decays to reach a more stable form.

Hall EJ, Giaccia AJ. Physics and chemistry of radiation absorption. In: Hall EJ, Giaccia AJ, eds. *Radiobiology for the Radiologist.* 7th ed. Philadelphia, PA: Lippincott Williams & Wilkins; 2012:3–11.

Question 8 *Describe the Compton scatter photon interaction.*

Answer 8

In a Compton scatter photon interaction, the incident x-ray photon interacts with a "free" outer shell electron, ejecting it from the nucleus as a fast electron, and continuing on as a scattered x-ray photon of lower energy. Part of the energy of the incident x-ray photon is imparted to the electron as kinetic energy, and the balance of energy is kept by the scattered x-ray photon. The initial photon may give 0% to 80% of its kinetic energy to the free electron, and this free electron causes ionization of other atoms and produces the chemical and biological effects seen.

Hall EJ, Giaccia AJ. Physics and chemistry of radiation absorption. In: Hall EJ, Giaccia AJ, eds. *Radiobiology for the Radiologist.* 7th ed. Philadelphia, PA: Lippincott Williams & Wilkins; 2012:3–11.

Question 9
What tissue and energy factors drive the probability of Compton scatter?

Question 10
Why are high-energy x-rays (MeV) favored over low-energy x-rays (keV) for treatment of most tumors in the body?

Question 11
Describe the photoelectric effect photon interaction. For what energy x-rays does photoelectric effect occur? What tissue and energy factors drive the probability of photoelectric effect?

Question 9 *What tissue and energy factors drive the probability of Compton scatter?*

Answer 9

Compton scatter is the most common interaction for x-rays in the therapeutic radiation energy range, dominating for energies between 25 keV and 23 MeV. The probability of Compton scatter is directly proportional to the electron density (electrons/gram) of the material and inversely proportional to the photon energy, and is independent of the Z (atomic number) of the material. This is the most common type of interaction seen at energies used in radiotherapy treatment. The mass absorption coefficient for the Compton process is independent of the atomic number of the absorbing material, unlike the photoelectric effect where it varies based on the atomic number and is proportional to Z^3.

Hall EJ, Giaccia AJ. Physics and chemistry of radiation absorption. In: Hall EJ, Giaccia AJ, eds. *Radiobiology for the Radiologist*. 7th ed. Philadelphia, PA: Lippincott Williams & Wilkins; 2012:3–11.

Question 10 *Why are high-energy x-rays (MeV) favored over low-energy x-rays (keV) for treatment of most tumors in the body?*

Answer 10

High-energy (MeV) x-rays are preferred for therapy since Compton scatter interactions predominate, leading to a nearly equal dose distribution in tissues of different Z (atomic numbers) such as bone, muscle, and soft tissue. Lower energy x-ray (keV) interactions in tissue are dominated by the photoelectric effect, which is dependent on the Z and is proportional to Z^3, leading to a higher energy deposition in high Z tissues such as bone.

Hall EJ, Giaccia AJ. Physics and chemistry of radiation absorption. In: Hall EJ, Giaccia AJ, eds. *Radiobiology for the Radiologist*. 7th ed. Philadelphia, PA: Lippincott Williams & Wilkins; 2012:3–11.

Question 11 *Describe the photoelectric effect photon interaction. For what energy x-rays does photoelectric effect occur? What tissue and energy factors drive the probability of photoelectric effect?*

Answer 11

In a photoelectric effect photon interaction, the incident x-ray photon interacts with an "inner" shell electron, ejecting it from the nucleus as a fast electron, and losing all of its energy to the electron. As outer shell electrons (or outside electrons) fill in the inner shell electron vacancy, characteristic x-rays are released. The kinetic energy of the ejected inner shell electron equals the energy of the incident x-ray photon ($h\nu$)—E_{bind}, where E_{bind} is binding energy of the inner shell electron.

The photoelectric effect is the most common interaction for x-rays in the diagnostic x-ray energy range, dominating for energies below 25 keV. The probability of the photoelectric effect is directly proportional to Z^3 (atomic number^3) and inversely proportional to E^3.

Hall EJ, Giaccia AJ. Physics and chemistry of radiation absorption. In: Hall EJ, Giaccia AJ, eds. *Radiobiology for the Radiologist*. 7th ed. Philadelphia, PA: Lippincott Williams & Wilkins; 2012:3–11.

Question 12
X-rays interact with tissue to produce fast electrons through Compton scatter. By what two mechanisms do fast electrons damage DNA?

Question 13
What predominant form of DNA damage is caused by x-rays and low linear energy transfer (LET) radiation versus high LET radiation?

Question 14
What is the theoretical maximum dose reduction factor for free radical scavengers when administered to decrease the biological effectiveness of low linear energy transfer (LET) radiation?

Question 15
What are the names in the sequence of events along with the time it takes for each event to occur going from low linear energy transfer (LET) radiation exposure to biological effect?

Question 12 *X-rays interact with tissue to produce fast electrons through Compton scatter. By what two mechanisms do fast electrons damage DNA?*

Answer 12

Fast electrons produce DNA damage in two general ways: (a) *direct action* where the fast electron itself directly damages the DNA, and (b) *indirect* action where the fast electron interacts with water molecules to produce free radicals which cause the damage to the DNA. It is estimated that 2/3 of the DNA damage from x-ray therapy is via indirect action.

Hall EJ, Giaccia AJ. Physics and chemistry of radiation absorption. In: Hall EJ, Giaccia AJ, eds. *Radiobiology for the Radiologist*. 7th ed. Philadelphia, PA: Lippincott Williams & Wilkins; 2012:3–11.

Question 13 *What predominant form of DNA damage is caused by x-rays and low linear energy transfer (LET) radiation versus high LET radiation?*

Answer 13

It is estimated that free radicals produced through indirect action cause approximately 2/3 of the DNA damage in low LET radiation and that direct action is the dominant form of DNA damage in high LET radiation.

Hall EJ, Giaccia AJ. Physics and chemistry of radiation absorption. In: Hall EJ, Giaccia AJ, eds. *Radiobiology for the Radiologist*. 7th ed. Philadelphia, PA: Lippincott Williams & Wilkins; 2012:3–11.

Question 14 *What is the theoretical maximum dose reduction factor for free radical scavengers when administered to decrease the biological effectiveness of low linear energy transfer (LET) radiation?*

Answer 14

Since 2/3 of the DNA damage from x-ray therapy is via indirect action, that is, formation of free radicals such as the hydroxyl radical, the theoretical maximum dose reduction factor for free radical scavengers is 3.

Hall EJ, Giaccia AJ. Physics and chemistry of radiation absorption. In: Hall EJ, Giaccia AJ, eds. *Radiobiology for the Radiologist*. 7th ed. Philadelphia, PA: Lippincott Williams & Wilkins; 2012:3–11.

Question 15 *What are the names in the sequence of events along with the time it takes for each event to occur going from low linear energy transfer (LET) radiation exposure to biological effect?*

Answer 15

There are six events which occur after low LET radiation exposure to tissue, leading to biological effects: (a) ionization (10^{-15} sec), (b) ion radical (10^{-10} sec), (c) free radical (10^{-9} sec), (d) DNA radicals (10^{-5} sec), (e) chemical reactions (minutes to days), and (f) biological effect (minutes to generations).

Hall EJ, Giaccia AJ. Physics and chemistry of radiation absorption. In: Hall EJ, Giaccia AJ, eds. *Radiobiology for the Radiologist*. 7th ed. Philadelphia, PA: Lippincott Williams & Wilkins; 2012:3–11.

Question 16
Compare and contrast the following particulate radiation: electrons, positrons, protons, neutrons, and alpha particles. What is their mass ratio?

Question 17
How does radon gas cause lung cancer?

Question 18
What are neutrons?

Question 16 *Compare and contrast the following particulate radiation: electrons, positrons, protons, neutrons, and alpha particles. What is their mass ratio?*

Answer 16

Electrons are small, negatively charged particles with a charge of −1 which are accelerated in a linear accelerator to near the speed of light and can be symbolized by either e− or β−. Positrons have the same mass as an electron but are a positively charged particle with a charge of +1 and are symbolized by β+. Positrons are antimatter and undergo an annihilation reaction when they encounter an electron, creating two 511 keV photons released "back-to-back" (i.e., 180° apart), forming the basis for positron emission tomography (PET) imaging. Protons are larger, positively charged particles with a charge of +1, are accelerated in a cyclotron to become useful energy for therapy, and are symbolized by p+. Neutrons have approximately the same mass as a proton but are neutral particles having no charge, are created in a nuclear reactor through high-speed collisions of deuterons or protons with a beryllium target in a particle accelerator, or by decay of man-made Californium-242, and can be symbolized by n. Neutrons interact with nuclei of atoms of the absorbing material and set in motion "fast recoil protons," alpha particles, and heavier nuclear fragments. Alpha particles are heavier, positively charged particles made up of two protons and two neutrons (i.e., Helium nucleus) with a charge of +2; they occur naturally during alpha decay of radioisotopes such as radium and uranium, and can be symbolized by α or He^{+2}. The mass ratio of these particles is ~1:1:2,000:2,000:8,000 for β −:β+:p+:n: α.

Hall EJ, Giaccia AJ. Physics and chemistry of radiation absorption. In: Hall EJ, Giaccia AJ, eds. *Radiobiology for the Radiologist*. 7th ed. Philadelphia, PA: Lippincott Williams & Wilkins; 2012:3–11.

Question 17 *How does radon gas cause lung cancer?*

Answer 17

Radon gas (Radon-222) is created when naturally occurring Radium-226 decays via alpha decay, creating radon gas and an alpha particle. Once radon gas is inhaled it will decay with a half-life of 3.8 days into radon gas "daughters," which are solids that become trapped in the lung. Once radon gas decays to Polonium-218 (Po-218) through alpha decay, then two additional alpha decays and two beta decays occur in less than 1 hour, resulting in Lead-2010 (Pb-210) which has a half-life of 22.3 years. High linear energy transfer (LET) alpha particle and low LET beta particle radiation to the lungs can lead to an estimated 10,000 to 20,000 cases of lung cancer each year in the United States.

Hall EJ, Giaccia AJ. Physics and chemistry of radiation absorption. In: Hall EJ, Giaccia AJ, eds. *Radiobiology for the Radiologist*. 7th ed. Philadelphia, PA: Lippincott Williams & Wilkins; 2012:3–11.

Question 18 *What are neutrons?*

Answer 18

Neutrons are particles with a mass similar to protons, but they do not carry an electrical charge. Because of their neutrality they are not able to be accelerated in an electrical device. Neutrons are created in two ways; first, if a charged particle accelerates to a high energy and hits an appropriate target material, and second, as a by-product of heavy radioactive atoms undergoing fission.

Hall EJ, Giaccia AJ. Physics and chemistry of radiation absorption. In Hall EJ, Giaccia AJ, eds. *Radiobiology for the Radiologist*. 7th ed. Philadelphia, PA: Lippincott Williams & Wilkins; 2012:3–11.

Question 19
Since neutrons are uncharged particles, how do they damage DNA?

Question 20
What is the difference between direct and indirect ionizing radiation?

Question 21
What are examples of low linear energy transfer (LET) and high LET radiation?

Question 22
What are heavy charged particles, and how may they be used for radiation therapy?

Question 19 *Since neutrons are uncharged particles, how do they damage DNA?*

Answer 19

Neutrons are uncharged, neutral particles and thus can penetrate deeply into tissue. Neutrons damage cells by indirect ionization through inelastic and elastic collisions with nuclei, setting into motion recoil protons, alpha particles, and heavy nuclei. Most of the neutron interactions in tissue are by elastic collisions with hydrogen atoms since hydrogen is the most abundant atom in tissue. Once neutron energies reach over 6 MeV, inelastic collisions occur and spallation products (alpha particles) are formed when high-energy neutrons collide with carbon and oxygen nuclei. For neutrons that are heavily ionizing, high linear energy transfer (LET) particles, direct action dominates with only a small percent of DNA damage occurring from the indirect action (creation of free radicals).

Hall EJ, Giaccia AJ. Physics and chemistry of radiation absorption. In: Hall EJ, Giaccia AJ, eds. *Radiobiology for the Radiologist.* 7th ed. Philadelphia, PA: Lippincott Williams & Wilkins; 2012:3–11.

Question 20 *What is the difference between direct and indirect ionizing radiation?*

Answer 20

Directly ionizing radiation particles are all charged particles that have sufficient energy to cause ionization. Examples of directly ionizing radiation are electrons, protons, alpha particles, and heavy nuclei. Indirectly ionizing radiation particles are uncharged and do not directly produce chemical and biological damage themselves but lead to the production of charged particles. Examples of indirectly ionizing radiation are x-rays, γ-rays, and neutrons.

Hall EJ, Giaccia AJ. Physics and chemistry of radiation absorption. In: Hall EJ, Giaccia AJ, eds. *Radiobiology for the Radiologist.* 7th ed. Philadelphia, PA: Lippincott Williams & Wilkins; 2012:3–11.

Question 21 *What are examples of low linear energy transfer (LET) and high LET radiation?*

Answer 21

Examples of low LET radiation are x-rays, electrons, and protons (excluding the Bragg peak). Examples of high LET radiation are alpha particles, neutrons, heavy charged particles, and the proton Bragg peak.

Hall EJ, Giaccia AJ. Physics and chemistry of radiation absorption. In: Hall EJ, Giaccia AJ, eds. *Radiobiology for the Radiologist.* 7th ed. Philadelphia, PA: Lippincott Williams & Wilkins; 2012:3–11.
Hall EJ, Giaccia AJ. Linear energy transfer and relative biologic effectiveness. In: Hall EJ, Giaccia AJ, eds. *Radiobiology for the Radiologist.* 7th ed. Philadelphia, PA: Lippincott Williams & Wilkins; 2012:104–113.

Question 22 *What are heavy charged particles, and how may they be used for radiation therapy?*

Answer 22

Heavy charged particles are nuclei of elements such as carbon, neon, argon, or even iron that has a positive charge because some or all of the electrons are stripped from them. These particles must be accelerated to very high energies (thousands of millions of volts). Only a few heavy charged particle radiotherapy facilities exist around the world.

Hall EJ, Giaccia AJ. Physics and chemistry of radiation absorption. In: Hall EJ, Giaccia AJ, eds. *Radiobiology for the Radiologist.* 7th ed. Philadelphia, PA: Lippincott Williams & Wilkins; 2012:3–11.

2

CELL SURVIVAL CURVES AND CELL DEATH

EHSAN H. BALAGAMWALA, C. MARC LEYRER, JEFFREY A. KITTEL, AND ALEX ALMASAN

Question 1
What is the most common mechanism of cell death induced by ionizing radiation?

Question 2
How is plating efficiency (PE) defined?

Question 3
What is the importance of calculating the surviving fraction?

Question 4
How does the shape of the cell survival curve differ based on whether sparsely ionizing radiation or densely ionizing radiation is utilized?

Turn page to see the answers.

Question 1 *What is the most common mechanism of cell death induced by ionizing radiation?*

Answer 1

Mitotic cell death is the most common mechanism for triggering cell death after exposure to ionizing radiation. The biochemical steps may overlap with those encountered during apoptosis (caspase activation, DNA laddering).

Chen Q, Chai Y, Mazumder S, et al. The late increase in free radical oxygen species during apoptosis is associated with cytochrome c release, caspase activation, and mitochondrial dysfunction. *Cell Death Differ.* 2003;10:323–334.
Vakifahmetoglu H, Olsson M, Zhivotovsky B. Death through a tragedy: mitotic catastrophe. *Cell Death Differ.* 2008;15:1153–1162.

Question 2 *How is plating efficiency (PE) defined?*

Answer 2

PE indicates the percentage of plated cells in a cell culture that grow into colonies. It is defined as:

$$PE = \frac{\text{Number of colonies counted}}{\text{Number of cells seeded}} \times 100$$

Hall EJ, Giaccia AJ. Cell survival curves (chap 3). In: Hall EJ, Giaccia AJ, eds. *Radiobiology for the Radiologist.* 7th ed. Philadelphia, PA: Lippincott Williams & Wilkins; 2012:135–153.

Question 3 *What is the importance of calculating the surviving fraction?*

Answer 3

The surviving fraction is important in generating cell survival curves. Cell survival curves plot the surviving fraction against dose. In the laboratory, experiments can be done to determine the impact of varying radiation dose on cell survival. The surviving fraction can be calculated using:

$$\text{Surviving Fraction} = \frac{\text{Colonies counted}}{\text{Cells seeded} \times (PE/100)}$$

Hall EJ, Giaccia AJ. Cell survival curves (chap 3). In: Hall EJ, Giaccia AJ, eds. *Radiobiology for the Radiologist.* 7th ed. Philadelphia, PA: Lippincott Williams & Wilkins; 2012:135–153.

Question 4 *How does the shape of the cell survival curve differ based on whether sparsely ionizing radiation or densely ionizing radiation is utilized?*

Answer 4

With sparsely ionizing (low linear energy transfer) radiation such as x-rays, the cell survival curve on a log-linear plot starts off as a straight line, indicating surviving fraction is an exponential function of dose. As radiation dose increases, the curve bends over a range of doses (until straightening out again at very high doses per fraction), indicating the radiation has become more effective at cell kill per unit dose increase at higher doses.

With densely ionizing (high linear energy transfer) radiation such as α-particles, the cell survival curve is linear from the origin, indicating that cell kill remains an exponential function of dose.

Hall EJ, Giaccia AJ. Cell survival curves (chap 3). In: Hall EJ, Giaccia AJ, eds. *Radiobiology for the Radiologist.* 7th ed. Philadelphia, PA: Lippincott Williams & Wilkins; 2012:135–153.

Question 5
What are the two most important biophysical models that explain the shape of cell survival curves?

Question 6
In the multitarget model of cell survival, what do the quantities D_0, D_1, D_q, and n represent?

Question 7
As the intrinsic radiosensitivity of cells increases, how does D_0 change?

Question 5 *What are the two most important biophysical models that explain the shape of cell survival curves?*

Answer 5

The two most important models are the multitarget model and the linear-quadratic model.

Hall EJ, Giaccia AJ. Cell survival curves. In: Hall EJ, Giaccia AJ, eds. *Radiobiology for the Radiologist*. 7th ed. Philadelphia, PA: Lippincott Williams & Wilkins; 2012:135–153.

Question 6 *In the multitarget model of cell survival, what do the quantities D_0, D_1, D_q and n represent?*

Answer 6

Both the multitarget model and the linear-quadratic model aim to explain the shape of the cell survival curve, which can be determined using *in vitro* experiments. In the multitarget model, D_1 is the initial slope of the curve and represents cell kill from single-hit events. D_0 is the final slope of the cell survival curve and represents cell kill from multiple-hit events. Both D_0 and D_1 represent the dose required to reduce the fraction of surviving cells to 0.37. Since the surviving fraction is on a logarithmic scale, the dose required to reduce the cell population by a given factor (0.37) is the same at all survival levels. The extrapolation number, *n*, is a measure of the width of the shoulder of the cell survival curve. D_q represents the quasi-threshold dose, which is the dose at which the discrete portion of the survival curve when extrapolated backwards cuts the dose axis at 100% survival. These three parameters are related by:

$$\log_e n = \frac{D_q}{D_0}$$

Hall EJ, Giaccia AJ. Cell survival curves. In: Hall EJ, Giaccia AJ, eds. *Radiobiology for the Radiologist*. 7th ed. Philadelphia, PA: Lippincott Williams & Wilkins; 2012:135–153.

Question 7 *As the intrinsic radiosensitivity of cells increases, how does D_0 change?*

Answer 7

Radiosensitive cells have a lower D_0 compared to radioresistant cells, which have a higher D_0.

Hall EJ, Giaccia AJ. Cell survival curves. In: Hall EJ, Giaccia AJ, eds. *Radiobiology for the Radiologist*. 7th ed. Philadelphia, PA: Lippincott Williams & Wilkins; 2012:135–153.

Question 8
In the linear-quadratic model, what do the quantities α and β represent?

Question 9
At what dose are the linear and quadratic components of cell kill equal to each other?

Question 8 *In the linear-quadratic model, what do the quantities α and β represent?*

Answer 8

The linear-quadratic model utilizes what we know about single- and double-stranded breaks to define the cell survival curve. Cell survival (S) is defined as:

$$S = e^{-\alpha D - \beta D^2}$$

α represents the component of cell kill that increases linearly with increasing dose (D). It can be conceptualized as a single photon causing two double-strand breaks, which can then lead to lethal chromosomal or chromatid aberrations. β represents the component of cell kill that increases proportionally with D^2, that is, quadratically with increasing dose. It can be conceptualized as two separate photons, each causing double-strand breaks, which can then lead to lethal chromosomal or chromatid aberrations.

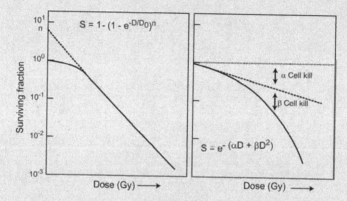

Figure 2.1 Graphic representation of the surviving fraction based as a function of dose.

Source: Reprinted with permission, Cleveland Clinic Center for Medical Art & Photography © 2014–2016. All Rights Reserved.

Hall EJ, Giaccia AJ. Cell survival curves. In: Hall EJ, Giaccia AJ, eds. *Radiobiology for the Radiologist*. 7th ed. Philadelphia, PA: Lippincott Williams & Wilkins; 2012:135–153.

Question 9 *At what dose are the linear and quadratic components of cell kill equal to each other?*

Answer 9

The linear and quadratic components are equal to each other when:

$$\alpha D = \beta D^2$$

or

$$D = \frac{\alpha}{\beta}$$

Hall EJ, Giaccia AJ. Cell survival curves (chap 3). In: Hall EJ, Giaccia AJ, eds. *Radiobiology for the Radiologist*. 7th ed. Philadelphia, PA: Lippincott Williams & Wilkins; 2012:135–153.

Question 10
What is the bystander effect?

Question 11
What is the most important type of cell death in irradiated cells? Do all cells undergo this type of cell death?

Question 12
In what cell types does apoptosis occur after irradiation?

Question 13
When a cell undergoes apoptosis, what is the characteristic fragment size of DNA?

Question 10 *What is the bystander effect?*

Answer 10

The bystander effect is the induction of biological effects in cells that are not directly targeted by ionizing radiation, but rather those that are in the vicinity of the targeted cells. At low radiation doses, the bystander effect may lead to radiation-induced effects in 30% of surrounding cells. It is interesting to note that the bystander effect is higher among cells that are connected to each other via gap-junctions and is lower (~5%–10%) when cells are sparsely plated in in vitro experiments.

Hall EJ, Giaccia AJ. Cell survival curves (chap 3). In: Hall EJ, Giaccia AJ, eds. *Radiobiology for the Radiologist*. 7th ed. Philadelphia, PA: Lippincott Williams & Wilkins; 2012:135–153.

Question 11 *What is the most important type of cell death in irradiated cells? Do all cells undergo this type of cell death?*

Answer 11

The most important type of cell death after irradiation is mitotic catastrophe. Mitotic catastrophe occurs when damaged chromosomes attempt to undergo mitosis; however, due to double-strand breaks as well as chromosomal aberrations such as rings, anaphase bridges, and dicentric chromosomes, mitosis cannot proceed and the cell undergoes mitotic catastrophe.

Hall EJ, Giaccia AJ. Cell survival curves. In: Hall EJ, Giaccia AJ, eds. *Radiobiology for the Radiologist*. 7th ed. Philadelphia, PA: Lippincott Williams & Wilkins; 2012:135–153.

Question 12 *In what cell types does apoptosis occur after irradiation?*

Answer 12

Although mitotic catastrophe is the predominant radiation-induced cell death mechanism, hematopoietic and lymphoid cells undergo apoptosis after irradiation.

Almasan A. Commitment to ionizing radiation-induced apoptosis. *Radiat Res*. 2000;153:347–350.
Vakifahmetoglu H, Olsson M, Zhivotovsky B. Death through a tragedy: mitotic catastrophe. *Cell Death Differ*. 2008;15:1153–1162.

Question 13 *When a cell undergoes apoptosis, what is the characteristic fragment size of DNA?*

Answer 13

As cells undergo apoptosis, the DNA is broken down into fragments of 185 base pairs (as a result of a nuclease cutting in the linker region of the nucleosome), to generate a "DNA ladder" that can be visualized following separation using gel electrophoresis.

Plesca D, Mazumder S, Almasan A. DNA damage-induced apoptosis. *Methods Enzymol*. 2008;446:107–122.

Question 14

In addition to apoptosis and mitotic catastrophe, cells under stress may undergo cell death by which other mechanism?

Question 15

What are the most important proteins responsible for cellular senescence?

Question 16

What is the impact of normal cell senescence on tumor growth?

Question 14 *In addition to apoptosis and mitotic catastrophe, cells under stress may undergo cell death by which other mechanism?*

Answer 14

Cells may also undergo cell death via autophagy, which is a self-digestive process. Autophagy is an evolutionarily conserved process in which parts of the cell are sequestered in organelles called autophagosomes, which ultimately fuse with lysosomes to lead to degradation of cellular proteins. Autophagy can also occur in situations of chronic stressful stimuli to cells. Defects in autophagy have been described in infections, neurodegeneration, aging, Crohn's disease, and heart disease, as well as in cancers. Autophagy in tumor cells is primarily a resistance/cell survival mechanism.

Klionsky DJ, Abdelmohsen K, Abe A, et al. Guidelines for the use and interpretation of assays for monitoring autophagy (3rd ed.). *Autophagy*. 2016;12:1–222. PMID: 26799652

Singh K, Matsuyama S, Drazba JA, Almasan A. Autophagy-dependent senescence in response to DNA damage and chronic apoptotic stress. *Autophagy*. 2012;8:236–251.

Question 15 *What are the most important proteins responsible for cellular senescence?*

Answer 15

The proteins p53 and Rb (primarily by regulating p21 and p16) are the most important proteins for senescence. Cellular senescence in primary cells leads to an irreversible cell cycle arrest that occurs due to shortening of telomeres through excessive cellular divisions, activation of oncogenes, or DNA damage due to oxidative stress. Mutations in p53 and Rb in tumor cells leads to loss of senescence in tumor cells; however, normal cells maintain such a response to oxidative stress.

Singh K, Matsuyama S, Drazba JA, Almasan A. Autophagy-dependent senescence in response to DNA damage and chronic apoptotic stress. *Autophagy*. 2012;8:236–251.

Question 16 *What is the impact of normal cell senescence on tumor growth?*

Answer 16

When normal cells undergo senescence, they may remain metabolically active; however, they are unable to continue their reproductive cycle. Although they are arrested in terms of growth, they may continue to contribute mitogens and cytokines to the cellular environment, which may ultimately promote tumor regrowth.

Hall EJ, Giaccia AJ. Cell survival curves (chap 3). In: Hall EJ, Giaccia AJ, eds. *Radiobiology for the Radiologist*. 7th ed. Philadelphia, PA: Lippincott Williams & Wilkins; 2012:135–153.

Question 17
Are cells more radiosensitive in interphase or during mitosis?

Question 18
What are two proteins that are important in recognizing double-stranded breaks in chromosomes?

Question 19
What is one mechanism responsible for the intrinsic radioresistance of cancer stem cells?

Question 20
What is the effective dose–survival curve?

Question 17 *Are cells more radiosensitive in interphase or during mitosis?*

Answer 17

Cells are more sensitive during mitosis. This is based on the finding that when evaluated during interphase, different cells have different levels of radiosensitivity. However, when the same cell lines are evaluated during mitosis, their radiosensitivities are very similar.

Hall EJ, Giaccia AJ. Radiosensitivity and cell age in the mitotic cycle (chap 4). In: Hall EJ, Giaccia AJ, eds. *Radiobiology for the Radiologist.* 7th ed. Philadelphia, PA: Lippincott Williams & Wilkins; 2012:135–153.

Question 18 *What are two proteins that are important in recognizing double-stranded breaks in chromosomes?*

Answer 18

Ku-70 and Ku-80 are important in recognizing double-stranded breaks, and by recruiting the DNA-dependent protein kinase (DNA-PK) initiate the non-homologous end joining DNA repair mechanism.

Chatterjee P, Choudhary GS, Alswillah T, et al. The TMPRSS2-ERG gene fusion blocks XRCC4-mediated non-homologous end joining repair and radiosensitizes prostate cancer cells to PARP inhibition. *Mol Cancer Ther.* 2015;14:1896–1906.

Hall EJ, Giaccia AJ. Molecular mechanisms of DNA and chromosome damage and repair (chap 2). In: Hall EJ, Giaccia AJ, eds. *Radiobiology for the Radiologist.* 7th ed. Philadelphia, PA: Lippincott Williams & Wilkins; 2012:135–153.

Question 19 *What is one mechanism responsible for the intrinsic radioresistance of cancer stem cells?*

Answer 19

In general, it is thought that cells that are more undifferentiated have increased sensitivity to radiation. However, this is not the case with cancer stem cells: cancer stem cells are in fact more radioresistant than "differentiated" cancer cells. It is thought that one mechanism of radioresistance in cancer stem cells is increased expression of free radical scavengers, which reduce levels of reactive oxygen species. Another mechanism is their higher capacity to repair DNA damage.

Hall EJ, Giaccia AJ. Molecular mechanisms of DNA and chromosome damage and repair (chap 2). In: Hall EJ, Giaccia AJ, eds. *Radiobiology for the Radiologist.* 7th ed. Philadelphia, PA: Lippincott Williams & Wilkins; 2012:135–153.

Question 20 *What is the effective dose–survival curve?*

Answer 20

Since radiotherapy is delivered most commonly using a fractionated regimen, the effective-dose survival curve represents the net effect of fractionated radiotherapy. Essentially, the shoulder part of the cell survival curve is repeated many times (since most daily fractionation schemes deliver <3 Gy per fraction). The effective survival curve is an exponential function of dose and hence it is a straight line on a log-linear plot.

Hall EJ, Giaccia AJ. Cell survival curves (chap 3). In: Hall EJ, Giaccia AJ, eds. *Radiobiology for the Radiologist.* 7th ed. Philadelphia, PA: Lippincott Williams & Wilkins; 2012:135–153.

Question 21

In a fractionated radiotherapy regimen, what is the effective D_0?

Question 22

In the multitarget model, what is D_{10}?

Question 21 *In a fractionated radiotherapy regimen, what is the effective* D_0?

Answer 21

The effective D_0 of a fractionated radiotherapy regimen is approximately 3 Gy for human cells.

Hall EJ, Giaccia AJ. Cell survival curves (chap 3). In: Hall EJ, Giaccia AJ, eds. *Radiobiology for the Radiologist*. 7th ed. Philadelphia, PA: Lippincott Williams & Wilkins; 2012:135–153.

Question 22 *In the multitarget model, what is* D_{10}?

Answer 22

D_0 represents the dose required to reduce the surviving fraction to 37%, whereas D_{10} represents the dose required to kill 90% of cells. It is represented by:

$$D_{10} = 2.3 \times D_0$$

Hall EJ, Giaccia AJ. Cell survival curves (chap 3). In: Hall EJ, Giaccia AJ, eds. *Radiobiology for the Radiologist*. 7th ed. Philadelphia, PA: Lippincott Williams & Wilkins; 2012:135–153.

3

DNA, CHROMOSOME AND CHROMATID DAMAGE, REPAIR, AND MEASUREMENT

EHSAN H. BALAGAMWALA, C. MARC LEYRER, JEFFREY A. KITTEL, AND ALEX ALMASAN

Question 1
What are the phases of mitosis?

Question 2
What are the important events during each phase of mitosis?

Turn page to see the answers.

Question 1 *What are the phases of mitosis?*

Answer 1

The distinct phases of mitosis are prophase, metaphase, anaphase, and telophase (Figure 3.1).

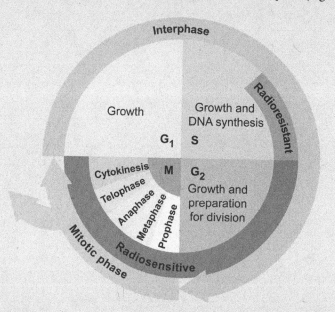

Figure 3.1 Representation of the phases of the cell cycle.

Source: Reprinted with permission, Cleveland Clinic Center for Medical Art & Photography © 2014–2016. All Rights Reserved.

Hall EJ, Giaccia AJ. Molecular mechanisms of DNA and chromosome damage and repair (chap 2). In: Hall EJ, Giaccia AJ, eds. *Radiobiology for the Radiologist.* 7th ed. Philadelphia, PA: Lippincott Williams & Wilkins; 2012:135–153.

Question 2 *What are the important events during each phase of mitosis?*

Answer 2

Prophase: The chromatin undergoes thickening and chromosomes condense into light coils. By the end of prophase, the chromosome is in its most condensed form.

Metaphase: Two events occur simultaneously during the metaphases—chromosomes move to the center of the cell and the spindle forms. Once the chromosomes are stabilized at the equator of the cell, their centromeres divide and metaphase is complete.

Anaphase: The chromosomes move on spindles to the poles of the cell.

Telophase: Chromosomes congregate at the poles and begin to uncoil. The nuclear membrane reappears (disappeared initially during the prophase) and the chromosomes continue to uncoil until the nucleus regains its characteristic interphase appearance.

Hall EJ, Giaccia AJ. Molecular mechanisms of DNA and chromosome damage and repair. In: Hall EJ, Giaccia AJ, eds. *Radiobiology for the Radiologist.* 7th ed. Philadelphia, PA: Lippincott Williams & Wilkins; 2012:135–153.

Question 3
What is the importance of telomeres?

Question 4
What enzyme can regenerate telomeres? What is its importance in cancer biology?

Question 5
What types of DNA damage are induced by radiation?

Question 6
What is the most lethal form of DNA damage and why?

Question 3 *What is the importance of telomeres?*

Answer 3

Telomeres cap and protect the ends of chromosomes. Telomeres are repetitive DNA sequences comprised of the TTAGGG (in humans) DNA sequence that vary in total length from 1.5 to 150 kb. With each replication cycle, telomeric DNA is lost. Once all telomeric DNA has been lost, vital DNA sequences are at risk for being lost; therefore, the cell undergoes senescence. It is estimated that a cell can divide between 40 and 60 times before undergoing senescence (called the Hayflick phenomenon).

Hall EJ, Giaccia AJ. Molecular mechanisms of DNA and chromosome damage and repair. In: Hall EJ, Giaccia AJ, eds. *Radiobiology for the Radiologist*. 7th ed. Philadelphia, PA: Lippincott Williams & Wilkins; 2012:135–153.

Question 4 *What enzyme can regenerate telomeres? What is its importance in cancer biology?*

Answer 4

Telomerase is a reverse transcriptase that contains an RNA component for the complementary sequence to the TTAGGG sequence repeats that it uses as a template to continually extend telomeres at the end of chromosomes. Telomerase is expressed in stem cells as well as cancer cells; however, it is not expressed at detectable levels in other normal human somatic tissues. Therefore, it is thought that immortalization and carcinogenesis are associated with telomerase expression. Approximately 90% of human cancer biopsies show expression of telomerase.

Hall EJ, Giaccia AJ. Molecular mechanisms of DNA and chromosome damage and repair. In: Hall EJ, Giaccia AJ, eds. *Radiobiology for the Radiologist*. 7th ed. Philadelphia, PA: Lippincott Williams & Wilkins; 2012:135–153.

Question 5 *What types of DNA damage are induced by radiation?*

Answer 5

Radiation therapy (RT) induces several types of DNA damage: base damage, single-strand breaks, and double-strand breaks (most common to least common). The majority of RT-induced DNA damage is repaired effectively; if the damage is not repaired correctly, the cells can undergo apoptosis or acquire mutation(s) that can lead to carcinogenesis.

Hall EJ, Giaccia AJ. Molecular mechanisms of DNA and chromosome damage and repair. In: Hall EJ, Giaccia AJ, eds. *Radiobiology for the Radiologist*. 7th ed. Philadelphia, PA: Lippincott Williams & Wilkins; 2012:135–153.

Question 6 *What is the most lethal form of DNA damage and why?*

Answer 6

The most lethal form of DNA damage is a double-stranded break (DSB). Single-strand breaks are of little biological consequence because the DNA repair mechanism utilizes the opposite strand to effectively and accurately repair the DNA damage. However, when a DSB occurs, DNA repair is more difficult. Unrepaired DSBs can lead to nonlethal DNA lesions such as deletions or translocations as well as the formation of lethal DNA lesions, including dicentrics, rings, and anaphase bridges.

Hall EJ, Giaccia AJ. Molecular mechanisms of DNA and chromosome damage and repair. In: Hall EJ, Giaccia AJ, eds. *Radiobiology for the Radiologist*. 7th ed. Philadelphia, PA: Lippincott Williams & Wilkins; 2012:135–153.

Question 7
Which phase of the cell cycle is the most radiosensitive?

Question 8
What are the basic repair mechanisms for single-strand breaks?

Question 9
In what phase of the cell cycles does homologous recombination repair (HRR) and nonhomologous end-joining (NHEJ) occur?

Question 10
What are the essential steps in nonhomologous end joining (NHEJ)?

Question 7 *Which phase of the cell cycle is the most radiosensitive?*

Answer 7

G2 and M phases of the cell cycle are the most sensitive phases of the cell cycle. This is because during these phases of the cell cycle, chromosomes are actively dividing and the DNA is more "exposed." In addition, cells may have already passed through the last cell cycle checkpoint so proceeding through replication results in "mitotic catastrophe."

Plesca D, Crosby ME, Gupta D, Almasan A. E2F4 function in G2: maintaining G2-arrest to prevent mitotic entry with damaged DNA. *Cell Cycle*. 2007;6:1147–1152.

Vakifahmetoglu H, Olsson M, Zhivotovsky B. Death through a tragedy: mitotic catastrophe. *Cell Death Differ*. 2008;15:1153–1162.

Question 8 *What are the basic repair mechanisms for single-strand breaks?*

Answer 8

Base excision repair (BER) and nucleotide excision repair (NER) are important single-strand break repair mechanisms. In BER, a nucleotide base is removed and it is synthesized using the opposite strand as a template. NER removes bulky adducts created most frequently by UV damage. NER occurs via global genome repair and transcription-coupled repair. Mutations in *BER* and *NER* genes do not lead to ionizing radiation sensitivity.

Hall EJ, Giaccia AJ. Molecular mechanisms of DNA and chromosome damage and repair. In: Hall EJ, Giaccia AJ, eds. *Radiobiology for the Radiologist*. 7th ed. Philadelphia, PA: Lippincott Williams & Wilkins; 2012:135–153.

Question 9 *In what phase of the cell cycles does homologous recombination repair (HRR) and nonhomologous end-joining (NHEJ) occur?*

Answer 9

HRR occurs primarily in the late S/G2 phase and NHEJ occurs in the G0/G1 phase of the cell cycle. While NHEJ is the predominant mechanism of radiation-induced DNA damage repair, it is suppressed in the late S and G2 phases of the cell cycle when HRR becomes possible due to the presence of sister chromatids.

Hall EJ, Giaccia AJ. Molecular mechanisms of DNA and chromosome damage and repair. In: Hall EJ, Giaccia AJ, eds. *Radiobiology for the Radiologist*. 7th ed. Philadelphia, PA: Lippincott Williams & Wilkins; 2012:135–153.

Question 10 *What are the essential steps in nonhomologous end joining (NHEJ)?*

Answer 10

The first step in cellular response to DNA double-strand breaks (DSB) is activation of a sensor, ATR (ATM and Rad3-related). ATM promotes the processing of broken DNA ends by phosphorylating H2AX to generate γ-H2AX that coats the DNA that surround the DSB. It also regulates other proteins involved, such as NBS/MRE11/Rad50s and 53BP1. NHEJ can be divided into five steps: DSB end recognition, recruitment of DNA-dependent protein kinase catalytic subunit (DNA-PKcs), end processing, fill-in synthesis or end bridging, end ligation. End recognition occurs when the Ku70/Ku80 heterodimer binds to the ends of DNA DSB. Ku recruits DNA-PKcs and Artemis, which have the ability (i.e., endonuclease activity) to perform end-processing. In the final step, ligation of nicked DNA ends is performed by a DNA ligase (DNA ligase IV in complex with XRCC4), which is also likely recruited by Ku.

Chatterjee P, Choudhary GS, Alswillah T, et al. The TMPRSS2-ERG gene fusion blocks XRCC4-mediated non-homologous end joining repair and radiosensitizes prostate cancer cells to PARP inhibition. *Mol Cancer Ther*. 2015;14:1896–1906.

Sharma A, Singh K, Almasan A. Gamma-H2AX as a marker for the DNA damage response. *Methods Mol Biol*. 2012;920:613–626.

Question 11
Mutations in *BRCA1/2* genes lead to deficiency in which DNA repair mechanism?

Question 12
Hereditary nonpolyposis colon cancer (HNPCC) is caused by mutation in which DNA repair mechanism?

Question 13
What is the difference between chromosome and chromatid aberrations?

Question 11 *Mutations in BRCA1/2 genes lead to deficiency in which DNA repair mechanism?*

Answer 11

BRCA1/2 genes are essential components of the homologous recombination repair (HRR). HRR occurs predominantly in the late S/G2 phase of the cell cycle. HRR requires a replicated undamaged chromatid or chromosome to serve as a template for DNA repair. During recombination, ATM phosphorylates BRCA1, which is then recruited to the site of a double-stranded break (DSB) which has been bound by the NBS/MRE11/Rad50s complex. MRE11 resects the damaged DNA, which serves as the binding site for Rad51. Rad51 displaces RPA to form a nucleofilament that is the essential driver of HRR, and then recruits Rad52, which protects against exonucleolytic degradation. The two invading ends serve as primers for DNA synthesis and form the so-called Holliday junctions. Once the gaps in nucleotide are filled, the Holliday junctions resolve, resulting in two identical double-stranded DNA strands. Mutations in HRR genes result in radiosensitivity and ensuing genomic instability.

Hall EJ, Giaccia AJ. Molecular mechanisms of DNA and chromosome damage and repair (chap 2). In: Hall EJ, Giaccia AJ, eds. *Radiobiology for the Radiologist*. 7th ed. Philadelphia, PA: Lippincott Williams & Wilkins; 2012:135–153.

Question 12 *Hereditary nonpolyposis colon cancer (HNPCC) is caused by mutation in which DNA repair mechanism?*

Answer 12

Mismatch repair (MMR). The MMR pathway detects and removes the incorrectly synthesized nucleotide base as well as small nucleotide insertion mismatches that can occur during DNA replication. First, the mismatch is identified by sensors that recruit MMR factors. Once the factors are recruited, the newly synthesized DNA strand harboring the mismatch is identified and the incorrect nucleotides are excised. Finally, the gap is filled and the DNA strand is joined together by ligases. Mutations in any of the *MMR* genes (MSH, MLH, PSM families of genes) can result in microsatellite instability and cancer (primarily of the colon).

Hall EJ, Giaccia AJ. Molecular mechanisms of DNA and chromosome damage and repair. In: Hall EJ, Giaccia AJ, eds. *Radiobiology for the Radiologist*. 7th ed. Philadelphia, PA: Lippincott Williams & Wilkins; 2012:135–153.

Question 13 *What is the difference between chromosome and chromatid aberrations?*

Answer 13

Different aberrations can occur depending on the phase of the cell cycle in which the cells are exposed to ionizing radiation. If cells are exposed to ionizing radiation during interphase or G1 phase prior to duplication of chromosomes, then a single strand of a chromatid develops a break that is duplicated during DNA replication—this is called a chromosome aberration. Lethal chromosome aberrations include dicentric chromosomes and rings.

When cells are exposed to ionizing radiation following DNA replication in the last S/G2 phase, the damage produced is called a chromatid aberration. Lethal chromatid aberrations include anaphase bridges.

Hall EJ, Giaccia AJ. Molecular mechanisms of DNA and chromosome damage and repair. In: Hall EJ, Giaccia AJ, eds. *Radiobiology for the Radiologist*. 7th ed. Philadelphia, PA: Lippincott Williams & Wilkins; 2012:135–153.

Question 14
What is a dicentric chromosome?

Question 15
What is a ring-type chromosomal aberration?

Question 14 *What is a dicentric chromosome?*

Answer 14

A dicentric chromosome is a chromosomal aberration produced by asymmetric exchange of DNA information that results in lethality. When chromosomal breaks are produced early in interphase, sticky ends result at the site of breakage. Therefore, if two nearby chromosomes suffer a break and they join, it results in one chromosome with two centromeres (dicentric chromosome) and another without centromeres at all (acentric chromosome). Acentric chromosomes are lost during DNA replication.

Hall EJ, Giaccia AJ. Molecular mechanisms of DNA and chromosome damage and repair. In: Hall EJ, Giaccia AJ, eds. *Radiobiology for the Radiologist.* 7th ed. Philadelphia, PA: Lippincott Williams & Wilkins; 2012:135–153.

Question 15 *What is a ring-type chromosomal aberration?*

Answer 15

This type of aberration occurs if the double-strand break (DSB) and the subsequent exchange of DNA information occur prior to DNA replication (interphase or G1 phase). After radiation-induced double-stranded breaks in interphase or G1 occur, two fragments can occur: one with a centromere and one without a centromere (acentric fragment). If the two ends of the fragment with a centromere are joined together, a ring structure results along with an acentric fragment. During mitosis, the acentric fragment is lost since it cannot interact with the spindle. After DNA replication, the ring chromosome aberration forms overlapping rings; because the rings cannot be separated they lead to the lethality of the cell (Figure 3.2).

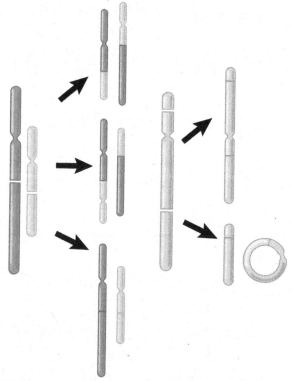

Figure 3.2 Graphic representation of a balanced translocation (left) and the formation of an acentric DNA fragment (right) that can be lost following mitosis.

Source: Reprinted with permission, Cleveland Clinic Center for Medical Art & Photography © 2014–2016. All Rights Reserved.

Hall EJ, Giaccia AJ. Molecular mechanisms of DNA and chromosome damage and repair (chap 2)..In: Hall EJ, Giaccia AJ, eds. *Radiobiology for the Radiologist.* 7th ed. Philadelphia, PA: Lippincott Williams & Wilkins; 2012:135–153.

Question 16
What is an anaphase bridge?

Question 17
What is a symmetric translocation?

Question 18
What is small interstitial deletion?

Question 19
What are the two most commonly utilized techniques to measure DNA damage?

Question 16 *What is an anaphase bridge?*

Answer 16

The anaphase bridge is a lethal chromatid aberration that occurs late in the cell cycle (G2 phase) after the chromosomes have replicated (which occurs in the S phase). If ionizing radiation leads to double-stranded breaks on the same side of the centromere but in both chromatid arms, the sticky ends may join, leading to a chromosome with one centromere and two arms joined together in the form of a ring as well as an acentric fragment. During mitosis, the chromosome is pulled toward the opposite spindle poles of the cell; however, the chromatids are attached to each other via the sticky ends and mitosis cannot proceed any further, resulting in mitotic cell death.

Hall EJ, Giaccia AJ. Molecular mechanisms of DNA and chromosome damage and repair. In: Hall EJ, Giaccia AJ, eds. *Radiobiology for the Radiologist*. 7th ed. Philadelphia, PA: Lippincott Williams & Wilkins; 2012:135–153.

Question 17 *What is a symmetric translocation?*

Answer 17

A symmetric translocation is a nonlethal chromosomal aberration that occurs during the G1 phase. When two chromosomes undergo double-stranded breaks and the broken ends are reciprocally transferred between chromosomes, it results in a symmetric translocation. This can lead to activation of certain genes such as *BCR/ABL* that has been implicated in malignancies including Burkitt lymphoma. Translocations could occur between different chromosomes or in the same chromosome (by deletion), as in the case of TMPRSS2-ERG that is common in prostate cancer.

Hall EJ, Giaccia AJ. Molecular mechanisms of DNA and chromosome damage and repair. In: Hall EJ, Giaccia AJ, eds. *Radiobiology for the Radiologist*. 7th ed. Philadelphia, PA: Lippincott Williams & Wilkins; 2012:135–153.

Question 18 *What is small interstitial deletion?*

Answer 18

A small interstitial deletion is also a nonlethal chromosomal aberration that occurs in an interphase chromosome. It occurs when two sets of double-stranded breaks occur on the same side of the centromere, resulting in a set of genes being deleted (they actually form an acentric ring and are lost during mitosis) and the rest of the chromosome rejoins. This type of chromosomal aberration can lead to carcinogenesis if the lost genetic material included a tumor suppressor gene. A deletion on human chromosome 21 can generate a TMPRSS2-ERG gene fusion that is found in the majority of prostate cancers.

Hall EJ, Giaccia AJ. Molecular mechanisms of DNA and chromosome damage and repair. In: Hall EJ, Giaccia AJ, eds. *Radiobiology for the Radiologist*. 7th ed. Philadelphia, PA: Lippincott Williams & Wilkins; 2012:135–153.

Question 19 *What are the two most commonly utilized techniques to measure DNA damage?*

Answer 19

Pulsed field gel electrophoresis (PFGE) and single-cell gel electrophoresis (comet assay) are the most common methods. γH2AX is a more recently, widely used surrogate for the DNA damage and its repair.

Hall EJ, Giaccia AJ. Molecular mechanisms of DNA and chromosome damage and repair. In: Hall EJ, Giaccia AJ, eds. *Radiobiology for the Radiologist*. 7th ed. Philadelphia, PA: Lippincott Williams & Wilkins; 2012:135–153.

Question 20
What is the pulsed field gel electrophoresis (PFGE) technique and how does it work?

Question 21
What is the single-cell electrophoresis (comet assay)?

Question 22
What is the radiation-induced nuclear foci assay?

Question 23
What test can be utilized to estimate the total dose of radiation exposure?

Question 20 *What is the pulsed field gel electrophoresis (PFGE) technique and how does it work?*

Answer 20

This is the most widely utilized technique to detect the induction and repair of DNA double-stranded breaks (DSB). This technique is based on electrophoresis and allows separation of DNA fragments based on size in the megabase pair range. The fragmentation of DNA is proportional to the dose of radiation.

Hall EJ, Giaccia AJ. Molecular mechanisms of DNA and chromosome damage and repair. In: Hall EJ, Giaccia AJ, eds. *Radiobiology for the Radiologist*. 7th ed. Philadelphia, PA: Lippincott Williams & Wilkins; 2012:135–153.

Question 21 *What is the single-cell electrophoresis (comet assay)?*

Answer 21

The comet assay has the advantage of detecting differences in DNA damage and repair at the single-cell level. Cells are exposed to ionizing radiation, embedded in agarose, and lysed under neutral buffer conditions to quantify induction and repair of DNA double-stranded breaks and in alkaline buffer conditions to quantify induction and repair of single-stranded DNA breaks. If the cells are undamaged, the DNA remains compact and there is no comet tail visible. If the DNA is damaged, the migration of DNA in agarose is directly proportional to the amount of DNA damage. This assay is excellent for detecting single-strand breaks and not as good for detecting DSB.

Hall EJ, Giaccia AJ. Molecular mechanisms of DNA and chromosome damage and repair. In: Hall EJ, Giaccia AJ, eds. *Radiobiology for the Radiologist*. 7th ed. Philadelphia, PA: Lippincott Williams & Wilkins; 2012:135–153.

Question 22 *What is the radiation-induced nuclear foci assay?*

Answer 22

When DNA is damaged by ionizing radiation, complexes of DNA damage signaling and DNA repair proteins localize to the site of DNA strand breaks in the nucleus of a cell. This assay can be done on both tissue sections as well as in individual cell preparations. Cells are incubated with an antibody against one of these proteins, for example, γH2AX or 53BP1 (primary antibody), which are proteins that localize to sites of DNA damage. A secondary antibody with a fluorescent tag is utilized to detect binding of the primary antibody. Most often this technique is utilized to measure DNA damage over time to reflect the kinetics of DNA repair (one can quantitate the number of foci/cell or the number of cells that are above a defined threshold, e.g., 5 or 10 foci).

Hall EJ, Giaccia AJ. Molecular mechanisms of DNA and chromosome damage and repair. In: Hall EJ, Giaccia AJ, eds. *Radiobiology for the Radiologist*. 7th ed. Philadelphia, PA: Lippincott Williams & Wilkins; 2012:135–153.

Question 23 *What test can be utilized to estimate the total dose of radiation exposure?*

Answer 23

The number of chromosomal aberrations can be measured in a sample of peripheral blood lymphocytes to estimate radiation exposure. The number of acentric chromosomal aberrations in these lymphocytes reflects the total dose received and can be measured within a few days to a few weeks after exposure. A dose response curve (aberrations per cell vs. absorbed dose) can be generated using in vitro cell cultures and the total radiation dose exposure can be estimated using this plot.

Hall EJ, Giaccia AJ. Molecular mechanisms of DNA and chromosome damage and repair. In: Hall EJ, Giaccia AJ, eds. *Radiobiology for the Radiologist*. 7th ed. Philadelphia, PA: Lippincott Williams & Wilkins; 2012:135–153.

4

RADIOSENSITIVITY AND THE DOSE-RATE EFFECT

BRIAN D. YARD AND MOHAMED E. ABAZEED

Question 1

What are the phases of the cell cycle?

Question 2

What phase of the cell cycle has the most variable length of time across various cell lines?

Question 3

What molecules regulate the transitions from one phase of the cell cycle to the next? How would you characterize them?

Question 4

What are the most radiosensitive phases of the cell cycle? What is the most resistant?

Turn page to see the answers.

Question 1 *What are the phases of the cell cycle?*

Answer 1

Proliferating mammalian cells have a cycle of DNA synthesis (S phase) followed by a pause or gap (G2), followed by mitosis (M phase), which is followed by another pause or gap (G1). If cells are not actively dividing, they are arrested in G.

Hall EJ, Giaccia AJ. Cell, tissue, and tumor kinetics. In: Hall EJ, Giaccia AJ, eds. *Radiobiology for the Radiologist.* 7th ed. Philadelphia, PA: Lippincott Williams & Wilkins; 2012:372–390.

Question 2 *What phase of the cell cycle has the most variable length of time across various cell lines?*

Answer 2

The most variable phase of the cell cycle is G1, which is typically the rate-determining step of the total cell cycle time across various cell lines. The other three phases (S, G2, and M) have limited variability among different cells.

Hall EJ, Giaccia AJ. Cell, tissue, and tumor kinetics. In: Hall EJ, Giaccia AJ, eds. *Radiobiology for the Radiologist.* 7th ed. Philadelphia, PA: Lippincott Williams & Wilkins; 2012:372–390.

Question 3 *What molecules regulate the transitions from one phase of the cell cycle to the next? How would you characterize them?*

Answer 3

The cell cycle is regulated by several cyclin-dependent kinases (Cdk), whose sequential activation preserves the temporal order of the cell cycle. Cdk enzymes are activated by cyclin and inactivated by Cdk inhibitory proteins. Cyclins and Cdk inhibitors are themselves regulated to ensure sequential and precise activation and deactivation.

Hall EJ, Giaccia AJ. Cell, tissue, and tumor kinetics. In: Hall EJ, Giaccia AJ, eds. *Radiobiology for the Radiologist.* 7th ed. Philadelphia, PA: Lippincott Williams & Wilkins; 2012:372–390.

Question 4 *What are the most radiosensitive phases of the cell cycle? What is the most resistant?*

Answer 4

Generally, the most radiosensitive phases of the cell cycle are M and G2. The most resistant phase is late S, presumably due to the ability to undergo homologous recombination. In slow replicating cells, early G1 is also considered to be radioresistant.

Hall EJ, Giaccia AJ. Cell, tissue, and tumor kinetics. In: Hall EJ, Giaccia AJ, eds. *Radiobiology for the Radiologist.* 7th ed. Philadelphia, PA: Lippincott Williams & Wilkins; 2012:372–390.

Question 5

How does the dependence of radiosensitivity on cell cycle phase apply to an asynchronously dividing population?

Question 6

What are the three categories of radiation-induced damage?

Question 7

What is an example of an experimental manipulation that can modify potentially lethal damage (PLD)?

Question 8

What is sublethal damage (SLD) and why is this type of damage important?

Question 5 *How does the dependence of radiosensitivity on cell cycle phase apply to an asynchronously dividing population?*

Answer 5

Cells replicating in culture are asynchronously dividing, that is, they are comprised of cells that are cycling independently of each other. The aforementioned experiments were conducted by various manipulations to "synchronize" these cells such that the population is cycling largely in sync. Virtually all tumors and normal tissue that is irradiated are comprised of asynchronously dividing populations. Therefore, unless the cells are arrested or timed such that they are in a particular phase of the cell cycle, either by chemical means or by "reassortment" (see the following), the dependence of radiosensitivity on cell cycle phases is not a major determinant of therapeutic radiosensitivity.

Hall EJ, Giaccia AJ. Cell, tissue, and tumor kinetics. In: Hall EJ, Giaccia AJ, eds. *Radiobiology for the Radiologist.* 7th ed. Philadelphia, PA: Lippincott Williams & Wilkins; 2012:372–390.

Question 6 *What are the three categories of radiation-induced damage?*

Answer 6

Lethal damage, potentially lethal damage (PLD), and sublethal damage (SLD) represent the three categories of radiation-induced damage. Lethal damage is irreparable and irreversible damage that leads to cell death. PLD is damage that can be modified by manipulation of the postirradiation environment to alter the degree of damage. Finally, SLD is damage that can be repaired.

Hall EJ, Giaccia AJ. Fractionated radiation and the dose-rate effect. In: Hall EJ, Giaccia AJ, eds. *Radiobiology for the Radiologist.* 7th ed. Philadelphia, PA: Lippincott Williams & Wilkins; 2012:67–85.

Question 7 *What is an example of an experimental manipulation that can modify potentially lethal damage (PLD)?*

Answer 7

Cells grown to stationary phase were either maintained in stationary phase for 6 or 12 hours or harvested immediately after irradiation. Survival curves were then measured for the three experimental conditions. Cells maintained in stationary phase were more resistant to radiation. In general, radiation resistance is enhanced when postirradiation conditions are suboptimal for growth. This is attributed to a delay in mitosis, which increases the probability of DNA damage repair prior to proceeding into mitosis.

Hall EJ, Giaccia AJ. Fractionated radiation and the dose-rate effect. In: Hall EJ, Giaccia AJ, eds. *Radiobiology for the Radiologist.* 7th ed. Philadelphia, PA: Lippincott Williams & Wilkins; 2012:67–85.
Little JB, Hahn GM, Frinde IE, et al. Repair of potentially lethal radiation damage in vitro and in vivo. *Radiology.* 1973;106:689–694.

Question 8 *What is sublethal damage (SLD) and why is this type of damage important?*

Answer 8

The experimental definition of SLD is that there is an increase in cell survival if a given dose of radiation is split into two equal fractions separated in time. If there is no repair occurring, the impact of a single fraction versus two equal fractions (e.g., 4 Gy vs. 2 × 2 Gy) should be zero to negligible. That is, the single fraction should decrease cellular survival as much as 2 × 2 Gy, if the other three "Rs" of reassortment, repopulation, and reoxygenation are held constant. In most experimental systems, this is not the case. By splitting a single fraction into two equal fractions, there are more cells that survive compared to the single fraction. This is compelling evidence for DNA repair. This repair and its optimal timing are important because it represents one of the main rationales for fractionation of radiation treatments, the repair of normal tissue.

Hall EJ, Giaccia AJ. Fractionated radiation and the dose-rate effect. In: Hall EJ, Giaccia AJ, eds. *Radiobiology for the Radiologist.* 7th ed. Philadelphia, PA: Lippincott Williams & Wilkins; 2012:67–85.

Question 9

How does sublethal damage (SLD) relate to the terminology of the linear-quadratic equation?

Question 10

What is synchrony and reassortment after irradiation?

Question 11

What is repopulation?

Question 12

What are the four "Rs" of radiobiology? How do they affect radiosensitivity?

Question 9 *How does sublethal damage (SLD) relate to the terminology of the linear-quadratic equation?*

Answer 9

There is a positive correlation between the extent of SLD and the size of the shoulder of the survival curve. If more cells survive after split dose treatment, the shoulder or the quadratic component (beta) is increased. Therefore, more SLD is associated with a large beta and therefore a low alpha/beta ratio.

Hall EJ, Giaccia AJ. Fractionated radiation and the dose-rate effect. In: Hall EJ, Giaccia AJ, eds. *Radiobiology for the Radiologist.* 7th ed. Philadelphia, PA: Lippincott Williams & Wilkins; 2012:67–85.

Question 10 *What is synchrony and reassortment after irradiation?*

Answer 10

After the first fraction of a two-fraction course of irradiation in a cell cycle, the asynchronous population of cells, the group of cells that are in the most resistant phases of the cell cycle, is the most likely to survive. This surviving fraction, therefore, has a trend toward being synchronized. As these synchronized cells recover and reenter the cell cycle, their sensitivity to the second fraction is dependent on the period of the cell cycle in which that fraction is delivered. If this fraction is delivered in the sensitive phases of the cell cycle (G2/M), there is significantly more cell death than if it were delivered in the more resistant phases (S phase).

Hall EJ, Giaccia AJ. Fractionated radiation and the dose-rate effect. In Hall EJ, Giaccia AJ, eds. *Radiobiology for the Radiologist.* 7th ed. Philadelphia, PA: Lippincott Williams & Wilkins; 2012:67–85.

Question 11 *What is repopulation?*

Answer 11

In rapidly dividing cell populations, if the time interval between the first and second fraction exceeds the cell cycle, there will be a greater number of cells due to proliferation or repopulation.

Hall EJ, Giaccia AJ. Fractionated radiation and the dose-rate effect. In Hall EJ, Giaccia AJ, eds. *Radiobiology for the Radiologist.* 7th ed. Philadelphia, PA: Lippincott Williams & Wilkins; 2012:67–85.

Question 12 *What are the four "Rs" of radiobiology? How do they affect radiosensitivity?*

Answer 12

The four "Rs" of radiobiology are repair, reassortment, repopulation, and reoxygenation. Repair and repopulation diminish the effects of radiation in tumors and enhance the survival of normal tissues. Reassortment and reoxygenation enhance the effects of radiation in tumors and can diminish the survival of normal tissues.

Hall EJ, Giaccia AJ. Fractionated radiation and the dose-rate effect. In: Hall EJ, Giaccia AJ, eds. *Radiobiology for the Radiologist.* 7th ed. Philadelphia, PA: Lippincott Williams & Wilkins; 2012:67–85.

Question 13
Which of the four "Rs" contributes to local control in stereotactic body radiation therapy (SBRT) treatments? Local failure?

Question 14
What is the impact of the dose-rate effect on survival after irradiation?

Question 15
What is the inverse dose-rate effect and what is this phenomenon attributed to?

Question 13 *Which of the four "Rs" contributes to local control in stereotactic body radiation therapy (SBRT) treatments? Local failure?*

Answer 13

The incomplete repair of sublethal damage (SLD) and the rapid delivery of a full regimen of radiation in a short period of time to prevent repopulation are main advantages of SBRT over fractionated treatment to achieve improved local control. It is unclear whether reassortment affects the biological effectiveness of SBRT. The lack of tumor reoxygenation can theoretically contribute to treatment failures after a short course of SBRT. It is not clear whether this occurs in practice.

Hall EJ, Giaccia AJ. Fractionated radiation and the dose-rate effect. In: Hall EJ, Giaccia AJ, eds. *Radiobiology for the Radiologist*. 7th ed. Philadelphia, PA: Lippincott Williams & Wilkins; 2012:67–85.

Question 14 *What is the impact of the dose-rate effect on survival after irradiation?*

Answer 14

The dose-rate effect is the principle that, as the dose rate of radiation delivery (Gy per minute) is reduced, the biological effect of a given dose is diminished. This is attributed to sublethal damage (SLD) repair during the prolonged radiation exposure interval. The magnitude of the dose-rate effect can vary substantially across cell lines. Cells that have a large initial shoulder have a larger dose-rate effect; this is largely attributed to their ability to undergo repair. As the dose rate is reduced, the survival curve becomes shallower and the shoulder decreases. Therefore, the survival curve approximates an exponential function of dose (or a straight line on a semi-log graph).

Hall EJ, Giaccia AJ. Fractionated radiation and the dose-rate effect. In: Hall EJ, Giaccia AJ, eds. *Radiobiology for the Radiologist*. 7th ed. Philadelphia, PA: Lippincott Williams & Wilkins; 2012:67–85.

Question 15 *What is the inverse dose-rate effect and what is this phenomenon attributed to?*

Answer 15

The inverse dose-rate effect occurs when decreasing the dose rate paradoxically results in increased cell death. This has been observed in HeLa cells and may also occur in other cells. This is attributed to the ability of cells to continue to cycle below a threshold dose rate. This converts an asynchronous population of cells to a synchronous population that accumulates at G2, the most sensitive phase of the cell cycle. Therefore, the lower dose rate results in greater cell kill than a higher-dose rate that does not allow this synchronization.

Hall EJ, Giaccia AJ. Fractionated radiation and the dose-rate effect. In: Hall EJ, Giaccia AJ, eds. *Radiobiology for the Radiologist*. 7th ed. Philadelphia, PA: Lippincott Williams & Wilkins; 2012:67–85.

5

RADIATION DAMAGE REPAIR AND MODELS FOR NORMAL TISSUES

ADITYA JULOORI, CHOAMEI XIANG, MICHAEL A. WELLER, AND JENNIFER S. YU

Question 1

What is the difference between lethal damage, potentially lethal damage, and sublethal damage?

Question 2

Why is a dividing cell more sensitive to radiation than a differentiated cell?

Question 3

What is the importance of the shoulder width on traditional curves for normal tissues?

Question 4

What is the difference between a structurally defined functional subunit (FSU) and a structurally undefined FSU?

Turn page to see the answers.

Question 1 *What is the difference between lethal damage, potentially lethal damage, and sublethal damage?*

Answer 1

Lethal damage from radiation is not reversible or reparable and leads to cell death. Potentially lethal damage can be modified by the conditions cells are placed in after being irradiated (observed in cell culture conditions). For example, this has been demonstrated in vitro by putting cells in saline for 6 hours after irradiation in order to plateau the growth curve—these cells then had a higher surviving fraction after radiotherapy than those cells that were not placed in these conditions after radiotherapy. It is hypothesized that tumors with relatively radioresistant histology like melanoma are able to repair this potentially lethal damage. Sublethal damage can be repaired in hours under normal conditions.

Hall EJ, Giaccia AJ. Radiation carcinogenesis. In: Hall EJ, Giaccia AJ, eds. *Radiobiology for the Radiologist*. 7th ed. Philadelphia, PA: Lippincott Williams & Wilkins; 2006:135–153.

Question 2 *Why is a dividing cell more sensitive to radiation than a differentiated cell?*

Answer 2

The dose of radiation needed to kill a dividing cell is less than that needed to kill a differentiated, nondividing cell. Cell death from radiation is primarily due to mitotic cell death. That is, DNA damage that is left unrepaired induces cells to die as the cell attempts to divide. In contrast, in differentiated cells, a higher dose of radiation is needed to kill cells or impair their function.

Hall EJ, Giaccia AJ. Clinical response of normal tissues. In: Hall EJ, Giaccia AJ, eds. *Radiobiology for the Radiologist*. 7th ed. Philadelphia, PA: Lippincott Williams & Wilkins; 2006:327–355.

Question 3 *What is the importance of the shoulder width on traditional curves for normal tissues?*

Answer 3

Various normal tissues have a wide range of radiosensitivities, with the shoulder length on survival curves being the principal variable. For example, jejunal crypt cells have a large shoulder while bone marrow stem cells have a limited shoulder. The shoulder length is larger for some tissues because of the inherent ability to repair potentially lethal damage.

Hall EJ, Giaccia AJ. Radiation carcinogenesis. In: Hall EJ, Giaccia AJ, eds. *Radiobiology for the Radiologist*. 7th ed. Philadelphia, PA: Lippincott Williams & Wilkins; 2006:135–153.

Question 4 *What is the difference between a structurally defined functional subunit (FSU) and a structurally undefined FSU?*

Answer 4

Structurally defined FSUs are self-contained and are independent of neighboring units. Clonogenic cells cannot travel between structurally defined FSUs. Examples include nephrons in the kidney or the lobules of the liver and acini in the lung. These structurally defined FSUs are depleted of clonogens with low doses of radiation. Structurally *undefined* FSUs differ in that clonogenic cells can migrate from one FSU to another in order to repopulate the FSU after irradiation. An example of this would be the spinal cord, the mucosa, and the skin.

Hall EJ, Giaccia AJ. Radiation carcinogenesis. In: Hall EJ, Giaccia AJ, eds. *Radiobiology for the Radiologist*. 7th ed. Philadelphia, PA: Lippincott Williams & Wilkins; 2006:135–153.

Question 5

What is Casarett's classification of tissue radiosensitivity based on?

Question 6

What is an H-type population according to the Michalowski classification?

Question 7

What is an F-type population according to the Michalowski classification?

Question 8

What is the role of TGF-β1 in radiation-induced fibrosis in normal tissue?

Question 5 *What is Casarett's classification of tissue radiosensitivity based on?*

Answer 5

Cells are divided into four major categories based on histopathological observations, from most sensitive to least resistant. Group I cells divide regularly with no differentiation (e.g., intestinal crypt cells). Group II cells divide regularly with some differentiation between divisions (e.g., myelocytes). Group III cells do not divide regularly and are variably differentiated (e.g., liver). Group IV cells do not divide and are highly differentiated (e.g., nerve cells).

Hall EJ, Giaccia AJ. Radiation carcinogenesis. In: Hall EJ, Giaccia AJ, eds. *Radiobiology for the Radiologist.* 7th ed. Philadelphia, PA: Lippincott Williams & Wilkins; 2006:135–153.
Rubin P, Casarett GW. *Clinical Radiation Pathology.* Vol. 1. Philadelphia, PA: WB Saunders; 1968.

Question 6 *What is an H-type population according to the Michalowski classification?*

Answer 6

These tissues follow a "hierarchical" model. These are fully functioning cells which are no longer dividing and are differentiated. Examples of tissues/cells that follow this hierarchical model are the bone marrow, the epidermis, and the intestinal epithelium.

Wheldon TE, Michalowski AS. Alternative models for the proliferative structure of normal tissues and their response to irradiation. *Br J Cancer.* 1986;7(suppl):382–385.

Question 7 *What is an F-type population according to the Michalowski classification?*

Answer 7

These tissues follow a "flexible" model. These tissues are in organs where the cells do not typically divide unless triggered to do so in response to damage. Examples of this type of tissue include liver, skin, and thyroid. These tissues have no hierarchy and no compartments.

Wheldon TE, Michalowski AS. Alternative models for the proliferative structure of normal tissues and their response to irradiation. *Br J Cancer.* 1986;7(suppl):382–385.

Question 8 *What is the role of TGF-β1 in radiation-induced fibrosis in normal tissue?*

Answer 8

TGF-β1 causes the proliferation of fibroblasts and helps differentiate epithelial cells into mesenchymal cells by epithelial-mesenchymal transition; it also causes upregulation of transcription of profibrotic genes.

Boothe DL, Coplowitz S, Greenwood E, et al. Transforming growth factor β-1 (TGF-β1) is a serum biomarker of radiation induced fibrosis in patients treated with intracavitary accelerated partial breast irradiation: preliminary results of a prospective study. *Int J Radiat Oncol Biol Phys.* 2013;87(5):1030–1036.

Question 9

How has the dose–response relationship for radiation exposure to skin been studied?

Question 10

What parts of the skin are damaged in early and late radiation dermatitis?

Question 11

What is the response of the hematopoietic system to radiation?

Question 12

What is the normal tissue response of the esophagus in response to radiation therapy?

Question 9 *How has the dose–response relationship for radiation exposure to skin been studied?*

Answer 9

Pig skin has been used in radiobiological experiments because of the similarity to human skin structure. Radiation of pig skin in experiments helped establish the timeline in which erythema and desquamation occurs in areas of irradiation. Late skin effects have also been studied in pig's skin. Often rodent skin is used because of the expense associated with the use of pig skin.

Fowler JR, Morgan RL, Silvester JA, Bewley DK, Turner BA. Experiments with fractionated x-ray treatment of the skin of pigs: 1. Fractionation up to 28 days. *Br J Radiol*. 1963;36:188–196.

Hall EJ, Giaccia AJ. Radiation carcinogenesis. In: Hall EJ, Giaccia AJ, eds. *Radiobiology for the Radiologist*. 7th ed. Philadelphia, PA: Lippincott Williams & Wilkins; 2006:135–153.

Question 10 *What parts of the skin are damaged in early and late radiation dermatitis?*

Answer 10

The epidermis is the outer layer of the skin and is composed of a basal layer of actively proliferating cells. This represents the site of early radiation reactions. The deeper layers, called the dermis, represent the site of late radiation dermatitis. It is formed by dense connective tissue and the vascular endothelial cell damage caused by radiation is the cause of the late reaction.

Hall EJ, Giaccia AJ. Radiation carcinogenesis. In: Hall EJ, Giaccia AJ, eds. *Radiobiology for the Radiologist*. 7th ed. Philadelphia, PA: Lippincott Williams & Wilkins; 2006:135–153.

Question 11 *What is the response of the hematopoietic system to radiation?*

Answer 11

Hematopoietic stem cells are very sensitive to radiation. Changes in peripheral blood count after irradiation reflect the life span of differentiated cells and the time to replenish those cells by stem/progenitor cells.

Hall EJ, Giaccia AJ. Clinical response of normal tissues. In: Hall EJ, Giaccia AJ, eds. *Radiobiology for the Radiologist*. 7th ed. Philadelphia, PA: Lippincott Williams & Wilkins; 2006:327–355.

Question 12 *What is the normal tissue response of the esophagus in response to radiation therapy?*

Answer 12

Similar to other mucosal surfaces, the esophageal mucosa is composed of rapidly dividing cells. After about 10 to 12 days of initiating therapy, patients begin experiencing acute esophagitis-characterized pain with swallowing. Late esophageal effects occur as a result of radiation damage to the deeper muscle levels of the esophagus.

Hall EJ, Giaccia AJ. Radiation carcinogenesis. In: Hall EJ, Giaccia AJ, eds. *Radiobiology for the Radiologist*. 7th ed. Philadelphia, PA: Lippincott Williams & Wilkins; 2006:135–153.

Question 13
How have early and late responses to irradiation of the lung been assessed in animal models?

Question 14
What are the manifestations of radiation-induced liver disease?

Question 15
What medication can be used to prevent the development of radiation-induced nephropathy?

Question 16
What is the reason for urinary symptoms following radiation exposure to the bladder during a course of radiotherapy?

Question 13 *How have early and late responses to irradiation of the lung been assessed in animal models?*

Answer 13

Breathing rate was assessed in mouse lungs after exposure of radiation. Increased breathing frequency at 4 to 6 months is reflective of pneumonitis. At roughly a year, increased breathing frequency is reflective of fibrosis.

Travis EL, Down JD, Holmes SJ, et al. Radiation pneumonitis and fibrosis in mouse lung assayed by respiratory frequency and histology. *Radiat Res.* 1980;84:133–142.
Travis EL, Vojnovic B, Davies EE, Hirst DG. A plethysmographic method for measuring function in locally irradiated mouse lung. *Br J Radiol.* 1979;52:67–74.

Question 14 *What are the manifestations of radiation-induced liver disease?*

Answer 14

Radiation-induced liver disease is a clinical syndrome characterized by elevated liver enzymes, ascites, and hepatomegaly, and typically occurs a few weeks to a few months after the completion of a fractionated radiotherapy regimen. The syndrome is pathologically characterized by central lobular venous congestion and the subsequent atrophy of hepatocytes next to the congested veins.

Lawrence TS, Robertson JM, Anscher MS, Jirtle RL, Ensminger WD, Fajardo LF. Hepatic toxicity resulting from cancer treatment. *Int J Radiat Oncol Biol Phys.* 1995;31:1237–1248.

Question 15 *What medication can be used to prevent the development of radiation-induced nephropathy?*

Answer 15

An important late side effect of renal irradiation is radiation nephropathy, which is characterized by hypertension, anemia, and proteinuria. Modulators of the renin-angiotensin system such as angiotensin-converting enzyme (ACE) inhibitors (like lisinopril) and angiotensin receptor antagonists (like losartan) have been effective as prophylactic agents.

Cohen EP, Hussain S, Moulder JE. Successful treatment of radiation nephropathy with angiotensin II blockade. *Int J Radiat Oncol Biol Phys.* 2003;55:190–193.
Robbins ME, Diz DI. Pathogenic role of the renin-angiotensin system in modulating radiation-induced late effects. *Int J Radiat Oncol Biol Phys.* 2006;64:6–12.

Question 16 *What is the reason for urinary symptoms following radiation exposure to the bladder during a course of radiotherapy?*

Answer 16

The superficial cells of the bladder have a long life span and are not renewed often. Thus, following irradiation, there is an extended interval before accelerated proliferation begins. As these cells are lost, there is a subsequent increase in frequency of irritation. With the absence of these surface cells, the urine in the bladder causes irritative symptoms.

Hall EJ, Giaccia AJ. Radiation carcinogenesis. In: Hall EJ, Giaccia AJ, eds. *Radiobiology for the Radiologist.* 7th ed. Philadelphia, PA: Lippincott Williams & Wilkins; 2006:135–153.

Question 17

What are the characteristics of spinal cord myelopathy after radiation?

Question 18

What is the relationship between the volume of spinal cord irradiated and the tolerance dose?

Question 19

What is the effect of radiation therapy on peripheral nerves?

Question 20

What is the importance of the latency period for cataract formation after radiation therapy?

Question 17 *What are the characteristics of spinal cord myelopathy after radiation?*

Answer 17

The dose–response relationship for the spinal cord can be made by observations of late damage that occurs after irradiation of the spinal cord in rats. Initial lesions are limited to white matter whereas late delayed injury may have a basis in vascular etiology. There is a long latency period to paralysis, from months to years. The impact of fractionation on spinal cord damage is significant, with an α/β ratio of about 1.5 Gy.

Hall EJ, Giaccia AJ. Radiation carcinogenesis. In: Hall EJ, Giaccia AJ, eds. *Radiobiology for the Radiologist*. 7th ed. Philadelphia, PA: Lippincott Williams & Wilkins; 2006:135–153.
Van der Kogel AJ. Radiation tolerance of the rat spinal cord: time–dose relationships. *Radiology*. 1977;122:505–509.
Van der Schueren E, Landuyt W, Ang KK, van der Kogel AJ. From 2 Gy to 1 Gy per fraction: sparing effect in rat spinal cord? *Int J Radiat Oncol Biol Phys*. 1988;14:297–300.

Question 18 *What is the relationship between the volume of spinal cord irradiated and the tolerance dose?*

Answer 18

The functional subunits (FSUs) of the spinal cord are arranged in a serial fashion. For small cord lengths, there is a significant dependence of the length of cord irradiated on the dose tolerance for white matter necrosis, with a higher dose tolerance for small lengths. As the length of spinal cord irradiated increases past a few centimeters, the tolerance of the cord is independent of length/volume.

Van der Kogel AJ. Central nervous system radiation injury in small animal models. In: Gutin PH, Leibel SA, Sheline GE, eds. *Radiation Injury to the Nervous System*. New York, NY: Raven Press; 1991:91–112.
Van der Kogel AJ. Effect of volume and localization on rat spinal cord tolerance. In: Fielden EM, Fowler JF, Hendry JH, Scott D, eds. *Radiation Injury to the Nervous System*. New York, NY: Taylor & Francis; 1987:352.

Question 19 *What is the effect of radiation therapy on peripheral nerves?*

Answer 19

Radiation injury to the peripheral nerves of the body is more common than damage to the spinal cord. It is generally believed that peripheral nerves have a higher radiation tolerance than the structures of the central nervous system (the spinal cord and the brain).

Hall EJ, Giaccia AJ. Radiation carcinogenesis. In: Hall EJ, Giaccia AJ, eds. *Radiobiology for the Radiologist*. 7th ed. Philadelphia, PA: Lippincott Williams & Wilkins; 2006:135–153.

Question 20 *What is the importance of the latency period for cataract formation after radiation therapy?*

Answer 20

One unique feature of the lens is that it does not have the ability to remove dead or damaged cells. The time period between irradiation and formation of a cataract, otherwise known as the latency period, is directly correlated to the dose of the radiation exposure.

Hall EJ, Giaccia AJ. Radiation carcinogenesis. In: Hall EJ, Giaccia AJ, eds. *Radiobiology for the Radiologist*. 7th ed. Philadelphia, PA: Lippincott Williams & Wilkins; 2006:135–153.

Question 21
How different is the radiosensitivity of bone or cartilage between children and adults?

Question 22
Are there any medications that have been shown to help treat radiation-induced fibrosis or osteoradionecrosis?

Question 23
What is the response of the vasculature to radiation?

Question 24
What is the mechanism of radiation-induced heart disease?

Question 21 *How different is the radiosensitivity of bone or cartilage between children and adults?*

Answer 21

Bone and cartilage in children are very sensitive to radiation. Doses as low as 10 Gy can reduce bone growth and result in short stature. Care should be taken to avoid the growth plate in children, if possible. In adults, radiation can contribute to osteonecrosis, particularly of the mandible and humeral/femoral head and neck.

Hall EJ, Giaccia AJ. Clinical response of normal tissues. In: Hall EJ, Giaccia AJ, eds. *Radiobiology for the Radiologist.* 7th ed. Philadelphia, PA: Lippincott Williams & Wilkins; 2006:327–355.

Question 22 *Are there any medications that have been shown to help treat radiation-induced fibrosis or osteoradionecrosis?*

Answer 22

Pentoxifylline has been shown to be effective in treating radiation-induced fibrosis and osteoradionecrosis. It is a phosphodiesterase inhibitor and increases blood flow while reducing inflammation and the innate immune response.

Delanian S, Lefaix JL. Current management for late normal tissue injury: radiation-induced fibrosis and necrosis. *Semin Radiat Oncol.* 2007; 17:99–107.
Essayan DM. Cyclic nucleotide phosphodiesterases. *J Allergy Clin Immunol.* 2001;108(5):671–680.

Question 23 *What is the response of the vasculature to radiation?*

Answer 23

Damage to blood vessels can contribute to late radiation effects. Late vascular damage can manifest as atherosclerosis, causing heart attacks and stroke, telangiectasias, arteriovenous malformations, and vessel wall necrosis that can cause aneurysm or rupture. Arteries and capillaries are more sensitive than veins to radiation.

Hall EJ, Giaccia AJ. Clinical response of normal tissues. In: Hall EJ, Giaccia AJ, eds. *Radiobiology for the Radiologist.* 7th ed. Philadelphia, PA: Lippincott Williams & Wilkins; 2006:327–355.

Question 24 *What is the mechanism of radiation-induced heart disease?*

Answer 24

Radiation exposure to the endothelial lining of vessels of the heart causes a cascade of inflammation that leads to arteriosclerosis and microvascular disruption. Arteries are of the most important concern in the development of cardiotoxicity. Use of systemic agents like Herceptin and doxorubicin potentiate this toxicity when administered in tandem with external beam radiation, particularly in breast cancer patients.

Schultz-Hector S, Trott KR. Radiation-induced cardiovascular diseases: is the epidemiologic evidence compatible with the radiobiologic data? *Int J Radiat Oncol Biol Phys.* 2007;67:10–18.

Question 25
What is the impact of radiation therapy on the heart?

Question 26
What is the therapeutic index in radiotherapy?

Question 27
What is the SOMA classification for late radiation toxicity?

Question 25 *What is the impact of radiation therapy on the heart?*

Answer 25

Acute pericarditis is the most common radiation-induced heart injury. Because the heart has a low alpha/beta ratio (roughly 1 Gy), the use of fractionation can effectively spare the normal heart. Late cardiotoxic effects are a reflection of fibrosis and can manifest as cardiomyopathy. This can occur slowly over years following radiotherapy.

Yusuf SW, Sami S, Daher IN. Radiation-induced heart disease: a clinical update. *Cardiol Res Pract.* 2011; 2011;9:1–9.

Question 26 *What is the therapeutic index in radiotherapy?*

Answer 26

The therapeutic index, or therapeutic ratio, is the ratio of a tumor's response to radiation compared to the associated normal tissue damage for that same amount of radiation. There are ways to modulate this ratio—such as using a radiosensitizer to improve the tumor control component. Another example of change is hyperfractionation, which helps better spare toxicity in normal late-responding tissues.

Hall EJ, Giaccia AJ. Radiation carcinogenesis. In: Hall EJ, Giaccia AJ, eds. *Radiobiology for the Radiologist.* 7th ed. Philadelphia, PA: Lippincott Williams & Wilkins; 2006:135–153.

Question 27 *What is the SOMA classification for late radiation toxicity?*

Answer 27

There is a specific classification for each organ in order to best understand the response to radiation. It is based on a subjective and objective description of the related toxicity, the management steps required, and the analytic tool used to better assess the tissue function, such as CT or MRI imaging.

Rubin P, Constine LS, Fajardo LF, et al., eds. Late effects of normal tissues consensus conference. San Francisco, CA, August 26–28, 1992. *Int J Radiat Oncol Biol Phys.* 1995;31:1049–1081.

6

HYPOXIA, OXYGEN, REOXYGENATION, AND ANGIOGENESIS

XINGJIANG YU, JENNIFER S. YU, AND ELI BAR

Question 1
What is tumor hypoxia?

Question 2
What are acute and chronic hypoxias?

Question 3
How does hypoxia contribute to tumor progression?

Question 4
What is the relationship between hypoxia and resistance to radiation? What is the oxygen fixation hypothesis?

Question 1 *What is tumor hypoxia?*

Answer 1

Hypoxia is a state of reduced oxygenation of tumor cells relative to their metabolic needs. Hypoxia is associated with poor prognosis. Hypoxic tumor cells are frequently found around necrotic areas away from blood vessels. Tumor cells have adapted to survive in hypoxia.

Brown JM. Hypoxia and tumor biology. *Methods Enzymol.* 2007;435:298–315.
Thomlinson RH, Gray LH. The histological structure of some human lung cancers and the possible implications for radiotherapy. *Brit J Cancer.* 1955;9:539–549.

Question 2 *What are acute and chronic hypoxias?*

Answer 2

Tumors may have regions of acute and chronic hypoxias. Acute hypoxia is the result of transient disruption of blood flow through tumor vasculature leading to reduced tissue oxygenation. Acute hypoxia may result from emboli or extrinsic compression of vessels.

In chronic hypoxia, cells that are located away from blood vessels receive less oxygen and nutrients by diffusion (oxygen diffusion distance is ≤70 to 200 microns and dependent on oxygen levels in the blood vessel).

Hall EJ, Giaccia AJ. Radiation carcinogenesis. In: Hall EJ, Giaccia AJ, eds. *Radiobiology for the Radiologist.* 7th ed. Philadelphia, PA: Lippincott Williams & Wilkins; 2006:135–153.
Wilson WR, Hay MP. Targeting hypoxia in cancer therapy. *Nat Rev Cancer.* 2011;11:393–410.

Question 3 *How does hypoxia contribute to tumor progression?*

Answer 3

As tumors proliferate, some cells become hypoxic due to their inadequate blood supply. Hypoxia promotes tumor angiogenesis, alters cellular metabolism, selects cells that bear mutations that favor survival (e.g., mutations in the tumor suppressor gene *p53*), downregulates programmed cell death (apoptosis), and facilitates invasion and metastasis. Hypoxic cancer cells are more resistant to radiation and some types of chemotherapy.

Liao D, Johnson RS. Hypoxia: a key regulator of angiogenesis in cancer. *Cancer Metastasis Rev.* 2007;26:281–290.

Question 4 *What is the relationship between hypoxia and resistance to radiation? What is the oxygen fixation hypothesis?*

Answer 4

Hypoxic tumor cells are more resistant to radiation.

The oxygen fixation hypothesis provides the explanation for why oxygen is a radiation sensitizer. X-rays produce free radicals that mediate most of the damage to cells and macromolecules. DNA lesions that are produced by x-rays with the chemical participation of oxygen pose a significant threat to cell survival because these lesions cannot be restored to an undamaged state. According to this hypothesis, oxygen sensitizes because these "nonrestorable" lesions ultimately increase the amount of stable DNA damage and thus the extent of lethality from a given dose.

Brown JM. Hypoxia and tumor biology. *Methods Enzymol.* 2007;435:298–315.
Hall EJ, Giaccia AJ. Radiation carcinogenesis. In: Hall EJ, Giaccia AJ, eds. *Radiobiology for the Radiologist.* 7th ed. Philadelphia, PA: Lippincott Williams & Wilkins; 2006:135–153.

Question 5
What is the oxygen enhancement ratio (OER)?

Question 6
What parameters affect the oxygen enhancement ratio (OER)?

Question 7
What is the relationship between hypoxia and resistance to chemotherapy?

Question 5 *What is the oxygen enhancement ratio (OER)?*

Answer 5

The OER is the ratio of doses needed to achieve the same biological effect under hypoxic and aerobic conditions. OER represents the enhancement of the therapeutic effect of ionizing radiation due to the presence of oxygen.

$$OER = \frac{D_0(\text{hypoxic})}{D_0(\text{aerobic})}$$

Hall EJ, Giaccia AJ. Radiation carcinogenesis. In: Hall EJ, Giaccia AJ, eds. *Radiobiology for the Radiologist*. 7th ed. Philadelphia, PA: Lippincott Williams & Wilkins; 2006:135–153.
Kunz M, Ibrahim SM. Molecular responses to hypoxia in tumor cells. *Mol Cancer*. 2003;17:2–23.

Question 6 *What parameters affect the oxygen enhancement ratio (OER)?*

Answer 6

- Intrinsic cellular sensitivity
- The quality of radiation (x-ray, neutron, alpha particle). Oxygen enhances cell killing for photons and electrons but not for neutrons or alpha particles
- pO_2 in tissues
- Duration of hypoxia
- Phase of the cell cycle (S-phase cells are more resistant to hypoxia)

Hall EJ, Giaccia AJ. Radiation carcinogenesis. In: Hall EJ, Giaccia AJ, eds. *Radiobiology for the Radiologist*. 7th ed. Philadelphia, PA: Lippincott Williams & Wilkins; 2006:135–153.
Sinclair WK. Cyclic x-ray responses in mammalian cells in vitro. *Radiat Res*. March 1968;33(3):620–643.
Sinclair WK, Morton RA. X-ray sensitivity during the cell generation cycle of cultured Chinese hamster cells. *Radiat Res*. 1966; 29:450–474.

Question 7 *What is the relationship between hypoxia and resistance to chemotherapy?*

Answer 7

1. Hypoxic regions exhibit reduced perfusion, thereby limiting drug efflux into the tumor. Tumor hypoxia can reduce cell cycling, thereby decreasing the efficacy of chemotherapy that targets proliferating cells.
2. Hypoxia can also reduce the efficacy of chemotherapy that is dependent on free radical formation (e.g., adriamycin, bleomycin).
3. Hypoxia is known to activate survival and multidrug-resistant pathways (including receptor tyrosine kinase signaling), thus providing intrinsic resistance to chemotherapy.
4. Hypoxia inhibits multiple apoptotic pathways, thus limiting the efficacy of chemotherapy which rely on activation of such pathways.
5. Hypoxia promotes genomic instability by inhibiting DNA repair to promote malignant progression and acquisition of resistance to radiation and chemotherapy (overexpression of MDR1 for example).

Huang LE, Yoo Y-G, Koshiji M, To KKW. Hypoxia Inhibits DNA Repair to Promote Malignant Progression, DNA Repair and Human Health. Vengrova S (Ed.). InTech; 2011.
Wilson WR, Hay MP. Targeting hypoxia in cancer therapy. *Nat Rev Cancer*. 2011;11:393–410.

Question 8

How can oxygen levels be evaluated in vivo?

Question 9

How does radiotherapy help to reoxygenate tumors?

Question 8 *How can oxygen levels be evaluated in vivo?*

Answer 8

Oxygen probe measurements (direct)

The Eppendorf oxygen electrode directly measures oxygen concentration. The probe can measure oxygen levels dynamically. Fiber-optic probes can indirectly measure oxygen concentration.

Markers of hypoxia (indirect)

Exogenous markers: Pimonidazole is a hypoxia marker, which forms adducts in hypoxic tumor cells and can be detected by immunohistochemistry. Radiolabeled 2-nitroimidazoles (EF5) and other redox-sensitive compounds can also be used.

Endogenous markers: carbonic anhydrase IX(CA9) and hypoxia-induced factors (HIF) can be detected by immunohistochemistry.

Wilson WR, Hay MP. Targeting hypoxia in cancer therapy, *Nat Rev Cancer*. 2011;11:393–410.

Question 9 *How does radiotherapy help to reoxygenate tumors?*

Answer 9

The inner core of the tumor is hypoxic while the cells at the periphery of the tumor are aerated. After irradiation, the aerated cells are predominantly killed off. The tumor mass is now smaller and the peripheral cells in this smaller tumor mass become aerated, leaving a smaller necrotic core. After another dose of radiation, the peripheral cells die and leave an even smaller necrotic core. The peripheral cells can become aerated and sensitized to the next fraction of irradiation. The cycle continues until the tumor cells are eliminated.

Hall EJ, Giaccia AJ. Radiation carcinogenesis. In: Hall EJ, Giaccia AJ, eds. *Radiobiology for the Radiologist*. 7th ed. Philadelphia, PA: Lippincott Williams & Wilkins; 2006:135–153.

Question 10

What are some cellular effects of hypoxia?

Question 11

What are some strategies to overcome tumor hypoxia in radiation therapy?

Question 10 *What are some cellular effects of hypoxia?*

Answer 10

- Gene/protein regulation: hypoxia-induced factor 1α (HIF1α, HIF2α, CA9, VEGF, EPO)
- Selection of apoptosis resistance: reduced p53 signaling
- Increased genomic instability: suppression of DNA repair pathways (mismatch repair, homologous recombination)
- Resistance to chemotherapy and radiotherapy (MDR1 expression)
- Increased glycolysis and inhibition of OXPHOS.
- Increased angiogenesis (VEGF)

Bristow RG, Hill RP. Hypoxia, DNA repair and genetic instability. *Nat Rev Cancer*. 2008;8(3):180–192.
Chi JT, Wang Z, Nuyten DS, et al. Gene expression programs in response to hypoxia: cell type specificity and prognostic significance in human cancers. *PLoS Med*. 2006;3(3):e47.
Kunz M, Ibrahim SM. Molecular responses to hypoxia in tumor cells. *Mol Cancer*. 2003;17:2–23.
Rodríguez-Jiménez FJ, Moreno-Manzano V, Lucas-Dominguez R, Sánchez-Puelles JM. Hypoxia causes downregulation of mismatch repair system and genomic instability in stem cells. *Stem Cells*. 2008;26(8):2052–2062.
Shannon AM, Bouchier-Hayes DJ, Condron CM, Toomey D. Tumour hypoxia, chemotherapeutic resistance and hypoxia-related therapies. *Cancer Treat Rev*. 2003;29(4):297–307.

Question 11 *What are some strategies to overcome tumor hypoxia in radiation therapy?*

Answer 11

a. Direct delivery of molecular oxygen to hypoxic regions:
   —Hyperbaric oxygenation
   —Red blood cell transfusion
   —Erythropoietin injection
   —ARCON

b. Radiosensitization by mimicking the effect of molecular oxygen:
   —Nitroimidazole derivatives: RSU-1069 and misonidazole.

c. Direct killing of hypoxic tumor cells:
   —Hypoxia cytotoxins, which are drugs that are reduced under hypoxic conditions to form toxic compounds or crosslink DNA, for example, tirapazamine, mitomycin C.
   —Gene therapy strategies: these target HIF1 positive tumor cells by delivering suicide genes (e.g., thymidine kinase) that become expressed under a hypoxia response element (HRE) promoter. Upon ganciclovir treatment, hypoxic cells expressing thymidine kinase are killed.

d. Hypoxia-inducible factor 1 (HIF1) inhibitors:
   —Suppression of radioresistant phenotype of hypoxic tumor cells by targeting the factor which orchestrates this phenotype: YC-1 decreases HIF1α levels and HIF1 target gene expression.

e. Radiation-induced reoxygenation of hypoxic tumor cells:
   —Fractionated radiation therapy.

Harada H. How can we overcome tumor hypoxia in radiation therapy? *J Radiat Res*. 2011;52(5):545–556.
Sun HL, Liu YN, Huang YT, et al. YC1 inhibits HIF1 expression in prostate cancer cells: contribution of AKT/NFKB signaling to HIF1 accumulation during hypoxia. *Oncogene*. 2007;26:3941–3951.

Question 12
What is angiogenesis?

Question 13
What is the relationship between hypoxia and angiogenesis?

Question 14
What is hypoxia-inducible factor 1 (HIF1) and how is it regulated?

Question 12 *What is angiogenesis?*

Answer 12

Angiogenesis is the formation of new blood vessels from preexisting vessels. Angiogenesis facilitates tumor growth, invasion, and metastasis.

Liao D, Johnson RS. Hypoxia: a key regulator of angiogenesis in cancer. *Cancer Metastasis Rev.* 2007;26:281–290.

Question 13 *What is the relationship between hypoxia and angiogenesis?*

Answer 13

Angiogenesis is directed by a delicate balance of activators and inhibitors. Hypoxia increases levels of activators (vascular endothelial growth factor [VEGF], fibroblast growth factor [FGF], epidermal growth factor [EGF], vascular endothelial growth factor receptor [VEGFR], platelet-derived growth factor receptor [PDGFR]) and decreases inhibitors (thrombospondin [TSP]) to promote angiogenesis. Hypoxia can regulate angiogenesis in hypoxia-induced factor (HIF) dependent and independent manners.

Liao D, Johnson RS. Hypoxia: a key regulator of angiogenesis in cancer. *Cancer Metastasis Rev.* 2007;26:281–290.

Question 14 *What is hypoxia-inducible factor 1 (HIF1) and how is it regulated?*

Answer 14

HIF1 is a transcription factor that regulates responses to hypoxia. It consists of an alpha and beta heterodimer. The HIF1α subunit is regulated by oxygen, whereas the HIF1β (ARNT; aryl hydrocarbon receptor nuclear translocator) subunit is not regulated by oxygen. Under normoxic conditions, HIF1α is targeted for degradation by the proteasome after its hydroxylation by one of three oxygen-sensitive, prolyl hydroxylases (PHD) and ubiquitylation by the VHL E3 ubiquitin ligase. Under hypoxic conditions, PHDs are not active. HIF1α is then stabilized and forms a complex with HIF1β to transactivate target genes including *VEGF/VEGFR*.

Liao D, Johnson RS. Hypoxia: a key regulator of angiogenesis in cancer. *Cancer Metastasis Rev.* 2007;26:281–290.

7

LINEAR ENERGY TRANSFER AND RELATIVE BIOLOGICAL EFFECTIVENESS

YVONNE PHAM AND CHIRAG SHAH

Question 1

What is the definition of linear energy transfer (LET)?

Question 2

What are two different methods to calculate linear energy transfer (LET)?

Question 3

What is considered high (densely ionizing) linear energy transfer (LET) radiation versus low (sparsely ionizing) LET radiation?

Question 4

What happens to the density of ionization and linear energy transfer (LET) as the energy increases within a certain particle type?

Turn page to see the answers.

Question 1 *What is the definition of linear energy transfer (LET)?*

Answer 1

LET is the average energy transferred per unit path length of travel within the local medium, expressed in kiloelectron volt (keV) per micrometer (μm). Energy deposition per path length varies widely due to the primary radiation and electrons set in motion; thus, LET is an average quantity.

Hall EJ, Giaccia AJ. Linear energy transfer and relative biologic effectiveness. In: Hall EJ, Giaccia AJ, eds. *Radiobiology for the Radiologist.* 7th ed. Philadelphia, PA: Lippincott Williams & Wilkins; 2012:104–113.

Question 2 *What are two different methods to calculate linear energy transfer (LET)?*

Answer 2

a. Track average: Obtained by dividing the track into equal lengths, calculating the energy transfer in each length, and deriving the average energy deposition.
   Example: /x x xx /xx   /xx x x / xx x /x   /xxxxx/
b. Energy average: Obtained by dividing the track into equal energy intervals, calculating the path length for each energy increment, and deriving the average of track lengths.
   Example: /xxxxx/xx x x x/xx xx x/x x x   x x   /x x x   xx/   xx xxx   /

Hall EJ, Giaccia AJ. Linear energy transfer and relative biologic effectiveness. In: Hall EJ, Giaccia AJ, eds. *Radiobiology for the Radiologist.* 7th ed. Philadelphia, PA: Lippincott Williams & Wilkins; 2012:104–113.

Question 3 *What is considered high (densely ionizing) linear energy transfer (LET) radiation versus low (sparsely ionizing) LET radiation?*

Answer 3

Radiation with LET values less than 10 keV/μm are considered low LET while radiation with LET values greater than 10 keV/μm are considered high LET.

Podgorsak, EB. Introduction to modern physics. In: Greenbaum E, ed. *Radiation Physics for Medical Physicists.* 2nd ed. New York, NY: Springer Science & Business Media; 2010:1–76.

Question 4 *What happens to the density of ionization and linear energy transfer (LET) as the energy increases within a certain particle type?*

Answer 4

The density of ionization and LET decreases as the energy increases for a given particle type. For example, 10 MeV protons have an LET of 4.7 keV/μm, whereas 150 MeV protons have an LET of 0.5 keV/μm.

Hall EJ, Giaccia AJ. Linear energy transfer and relative biologic effectiveness. In: Hall EJ, Giaccia AJ, eds. *Radiobiology for the Radiologist.* 7th ed. Philadelphia, PA: Lippincott Williams & Wilkins; 2012:104–113.

Question 5
What are some linear energy transfer (LET) values for different radiation types?

Question 6
What does a unit of gray (Gy) represent?

Question 5 *What are some linear energy transfer (LET) values for different radiation types?*

Answer 5

LET Values	
Radiation Type	**LET (keV/μm)**
Cobalt-60 γ-rays	0.2
250-kV x-rays	2.0
1 MeV electrons	0.25
10 keV electrons	2.3
150 MeV proton	0.5
2 MeV proton	17
14 MeV neutrons	12
100 MeV carbon ion	160
2.5 MeV α-particle	166
75 MeV argon ion	250
2 GeV Fe ions	1,000

Hall EJ, Giaccia AJ. Linear energy transfer and relative biologic effectiveness. In: Hall EJ, Giaccia AJ, eds. *Radiobiology for the Radiologist*. 7th ed. Philadelphia, PA: Lippincott Williams & Wilkins; 2012:104–113.

Podgorsak EB. Introduction to modern physics. In: Greenbaum E, ed. *Radiation Physics for Medical Physicists*. 2nd ed. New York, NY: Springer Science & Business Media; 2010:1–76.

Question 6 *What does a unit of gray (Gy) represent?*

Answer 6

Gy is the International System of Units (SI) unit used to measure the amount of energy deposited into a mass of certain material from ionizing radiation. 1 Gy = 1 J/kg. Two different types of radiation with equivalent doses in Gy, however, do not have the same degree of biological effect. For example, 1 Gy of neutrons will have a different biological effect compared to 1 Gy of protons.

Hall EJ, Giaccia AJ. Linear energy transfer and relative biologic effectiveness. In: Hall EJ, Giaccia AJ, eds. *Radiobiology for the Radiologist*. 7th ed. Philadelphia, PA: Lippincott Williams & Wilkins; 2012:104–113.

Question 7

What is the definition of relative biological effectiveness (RBE)?

Question 8

The dose required to give a surviving fraction of 0.5 for a cell population is 8 Gy with neutrons versus 12 Gy for 250-kV x-rays. What is the relative biological effectiveness (RBE) for neutrons in this scenario?

Question 9

What is the relationship between linear energy transfer (LET) and relative biological effectiveness (RBE)?

Question 10

Why does a linear energy transfer (LET) of approximately 100 keV/μm produce the highest relative biological effectiveness (RBE)?

Question 7 *What is the definition of relative biological effectiveness (RBE)?*

Answer 7

According to the National Bureau of Standards in 1954, RBE is defined by using 250-kV x-rays as the standard and is the ratio of D_{250}/D_r, where D_{250} is the dose of 250-kV x-rays and D_r is the dose of some test radiation that is required to produce an equal biological effect.

$$\text{RBE} = \frac{D_{250}}{D_r}$$

Hall EJ, Giaccia AJ. Linear energy transfer and relative biologic effectiveness. In: Hall EJ, Giaccia AJ, eds. *Radiobiology for the Radiologist.* 7th ed. Philadelphia, PA: Lippincott Williams & Wilkins; 2012:104–113.

Question 8 *The dose required to give a surviving fraction of 0.5 for a cell population is 8 Gy with neutrons versus 12 Gy for 250-kV x-rays. What is the relative biological effectiveness (RBE) for neutrons in this scenario?*

Answer 8

The calculation of RBE = D_{250}/D_r = 12 Gy/8 Gy = 1.5

Hall EJ, Giaccia AJ. Linear energy transfer and relative biologic effectiveness. In: Hall EJ, Giaccia AJ, eds. *Radiobiology for the Radiologist.* 7th ed. Philadelphia, PA: Lippincott Williams & Wilkins; 2012:104–113.

Question 9 *What is the relationship between linear energy transfer (LET) and relative biological effectiveness (RBE)?*

Answer 9

As LET increases, RBE increases due to increased deposition of energy. The peak RBE is reached at an LET of 100 keV/μm. Beyond this, the RBE falls.

Hall EJ, Giaccia AJ. Linear energy transfer and relative biologic effectiveness. In: Hall EJ, Giaccia AJ, eds. *Radiobiology for the Radiologist.* 7th ed. Philadelphia, PA: Lippincott Williams & Wilkins; 2012:104–113.

Question 10 *Why does a linear energy transfer (LET) of approximately 100 keV/μm produce the highest relative biological effectiveness (RBE)?*

Answer 10

100 keV/μm correlates with the diameter of the DNA double helix. Radiation with this LET has the highest chance of causing double-strand breaks, the most biologically significant lesion in chromosomes caused by radiation.

Hall EJ, Giaccia AJ. Linear energy transfer and relative biologic effectiveness. In: Hall EJ, Giaccia AJ, eds. *Radiobiology for the Radiologist.* 7th ed. Philadelphia, PA: Lippincott Williams & Wilkins; 2012:104–113.

Question 11
What types of radiation have the optimal linear energy transfer (LET) of 100 keV/μm?

Question 12
How is linear energy transfer (LET) affected by the density of ionization for a certain type of radiation?

Question 13
Does relative biological effectiveness (RBE) increase or decrease when a fractionated radiation regimen is used?

Question 14
What factors affect relative biological effectiveness (RBE)?

Question 11 *What types of radiation have the optimal linear energy transfer (LET) of 100 keV/µm?*

Answer 11

Neutrons of a few hundred keV, low-energy protons, and alpha particles have the optimal LET of 100 keV/µm.

Hall EJ, Giaccia AJ. Linear energy transfer and relative biologic effectiveness. In: Hall EJ, Giaccia AJ, eds. *Radiobiology for the Radiologist*. 7th ed. Philadelphia, PA: Lippincott Williams & Wilkins; 2012:104–113.

Question 12 *How is linear energy transfer (LET) affected by the density of ionization for a certain type of radiation?*

Answer 12

If the radiation type is too sparsely ionizing with a low LET (below 100 keV/µm), there is a smaller chance of producing double-strand breaks. In contrast, if the radiation type is very densely ionizing (e.g., 300 keV/µm), the chance of producing double-strand breaks is high but there is extra unnecessary energy deposition, making it less efficient per unit dose to produce the same biological effect. Generally speaking, densely ionizing radiation includes neutrons, protons, alpha particles, pi-mesons, and other heavy particles such as those encountered in space by astronauts. However, as the energy increases within a particular radiation type, the LET decreases and these radiation types can become more sparsely ionizing.

Hall EJ, Giaccia AJ. Linear energy transfer and relative biologic effectiveness. In: Hall EJ, Giaccia AJ, eds. *Radiobiology for the Radiologist*. 7th ed. Philadelphia, PA: Lippincott Williams & Wilkins; 2012:104–113.

Question 13 *Does relative biological effectiveness (RBE) increase or decrease when a fractionated radiation regimen is used?*

Answer 13

The RBE for certain types of radiation, such as neutrons, will increase with a more fractionated regimen. This is due to the broader shoulder of the x-ray dose–response curve compared to the smaller repeated shoulder of the neutron curve; therefore, a larger dose of x-rays is needed to produce the same biological effect in a fractionated regimen compared to a single fraction regimen. Since neutrons have little or no shoulder on the dose–response curve, this increases the RBE for this type of radiation in a fractionated regimen versus a single exposure.

Hall EJ, Giaccia AJ. Linear energy transfer and relative biologic effectiveness. In: Hall EJ, Giaccia AJ, eds. *Radiobiology for the Radiologist*. 7th ed. Philadelphia, PA: Lippincott Williams & Wilkins; 2012:104–113.

Question 14 *What factors affect relative biological effectiveness (RBE)?*

Answer 14

Factors that affect RBE include radiation type, LET, total radiation dose, number of dose fractions, dose rate, and type of tissue irradiated.

Hall EJ, Giaccia AJ. Linear energy transfer and relative biologic effectiveness. In: Hall EJ, Giaccia AJ, eds. *Radiobiology for the Radiologist*. 7th ed. Philadelphia, PA: Lippincott Williams & Wilkins; 2012:104–113.

Question 15
How does relative biological effectiveness (RBE) depend on the type of tissue irradiated?

Question 16
What is the relationship between linear energy transfer (LET) and the oxygen enhancement ratio (OER)?

Question 17
For a given radiation type with a higher linear energy transfer (LET) value than that of x-rays, how does the relative biological effectiveness (RBE) change in a hypoxic setting compared to an aerated setting?

Question 18
At what linear energy transfer (LET) range does relative biological effectiveness (RBE) change the most?

Question 15 *How does relative biological effectiveness (RBE) depend on the type of tissue irradiated?*

Answer 15

Tissues that are able to accumulate and repair large amounts of sublethal radiation damage have large shoulders on survival curves. These tissues require larger doses of x-rays to produce the same biological effect (relative to higher LET particles with smaller shoulders) and thus have larger RBE values.

Hall EJ, Giaccia AJ. Linear energy transfer and relative biologic effectiveness. In: Hall EJ, Giaccia AJ, eds. *Radiobiology for the Radiologist*. 7th ed. Philadelphia, PA: Lippincott Williams & Wilkins; 2012:104–113.

Question 16 *What is the relationship between linear energy transfer (LET) and the oxygen enhancement ratio (OER)?*

Answer 16

OER is defined as the ratio of radiation dose required to produce a given effect in the absence of oxygen to the dose required to produce the same effect in the presence of oxygen. As LET increases (↑), the OER decreases (↓) since higher LET radiation is less affected by the absence of oxygen.

Hall EJ, Giaccia AJ. Linear energy transfer and relative biologic effectiveness. In: Hall EJ, Giaccia AJ, eds. *Radiobiology for the Radiologist*. 7th ed. Philadelphia, PA: Lippincott Williams & Wilkins; 2012:104–113.

Question 17 *For a given radiation type with a higher linear energy transfer (LET) value than that of x-rays, how does the relative biological effectiveness (RBE) change in a hypoxic setting compared to an aerated setting?*

Answer 17

The RBE increases in a hypoxic setting compared to an aerated setting. This is a consequence of requiring a higher x-ray dose to produce the same biological effect in a hypoxic setting relative to a radiation type (with a higher LET) that is less affected by the presence or absence of oxygen.

Hall EJ, Giaccia AJ. Linear energy transfer and relative biologic effectiveness. In: Hall EJ, Giaccia AJ, eds. *Radiobiology for the Radiologist*. 7th ed. Philadelphia, PA: Lippincott Williams & Wilkins; 2012:104–113.

Question 18 *At what linear energy transfer (LET) range does relative biological effectiveness (RBE) change the most?*

Answer 18

An LET range between 20 and 100 keV/μm shows the greatest RBE change.

Hall EJ, Giaccia AJ. Linear energy transfer and relative biologic effectiveness. In: Hall EJ, Giaccia AJ, eds. *Radiobiology for the Radiologist*. 7th ed. Philadelphia, PA: Lippincott Williams & Wilkins; 2012:104–113.

Question 19

Is the relative biological effectiveness (RBE) for heavy charged particles smaller or larger at the end of the track?

Question 20

For a given radiation type with a higher linear energy transfer (LET) value than that of x-rays, how does relative biological effectiveness (RBE) depend on dose rate?

Question 21

How does linear energy transfer (LET) relate to the α/β ratio?

Question 19 *Is the relative biological effectiveness (RBE) for heavy charged particles smaller or larger at the end of the track?*

Answer 19

The RBE for charged particles is small at the beginning of the track, increases slowly with depth, and is greatest in the Bragg peak region where there is maximum dose deposition by the charged particle near the end of its path.

Hall EJ, Giaccia AJ. Linear energy transfer and relative biologic effectiveness. In: Hall EJ, Giaccia AJ, eds. *Radiobiology for the Radiologist*. 7th ed. Philadelphia, PA: Lippincott Williams & Wilkins; 2012:104–113.

Question 20 *For a given radiation type with a higher linear energy transfer (LET) value than that of x-rays, how does relative biological effectiveness (RBE) depend on dose rate?*

Answer 20

As dose rate decreases, RBE increases since there is more time for repair and a larger dose of x-rays is needed to produce the same biological effect relative to high LET particles, which are less affected by changes in dose rate.

Hall EJ, Giaccia AJ. Linear energy transfer and relative biologic effectiveness. In: Hall EJ, Giaccia AJ, eds. *Radiobiology for the Radiologist*. 7th ed. Philadelphia, PA: Lippincott Williams & Wilkins; 2012:104–113.

Question 21 *How does linear energy transfer (LET) relate to the α/β ratio?*

Answer 21

Based on the linear-quadratic model of cell survival, the α/β ratio represents the dose where cell killing due to the linear and quadratic components are equal. The α parameter represents single-event cell killing caused by double-stranded breaks while the β parameter represents multiple-event cell killing. As LET increases toward 100 keV/μm, the α/β ratio increases due primarily to an increase in the α parameter and double-stranded breaks.

Hall EJ, Giaccia AJ. Linear energy transfer and relative biologic effectiveness. In: Hall EJ, Giaccia AJ, eds. *Radiobiology for the Radiologist*. 7th ed. Philadelphia, PA: Lippincott Williams & Wilkins; 2012:104–113.

8

ASSAYS FOR CELL, TISSUE, AND SOLID TUMORS

C. MARC LEYRER, EHSAN H. BALAGAMWALA, AND CAMILLE BERRIOCHOA

Question 1

What is a vector?

Question 2

What are the different types of vectors?

Question 3

What is the difference between an adenovirus and a retrovirus?

Question 4

What is the purpose of agarose gel electrophoresis, and which charge does the DNA move toward?

Turn page to see the answers.

Question 1 *What is a vector?*

Answer 1

A vector is a self-replicating DNA molecule, which artificially carries a foreign DNA into a host cell where it can be replicated and/or expressed.

Hall EJ, Giaccia AJ. Molecular techniques in radiobiology. In: Hall EJ, Giaccia AJ, eds. *Radiobiology for the Radiologist*. 6th ed. Philadelphia, PA: Lippincott Williams & Wilkins; 2006:240–273.

Question 2 *What are the different types of vectors?*

Answer 2

a. Plasmid—circular DNA molecules that can contain a piece of foreign DNA, which can reside and replicate inside bacteria independent of the host chromosome. Limited to small DNA inserts up to 10,000 base pairs (bp).
b. Bacteriophage—a virus that infects and replicates within bacteria with the central portion deleted and foreign DNA inserted. Can accommodate larger DNA fragments than plasmids, up to 24,000 bp.
c. Bacterial artificial chromosomes (BACs)—a DNA construct used for transforming and cloning in bacteria (usually *Escherichia coli*) with large DNA fragments up to 300,000 bp.
d. Viruses—most efficient vector for gene transfer and similar to how a bacteriophage integrates DNA into a bacteria but also effective in mammalian cells. Generally, genetically engineered viruses integrate noninfectious viral DNA (adenovirus) or RNA (retrovirus).

Brown TA. Vectors for gene cloning: plasmids and bacteriophage (chap 2). In: Brown TA, ed. *Gene Cloning and DNA Analysis: An Introduction*. 6th ed. Oxford/Hoboken, NJ: Wiley-Blackwell; 2010:14–27.
Hall EJ, Giaccia AJ. Molecular techniques in radiobiology. In: Hall EJ, Giaccia AJ, eds. *Radiobiology for the Radiologist*. 6th ed. Philadelphia, PA: Lippincott Williams & Wilkins; 2006:240–273.

Question 3 *What is the difference between an adenovirus and a retrovirus?*

Answer 3

Retroviruses integrate the viral RNA into the DNA by reverse transcription to DNA, which is then integrated to the host DNA through an integrase enzyme. This method requires active division of the host cell for replication. An adenovirus contains double-stranded DNA, which is not integrated into the host DNA. It instead uses the host cell's enzymes and proteins for replication.

Brown TA. Vectors for gene cloning: plasmids and bacteriophage. In: Brown TA, ed. *Gene Cloning and DNA Analysis: An Introduction*. 6th ed. Wiley-Blackwell; 2010:14–27.
Hall EJ, Giaccia AJ. Molecular techniques in radiobiology. In: Hall EJ, Giaccia AJ, eds. *Radiobiology for the Radiologist*. 6th ed. Philadelphia, PA: Lippincott Williams & Wilkins; 2006:240–273.

Question 4 *What is the purpose of agarose gel electrophoresis, and which charge does the DNA move toward?*

Answer 4

It allows the separation of multiple differing DNA fragments based on the size when under a constant charge. It takes advantage of the negative charge on DNA, which moves from the negative pole toward the positive pole at a rate that is dependent on the size of the DNA.

Hall EJ, Giaccia AJ. Molecular techniques in radiobiology. In: Hall EJ, Giaccia AJ, eds. *Radiobiology for the Radiologist*. 6th ed. Philadelphia, PA: Lippincott Williams & Wilkins; 2006:240–273.

Question 5

What is the process of polymerase chain reactions (PCR)?

Question 6

What is an exonuclease?

Question 7

What is an endonuclease?

Question 8

What are restriction endonucleases?

Question 5 *What is the process of polymerase chain reactions (PCR)?*

Answer 5

a. Identify the section of dsDNA sequence requiring amplification and create a primer corresponding to the 5′ end of the dsDNA.
b. Combine the two primers and the DNA sample to be amplified with a heat-stable Taq DNA polymerase and an excess amount of the four deoxyribonucleotide triphosphates.
c. Heat the sample to 94°C to denature the dsDNA.
d. Cool to ~50°C to allow the primers to anneal to the complementary sequence on the DNA.
e. Heat the sample to 72°C, which is the optimal temperature for the Taq polymerase to allow for extension from the primers along the DNA strand, creating a new dsDNA.
f. This process is repeated 25 to 35 times to create millions of copies of a specific DNA fragment.

Hall EJ, Giaccia AJ. Molecular techniques in radiobiology. In: Hall EJ, Giaccia AJ, eds. *Radiobiology for the Radiologist.* 6th ed. Philadelphia, PA: Lippincott Williams & Wilkins; 2006:240–273.

Question 6 *What is an exonuclease?*

Answer 6

An exonuclease is an enzyme that cleaves nucleotides at one end of a polynucleotide chain by hydrolysis, which breaks phosphodiester bonds at the 3′ or 5′ position.

Hall EJ, Giaccia AJ. Molecular techniques in radiobiology. In: Hall EJ, Giaccia AJ, eds. *Radiobiology for the Radiologist.* 6th ed. Philadelphia, PA: Lippincott Williams & Wilkins; 2006:240–273.

Question 7 *What is an endonuclease?*

Answer 7

An endonuclease is an enzyme that cleaves the phosphodiester bonds in the middle of a polynucleotide chain.

Hall EJ, Giaccia AJ. Molecular techniques in radiobiology. In: Hall EJ, Giaccia AJ, eds. *Radiobiology for the Radiologist.* 6th ed. Philadelphia, PA: Lippincott Williams & Wilkins; 2006:240–273.

Question 8 *What are restriction endonucleases?*

Answer 8

This endonuclease cleaves at or near a specific DNA sequence. This is usually a short 4 to 8 nucleotide site and usually a palindromic sequence. A palindromic sequence is one which is read the same way if evaluated in either direction along the DNA.

Hall EJ, Giaccia AJ. Molecular techniques in radiobiology. In: Hall EJ, Giaccia AJ, eds. *Radiobiology for the Radiologist.* 6th ed. Philadelphia, PA: Lippincott Williams & Wilkins; 2006:240–273.

Question 9

What is the difference between a Southern, Northern, and Western blot?

Question 10

What is chromosome walking?

Question 11

What is homologous recombination and how is it utilized in genomic analysis?

Question 12

What are two common mechanisms used to select clones containing a knockout event?

Question 9 *What is the difference between a Southern, Northern, and Western blot?*

Answer 9

a. A Southern blot is used to determine specific DNA fragments in DNA samples.

b. A Northern blot is used to determine gene expression of RNA (or mRNA) in a sample.

c. A Western blot is used to identify and quantify specific proteins within a mixture of proteins.

A helpful mnemonic is SNoW DRoP: **S**outhern/**DNA**, **N**orthern/**RNA**, **W**estern/**Protein**.

Hall EJ, Giaccia AJ. Molecular techniques in radiobiology. In: Hall EJ, Giaccia AJ, eds. *Radiobiology for the Radiologist*. 6th ed. Philadelphia, PA: Lippincott Williams & Wilkins; 2006:240–273.

Question 10 *What is chromosome walking?*

Answer 10

Chromosome walking is a technique used to isolate a specific, yet unknown, gene of interest on a known chromosomal arm. It requires identification of adjacent DNA sequences on either side of the unknown gene, known as flanking marker genes. Short complementary strands are then sequenced toward the unknown gene with a new marker gene identified for further "walking" toward the gene of interest. This "walking" of overlapping sequences is completed for the area between the known markers to identify the unknown gene of interest.

Hall EJ, Giaccia AJ. Molecular techniques in radiobiology. In: Hall EJ, Giaccia AJ, eds. *Radiobiology for the Radiologist*, 6th ed. Philadelphia, PA: Lippincott Williams & Wilkins; 2006:240–273.

Question 11 *What is homologous recombination and how is it utilized in genomic analysis?*

Answer 11

Homologous recombination is a cellular mechanism that allows for repair of one chromosome using the template of the complementary chromosome. This can be utilized to remove/alter, or "knockout," a particular gene of interest.

Hall B, Limaye A, Kulkarni AB. Overview: generation of gene knockout mice. *Curr Protoc Cell Biol*. Chapter 19, 2009;Unit 19.12:1–17. doi:10.1002/0471143030.cb1912s44

Hall EJ, Giaccia AJ. Molecular techniques in radiobiology. In: Hall EJ, Giaccia AJ, eds. *Radiobiology for the Radiologist*. 6th ed. Philadelphia, PA: Lippincott Williams & Wilkins; 2006:240–273.

Question 12 *What are two common mechanisms used to select clones containing a knockout event?*

Answer 12

a. Neomycin resistance (*neoR*) and sensitivity to gancyclovir (*tk*) are commonly used. If these genes are randomly inserted into the genome, then they are both expressed, leading to *neoR* and *tk*. If a homologous recombination event occurs around the selected gene of interest, then the *tk* gene is not incorporated, leading to neomycin and gancyclovir resistance.

Hall B, Limaye A, Kulkarni AB. Overview: generation of gene knockout mice. *Curr Protoc Cell Biol*. chap 19, 2009; Unit 19.12:1–17. doi:10.1002/0471143030.cb1912s44

Hall EJ, Giaccia AJ. Molecular techniques in radiobiology. In: Hall EJ, Giaccia AJ, eds. *Radiobiology for the Radiologist*. 6th ed. Philadelphia, PA: Lippincott Williams & Wilkins; 2006:240–273.

Question 13

How do you confirm the homozygous deletion of the gene of interest once a knockout model is created?

Question 14

Describe two ways by which RNA can interfere with gene expression.

Question 15

What does fluorescence in situ hybridization (FISH) detect?

Question 16

What is a reporter gene?

Question 13 *How do you confirm the homozygous deletion of the gene of interest once a knockout model is created?*

Answer 13
PCR or Southern blotting can confirm the loss.

Hall EJ, Giaccia AJ. Molecular techniques in radiobiology. In: Hall EJ, Giaccia AJ, eds. *Radiobiology for the Radiologist*. 6th ed. Philadelphia, PA: Lippincott Williams & Wilkins; 2006:240–273.

Question 14 *Describe two ways by which RNA can interfere with gene expression.*

Answer 14
a. Short-interfering RNAs (SiRNAs)—short RNA nucleotides (21–25 nucleotides in length), which interact with the RNA-silencing complex (RISC) and allows for targeting of the specific complementary RNA sequence. The RISC will then cleave and silence the targeted RNA.
b. Short hairpin RNA (small hairpin RNA or shRNA)—expression vectors are used to introduce shRNA, which contain a tight hairpin turn in the RNA; these are processed by Dicer (a cytoplasmic nuclease) into dsRNA. The dsRNA then interacts with RISC and causes silencing of the targeted RNA sequence.

Hall EJ, Giaccia AJ. Molecular techniques in radiobiology. In: Hall EJ, Giaccia AJ, eds. *Radiobiology for the Radiologist*. 6th ed. Philadelphia, PA: Lippincott Williams & Wilkins; 2006:240–273.

Question 15 *What does fluorescence in situ hybridization (FISH) detect?*

Answer 15
FISH is a cytogenetic technique that detects the presence or absence of specific DNA sequences on chromosomes with a fluorescent DNA or RNA probe. Microscopy can then be used to determine where on the chromosome the fluorescent probe is bound.

Hall EJ, Giaccia AJ. Molecular techniques in radiobiology. In: Hall EJ, Giaccia AJ, eds. *Radiobiology for the Radiologist*. 6th ed. Philadelphia, PA: Lippincott Williams & Wilkins; 2006:240–273.

Question 16 *What is a reporter gene?*

Answer 16
A reporter gene is a gene that can be added to a known regulatory or promotor sequence of DNA. This then conveys a particular characteristic and allows for easy identification and/or measuring of the organism when the gene of interest is expressed.

Hall EJ, Giaccia AJ. Molecular techniques in radiobiology. In: Hall EJ, Giaccia AJ, eds. *Radiobiology for the Radiologist*. 6th ed. Philadelphia, PA: Lippincott Williams & Wilkins; 2006:240–273.

Question 17

What are the common types of reporter genes?

Question 18

What is promotor bashing?

Question 19

What is the difference between the contents of a genomic, complementary DNA (cDNA), and expression library?

Question 20

What protein when detected allows for quantification of repair of double-stranded DNA breaks?

Question 17 *What are the common types of reporter genes?*

Answer 17

a. β-galactosidase—involves the *lacZ* gene, which creates a blue hue to the organism.
b. Chloramphenicol acetyltransferase—using the *cat* gene, it allows for resistance to chloramphenicol.
c. Green fluorescent protein—uses the jellyfish green fluorescent protein (*gfp*), which creates a green glow under blue light (510 nm).
d. Firefly luciferase—allows for light/photon emission of the particular organism, which can be subsequently detected and quantified.
e. Red fluorescent protein—causes a red glow under blue, green, or yellow light (588 nm).

Gibco. Reporter gene assays (chap 5). In *Gibco Cell Culture Basics Handbook*. Thermo Fisher Scientific, Inc.; 2015:63–65. https://www.thermofisher.com/us/en/home/references/gibco-cell-culture-basics.html
Hall EJ, Giaccia AJ. Molecular techniques in radiobiology. In: Hall EJ, Giaccia AJ, eds. *Radiobiology for the Radiologist*. 6th ed. Philadelphia, PA: Lippincott Williams & Wilkins; 2006:240–273.

Question 18 *What is promotor bashing?*

Answer 18

Promoter bashing is a technique used to identify the importance of a promotor gene in relation to a particular gene of interest. After identification, mutations are created in the promotor gene and expression levels of the gene of interest are subsequently evaluated.

Hall EJ, Giaccia AJ. Molecular techniques in radiobiology. In: Hall EJ, Giaccia AJ, eds. *Radiobiology for the Radiologist*. 6th ed. Philadelphia, PA: Lippincott Williams & Wilkins; 2006:240–273.

Question 19 *What is the difference between the contents of a genomic, complementary DNA (cDNA), and expression library?*

Answer 19

a. A genomic library is a set of clones containing DNA fragments, which make up the entire genome.
b. cDNA libraries contain mRNA expressed at a particular time, which has been converted back into its complementary DNA by reverse transcriptase. This represents the section of DNA undergoing transcription at a particular time point.
c. An expression library contains DNA fragments and the ability to create the encoded proteins, which can be detected by antibodies.

Hall EJ, Giaccia AJ. Molecular techniques in radiobiology. In: Hall EJ, Giaccia AJ, eds. *Radiobiology for the Radiologist*. 6th ed. Philadelphia, PA: Lippincott Williams & Wilkins; 2006:240–273.

Question 20 *What protein when detected allows for quantification of repair of double-stranded DNA breaks?*

Answer 20

H2AX is a histone that resides throughout the nucleus and becomes phosphorylated into γ-H2AX in a region of double-stranded breaks. This allows for quantification of repair.

Hall EJ, Giaccia AJ. Molecular techniques in radiobiology. In: Hall EJ, Giaccia AJ, eds. *Radiobiology for the Radiologist*. 6th ed. Philadelphia, PA: Lippincott Williams & Wilkins; 2006:240–273.

Question 21

How is a spotted microarray created?

Question 22

What is the difference between a spotted and oligonucleotide (or in situ) microarray?

Question 23

What is a restriction fragment length polymorphism (RFLP)?

Question 24

What is single-stranded conformation polymorphism (SSCP)?

Question 21 *How is a spotted microarray created?*

Answer 21

RNA is extracted and converted to cDNA through reverse transcription. A nucleotide, which allows for fluorescent detection, is attached to the cDNA and then hybridized to the microarray.

Hall EJ, Giaccia AJ. Molecular techniques in radiobiology. In: Hall EJ, Giaccia AJ, eds. *Radiobiology for the Radiologist*. 6th ed. Philadelphia, PA: Lippincott Williams & Wilkins; 2006:240–273.

Question 22 *What is the difference between a spotted and oligonucleotide (or in situ) microarray?*

Answer 22

In a spotted microarray, the probes are created prior to hybridization on the surface of the microarray and subsequently deposited on specific spots of a grid. An oligonucleotide microarray is where the probes (or oligonucleotides) are synthesized directly on the surface of the microarray one nucleotide at a time.

Hall EJ, Giaccia AJ. Molecular techniques in radiobiology. In: Hall EJ, Giaccia AJ, eds. *Radiobiology for the Radiologist*. 6th ed. Philadelphia, PA: Lippincott Williams & Wilkins; 2006:240–273.

Question 23 *What is a restriction fragment length polymorphism (RFLP)?*

Answer 23

RFLP involves differences in DNA conformation due to differing restriction fragments. These can be used to determine the difference between multiple similar DNA sequences, which could result from deletions/insertions, point mutations, or tandem repeats. A restriction enzyme is used to fragment a DNA sequence, resulting in restriction fragments. This is then separated by gel electrophoresis. The difference in length and separation can be used to identify variations in the sequence.

Hall EJ, Giaccia AJ. Molecular techniques in radiobiology. In: Hall EJ, Giaccia AJ, eds. *Radiobiology for the Radiologist*. 6th ed. Philadelphia, PA: Lippincott Williams & Wilkins; 2006:240–273.

Question 24 *What is single-stranded conformation polymorphism (SSCP)?*

Answer 24

It is difficult to determine the difference between lengths of two ssDNA molecules with a single base-pair difference such as in SSCP. However, due to the different sequences, the two ssDNA strands form a unique structural state due to the difference in DNA sequence, which can then be separated on a neutral polyacrylamide gel electrophoresis (PAGE).

Hall EJ, Giaccia AJ. Molecular techniques in radiobiology. In: Hall EJ, Giaccia AJ, eds. *Radiobiology for the Radiologist*. 6th ed. Philadelphia, PA: Lippincott Williams & Wilkins; 2006:240–273.
Orita M, Iwahana H, Kanazawa H, Hayashi K, Sekiya T. Detection of polymorphisms of human DNA by gel electrophoresis as single-strand conformation polymorphisms. *Proc Natl Acad Sci USA*. 1989;86(8):2766–2770.

Question 25
What is the significance of the Cy5:Cy3 ratio in comparative genome hybridization (CGH)?

Question 26
What is Electrophoretic Mobility Shift Assay (EMSA or gel shift assay)?

Question 27
What does chromatin immunoprecipitation (ChIP) determine and how does it work?

Question 25 *What is the significance of the Cy5:Cy3 ratio in comparative genome hybridization (CGH)?*

Answer 25

A high Cy5:Cy3 ratio corresponds with regions of the genome that are amplified in a specific cancer cell. A low Cy5:Cy3 ratio corresponds with regions of the genome with chromosomal deletions.

Bilban M, Buehler LK, Head S, Desoye G, Quaranta V. Normalizing DNA microarray data. *Curr Issues Mol Biol.* 2002;4(2):57–64.

Hall EJ, Giaccia AJ. Molecular techniques in radiobiology. In: Hall EJ, Giaccia AJ, eds. *Radiobiology for the Radiologist.* 6th ed. Philadelphia, PA: Lippincott Williams & Wilkins; 2006:240–273.

Question 26 *What is Electrophoretic Mobility Shift Assay (EMSA or gel shift assay)?*

Answer 26

EMSA is used to determine if certain proteins are binding to a specific DNA or RNA sequence and sometimes if more than one protein is required. This is utilized to identify specific DNA sequences bound by transcription factors, DNA replication/repair, and RNA modification.

Hall EJ, Giaccia AJ. Molecular techniques in radiobiology. In: Hall EJ, Giaccia AJ, eds. *Radiobiology for the Radiologist.* 6th ed. Philadelphia, PA: Lippincott Williams & Wilkins; 2006:240–273.

Question 27 *What does chromatin immunoprecipitation (ChIP) determine and how does it work?*

Answer 27

ChIP shows which sequence of DNA a particular protein interacts with. The proteins under investigation are crosslinked in vivo with formaldehyde or UV light. The DNA is then sheared into smaller fragments and the protein-bound segments are separated by immunoprecipitation from the nonbound sequences. The separated fragments can then be purified, amplified, and sequenced.

Hall EJ, Giaccia AJ. Molecular techniques in radiobiology. In: Hall EJ, Giaccia AJ, eds. *Radiobiology for the Radiologist.* 6th ed. Philadelphia, PA: Lippincott Williams & Wilkins; 2006:240–273.

9

MOLECULAR TECHNIQUES, ASSAY SYSTEMS, AND SIGNALING IN RADIOBIOLOGY

KAILIN YANG AND JENNIFER S. YU

Question 1

What is cytogenetics and how is a cytogenetic study performed?

Question 2

What is used to detect specific DNA sequences in fluorescence in situ hybridization (FISH)?

Question 1 *What is cytogenetics and how is a cytogenetic study performed?*

Answer 1

Cytogenetics is the study of chromosome number and structure. The first step of a cytogenetic study is the preparation of chromosome spreads by mechanically rupturing metaphase cells that are hypotonically swollen. The chromosomes are spread across a small region on a microscope slide and stained. These stained chromosomes are individually recognized and classified. Traditional Q-banding used alkylating fluorochromes to stain chromosomes. Modern banding techniques can generate 300 to 850 bands across all chromosomes of the human genome. Traditional cytogenetics can be complemented with fluorescence in situ hybridization (FISH) and genomic microarray analysis (Figure 9.1).

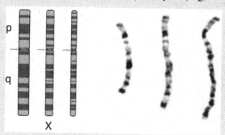

Figure 9.1 Ideograms and photomicrographs of the X chromosome (from left to right: metaphase, prometaphase, and prophase).

Source: Figure 9.1 from Nussbaum RL, McInnes RR, Willard HF. *Thompson & Thompson Genetics in Medicine.* 8th ed. Philadelphia; PA: Elsevier, 2016:57–74.

Spellman PT, Costello JF, Gray JW. Cancer genomics. In: Mendelsohn J, Howley PM, Israle MA, Gray JW, Thompson CB, eds. *The Molecular Basis of Cancer.* 3rd ed. Philadelphia, PA: Saunders/Elsevier; 2008:267–282.

Question 2 *What is used to detect specific DNA sequences in fluorescence in situ hybridization (FISH)?*

Answer 2

FISH is used to visually detect a specific genomic region under the microscope. It can be performed on either a metaphase spread (as in a cytogenetic study) or interphase nuclei, in which the chromatin is condensed. FISH uses fluorescently labeled, single-stranded DNA probes. The probe hybridizes to the complementary genomic region. FISH can be used to detect copy number variation and chromosomal structural aberrations in cancer cells (Figure 9.2).

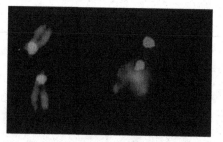

Figure 9.2 FISH study using centromere enumeration probe (CEP) for chromosome 12. Left: pair of chromosome 12 showing two hybridization signals in red in the centromeric area. Right: interphase cell showing two tight signals in interphase cell consistent with normal disomy.

Source: Figure 9.2 from Najfeld V. *Hematology: Basic Principles and Practice.* 6th ed. Philadelphia, PA: Saunders/Elsevier; 2013:728–780.

Spellman PT, Costello JF, Gray JW. Cancer genomics. In: Mendelsohn J, Howley PM, Israle MA, Gray JW, Thompson CB, eds. *The Molecular Basis of Cancer.* 3rd ed. Philadelphia, PA: Saunders/Elsevier; 2008:267–282.

Question 3

What is the basic mechanism of Sanger sequencing?

Question 3 *What is the basic mechanism of Sanger sequencing?*

Answer 3

Sanger sequencing is the mainstay of traditional sequencing methodology used to detect mutations in a specific gene. The DNA template to be sequenced is subjected to a modified version of the polymerase chain reaction (PCR): standard deoxynucleotides (dNTPs: dATP, dTTP, dCTP, dGTP), DNA primer, and DNA polymerase are added to the DNA template, and the mixture is divided into four separate PCRs. To each reaction, a different fluorescently labeled dideoxynucleotide (ddATP, ddTTP, ddCTP, ddGTP) is added at a low concentration to terminate the DNA elongation. The DNA population of each modified PCR reaction is a mixture of DNA fragments of different lengths labeled with a fluorescent dideoxynucleotide at one end. Electrophoresis is then performed for each of the four DNA populations, to generate a chromatogram to decode a full sequence of the original DNA template (Figure 9.3).

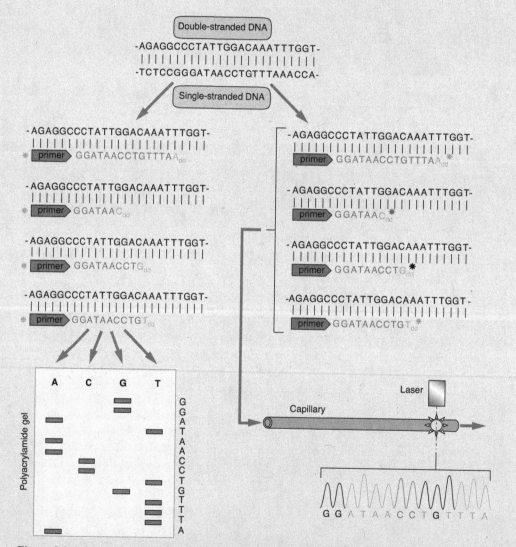

Figure 9.3 Schematic presentation of Sanger DNA sequencing, using chain termination method.

Source: Figure 9.3 from Pitt AR, Kolch W. *Medical Biochemistry*. 4th ed. Philadelphia, PA: Saunders/Elsevier; 2014:466–485.

Spellman PT, Costello JF, Gray JW. Cancer genomics. In: Mendelsohn J, Howley PM, Israle MA, Gray JW, Thompson CB, eds. *The Molecular Basis of Cancer*. 3rd ed. Philadelphia, PA: Saunders/Elsevier; 2008:267–282.

Question 4
What is DNA methylation? What methods have been developed to study DNA methylation status in cancer cells?

Question 5
What molecular methods can be used to monitor apoptosis following therapy?

Question 6
What is the phenotypical consequence of congenital mutations impairing the function of a DNA damage response gene?

Question 4 *What is DNA methylation? What methods have been developed to study DNA methylation status in cancer cells?*

Answer 4

DNA methylation is defined as the addition of methyl group onto DNA itself, specifically to the cytosine base to form 5-methylcytosine. Such cytosine is usually followed with guanine at its 3' end, forming a CpG island for methylation. This reaction is catalyzed by DNA methyltransferase. Cells use DNA methylation as a form of epigenetic regulation on gene expression. In cancers, an aberrant pattern of DNA methylation modulates gene expression to promote tumorigenesis and resistance to treatment. Several methodologies have been developed to detect DNA methylation, including methylation-specific PCR at a single gene, restriction-landmark genomic scanning, microarray-based DNA methylation analysis, and reduced-representation bisulfite sequencing. The method of reduced-representation bisulfite sequencing uses a combination of restriction enzymes and bisulfite sequencing to detect DNA methylation on the genome. Bisulfite treatment of DNA converts unmethylated cytosine nucleotide into uracil, while 5-methylcytosine is not affected. Sophisticated bioinformatics analysis is then performed to interpret the methylation status based on the sequencing results from bisulfite-treated DNA samples.

Spellman PT, Costello JF, Gray JW. Cancer genomics. In: Mendelsohn J, Howley PM, Israle MA, Gray JW, Thompson CB, eds. *The Molecular Basis of Cancer*. 3rd ed. Philadelphia, PA: Saunders/Elsevier; 2008:267–282.

Question 5 *What molecular methods can be used to monitor apoptosis following therapy?*

Answer 5

Phosphatidylserine is externalized to the extracellular side of the plasma membrane on the cells undergoing the early phase of apoptosis. Annexin V is a calcium-dependent phospholipid which binds to phosphatidylserine with high affinity and specificity. Therefore, fluorescent-labeled or radiolabeled annexin V has been used to monitor apoptosis of tumor cells following therapy. This is usually performed using flow cytometry to detect annexin V on the extracellular side of the plasma membrane.

Cleaved caspase 3, which is the active form, is another marker for apoptosis. Cleaved caspase can be detected using Western blot, as it exhibits a smaller molecular weight compared to its inactive zymogen form.

The terminal deoxynucleotidyl transferase dUTP nick end-labeling (TUNEL) assay detects DNA fragmentation by labeling the terminal end of nucleic acids. As a cell goes through apoptosis, activation of endonucleases generates short DNA fragments, which can be readily detected using TUNEL assay.

Yaghoubi SS, Gambhir SS. Imaging and cancer. In: Mendelsohn J, Howley PM, Israle MA, Gray JW, Thompson CB, eds. *The Molecular Basis of Cancer*. 3rd ed. Philadelphia, PA: Saunders/Elsevier; 2008:309–324.

Question 6 *What is the phenotypical consequence of congenital mutations impairing the function of a DNA damage response gene?*

Answer 6

Patients carrying germline mutations in genes involved in DNA damage response and repair pathways will develop various cancer-prone syndromes, which are characterized by hypersensitivity to DNA damage (including radiation) and genomic instability.

Hall EJ, Giaccia AJ. Cancer biology. In: Hall EJ, Giaccia AJ, eds. *Radiobiology for the Radiologists*. 7th ed. Philadelphia, PA: Lippincott Williams & Wilkins; 2012:274–303.

Question 7

What is the typical characteristic of patients with ataxia telangiectasia (AT)?

Question 8

How do mutations in ataxia telangiectasia mutated (ATM) kinase cause radioresistant DNA synthesis?

Question 9

Why do Seckel syndrome patients not appear to be radiosensitive?

Question 10

Which genes are mutated in murine and human severe combined immunodeficiency (SCID) syndrome, respectively?

Question 7 *What is the typical characteristic of patients with ataxia telangiectasia (AT)?*

Answer 7

AT is a rare autosomal recessive genetic disease that results from mutations in the *ATM* gene. The prototypical cerebellar ataxia is caused by progressive loss of Purkinje cells in the cerebellum; affected patients also present with oculocutaneous telangiectasias. These patients are immune deficient with a higher susceptibility to develop cancer. Fibroblasts and lymphocytes derived from AT patients demonstrate hypersensitivity to ionizing radiation.

Hall EJ, Giaccia AJ. Cancer biology. In: Hall EJ, Giaccia AJ, eds. *Radiobiology for the Radiologists*. 7th ed. Philadelphia, PA: Lippincott Williams & Wilkins; 2012:274–303.

Question 8 *How do mutations in ataxia telangiectasia mutated (ATM) kinase cause radioresistant DNA synthesis?*

Answer 8

ATM protein is a serine/threonine kinase that mediates cellular responses to DNA double-strand breaks. At the G1/S checkpoint in response to DNA damage (such as radiation), ATM phosphorylates p53, leading to p53 protein stabilization and transactivation of its target gene, *p21*. p21 is a cell cycle inhibitor that arrests cells at the G1/S checkpoint. Mutation of the ATM gene, as seen in AT patients, fails to activate p21 and leads to cell cycle progression into S phase in response to radiation. The phenomenon of radioresistant DNA synthesis is a distinctive hallmark of AT cells.

Hall EJ, Giaccia AJ. Cancer biology. In: Hall EJ, Giaccia AJ, eds. *Radiobiology for the Radiologists*. 7th ed. Philadelphia, PA: Lippincott Williams & Wilkins; 2012:274–303.

Question 9 *Why do Seckel syndrome patients not appear to be radiosensitive?*

Answer 9

Seckel syndrome is a rare autosomal recessive disorder characterized with microcephaly and other developmental abnormalities. Seckel syndrome is caused by mutations in the *ATR* gene, another member in the phosphatidylinositol 3-kinase-related kinase (PIKK) family including *ATM*. Unlike *ATM*, *ATR* is an essential gene in mammalian cells. Therefore, mutation in *ATR* found in Seckel patients does not completely abolish *ATR* activity, but rather reduces its absolute quantity. The residual ATR activity observed in Seckel patients probably explains why they do not appear to be radiosensitive.

Hall EJ, Giaccia AJ. Cancer biology. In: Hall EJ, Giaccia AJ, eds. *Radiobiology for the Radiologists*. 7th ed. Philadelphia, PA: Lippincott Williams & Wilkins; 2012:274–303.

Question 10 *Which genes are mutated in murine and human severe combined immunodeficiency (SCID) syndrome, respectively?*

Answer 10

DNA-dependent protein kinase catalytic subunit (DNA-PKcs), the third member of the phosphatidylinositol 3-kinase-related kinase (PIKK) family involved in DNA damage response, plays an essential role in nonhomologous end joining (NHEJ). Mutation in DNA-PKcs causes murine SCID. Mutation in Artemis, which encodes a target protein of DNA-PKcs, causes human SCID. Cells derived from human SCID patients demonstrate hypersensitivity to radiation and genomic instability.

Hall EJ, Giaccia AJ. Cancer biology. In: Hall EJ, Giaccia AJ, eds. *Radiobiology for the Radiologists*. 7th ed. Philadelphia, PA: Lippincott Williams & Wilkins; 2012:274–303.

Question 11
Which gene is defective in Ataxia-Telangiectasia-Like Disorder (ATLD)?

Question 12
What is the molecular function of Nijmegen Breakage Syndrome 1 protein (NBS1) in the DNA damage response?

Question 13
What is the key molecular event in the Fanconi anemia (FA) pathway?

Question 14
What are the phenotypical manifestations of patients with Bloom syndrome (BLM)?

Question 11 *Which gene is defective in Ataxia-Telangiectasia-Like Disorder (ATLD)?*

Answer 11

MRE11 is the gene mutated in ATLD. In response to radiation, MRE11 forms a complex with Rad50 and NBS (MRN complex), which functions in double-strand break repair through activating ATM kinase. MRE11 also possesses nuclease activity, which resects double-strand break ends to promote repair through homologous recombination. Cells derived from ATLD patients exhibit both radiation sensitivity and defects in cell cycle checkpoint response following radiation.

Hall EJ, Giaccia AJ. Cancer biology. In: Hall EJ, Giaccia AJ, eds. *Radiobiology for the Radiologists*. 7th ed. Philadelphia, PA: Lippincott Williams & Wilkins; 2012:274–303.

Question 12 *What is the molecular function of Nijmegen Breakage Syndrome 1 protein (NBS1) in the DNA damage response?*

Answer 12

NBS1 is encoded by the gene mutated in Nijmegen Breakage Syndrome, a rare autosomal recessive congenital disorder causing chromosomal instability. In response to double-strand breaks, NBS1 forms a complex with Rad50 and MRE11, which functions in DNA repair as a nuclease. NBS1 is also a direct kinase substrate of ATM, and mediates the activation of ATM checkpoint response.

Hall EJ, Giaccia AJ. Cancer biology. In: Hall EJ, Giaccia AJ, eds. *Radiobiology for the Radiologists*. 7th ed. Philadelphia, PA: Lippincott Williams & Wilkins; 2012:274–303.

Question 13 *What is the key molecular event in the Fanconi anemia (FA) pathway?*

Answer 13

FA is a recessive disorder characterized by chromosomal instability, sensitivity to interstrand DNA crosslinks, and, in certain cases, sensitivity to ionizing radiation. Most of the FA proteins form a large E3 ubiquitin ligase complex. Upon DNA damage, the FA core E3 ligase monoubiquitinates the FANCD2 (Fanconi anemia complementation group D2) protein. Monoubiquitinated FANCD2 then localizes to foci containing BRCA2 and function in DNA damage response by recruiting downstream repair enzymes.

Hall EJ, Giaccia AJ. Cancer biology. In: Hall EJ, Giaccia AJ, eds. *Radiobiology for the Radiologists*. 7th ed. Philadelphia, PA: Lippincott Williams & Wilkins; 2012:274–303.

Question 14 *What are the phenotypical manifestations of patients with Bloom syndrome (BLM)?*

Answer 14

BLM is caused by congenital mutations in BLM helicase, a member of the RecQ helicase family that functions as DNA helicases that unwind DNA 3' to 5' in an ATP-dependent manner together with 3' to 5' exonuclease activity. Patients with BLM are highly sensitive to sunlight, and also demonstrate dwarfism, immunodeficiency, male sterility, and elevated level of sister chromatid exchange (SCE).

Hall EJ, Giaccia AJ. Cancer biology. In: Hall EJ, Giaccia AJ, eds. *Radiobiology for the Radiologists*. 7th ed. Philadelphia, PA: Lippincott Williams & Wilkins; 2012:274–303.

Question 15

In addition to cancer, what other medical issues do Werner syndrome (WS) patients suffer from?

Question 16

What are the clinical characterizations of patients with Rothmund–Thompson syndrome (RTS)?

Question 17

What are the roles for early and late response genes in mediating the cellular effects of radiation?

Question 18

How does DNA damage induce the production of ceramide?

Question 15 *In addition to cancer, what other medical issues do Werner syndrome (WS) patients suffer from?*

Answer 15

Besides predisposition to cancer development, WS patients also exhibit accelerated aging, which is characterized by age-related diseases including diabetes, osteoporosis, and atherosclerotic cardiovascular disease. WS ATP-dependent helicase, another member of the RecQ helicase family, is mutated in WS patients. At the molecular level, susceptibility to cancer and premature aging are probably caused by elevated levels of genomic instability.

Hall EJ, Giaccia AJ. Cancer biology. In: Hall EJ, Giaccia AJ, eds. *Radiobiology for the Radiologists*. 7th ed. Philadelphia, PA: Lippincott Williams & Wilkins; 2012:274–303.

Question 16 *What are the clinical characterizations of patients with Rothmund–Thompson syndrome (RTS)?*

Answer 16

Mutation in *RECQL4* gene encoding ATP-dependent DNA helicase Q4 causes in RTS. RTS patients exhibit growth deficiency, photosensitivity, early greying and hair loss, juvenile cataracts, and skeletal dysplasia. They are also highly susceptible to develop cancer, particularly osteogenic sarcoma, due to an elevated level of chromosomal instability.

Hall EJ, Giaccia AJ. Cancer biology. In: Hall EJ, Giaccia AJ, eds. *Radiobiology for the Radiologists*. 7th ed. Philadelphia, PA: Lippincott Williams & Wilkins; 2012:274–303.

Question 17 *What are the roles for early and late response genes in mediating the cellular effects of radiation?*

Answer 17

Ionizing radiation activates early response genes, such as *Ras* and *Raf*, which mimic the signaling response of mitogenic activation of quiescent cells. The activation of early response genes contributes to radiation resistance through facilitating DNA repair and cell cycle arrest. Early response genes also provide a mechanism for secondary stimulation of late response genes, such as *TNF-α, PDGF, FGF*, and *IL-1*. Induction of late response genes promote cellular adjustment to the change in microenvironment. Late response genes also mediate cellular response (such as apoptosis) after radiation treatment.

Hall EJ, Giaccia AJ. Cancer biology. In: Hall EJ, Giaccia AJ, eds. *Radiobiology for the Radiologists*. 7th ed. Philadelphia, PA: Lippincott Williams & Wilkins; 2012:274–303.

Question 18 *How does DNA damage induce the production of ceramide?*

Answer 18

The intracellular production of ceramide is a potent activator of the caspase cascade to induce apoptosis. The production of ceramide in response to DNA damage is mediated through two major pathways: first, ionizing radiation and DNA-damaging agents activate acid sphingomyelinase (ASMase) to hydrolyze sphingomyelin to form ceramide. This process consumes up to 50% of the total cellular store of sphingomyelin to produce ceramide. Second, ceramide synthase can directly synthesize ceramide, in a process that is negatively regulated by ATM kinase.

Hall EJ, Giaccia AJ. Cancer biology. In: Hall EJ, Giaccia AJ, eds. *Radiobiology for the Radiologists*. 7th ed. Philadelphia, PA: Lippincott Williams & Wilkins; 2012:274–303.

Question 19

What is the preferred assay in evaluating the effectiveness of radiation therapy?

Question 20

What methodology can be used to monitor DNA damage after radiation?

Question 19 *What is the preferred assay in evaluating the effectiveness of radiation therapy?*

Answer 19

Long-term clonogenic assay is a critical component in measuring the effectiveness of radiation therapy and radiation sensitizers. For moderate DNA damage, it might take as many as nine mitoses to cause cellular death. Therefore, a long-term clonogenic assay is a more reliable method to measure cell survival after radiation compared to a short-term assay (e.g., apoptosis).

Woodward WA, Cox JD. Molecular basis of radiation therapy. In: Mendelsohn J, Howley PM, Israle MA, Gray JW, Thompson CB, eds. *The Molecular Basis of Cancer*. 3rd ed. Philadelphia, PA: Saunders/Elsevier; 2008:593–604.

Question 20 *What methodology can be used to monitor DNA damage after radiation?*

Answer 20

Radiation-induced double-strand breaks are marked by γ-H2AX, a phosphorylated histone H2A variant. The phosphorylation process of H2AX is mediated by the concerted action of the DNA damage response pathway, particularly the phosphatidylinositol 3-kinase-related kinase (PIKK) family kinase ATM. The resolution of γ-H2AX foci correlates with the effectiveness of DNA repair. Therefore, staining the nuclei with anti-γ-H2AX antibody followed with immunofluorescence detection is a viable method to monitor induction and repair of DNA damage after radiation. Another method to monitor DNA damage is comet assay, which uses single-cell gel electrophoresis to measure DNA strand breaks. Cells were embedded in agarose on a microscope slide. They were then lysed to form nucleoids, which are composed of supercoiled DNA. Electrophoresis was then performed, resulting in structures resembling comets. These comet-shape structures could be visualized with fluorescence microscopy.

Woodward WA, Cox JD. Molecular basis of radiation therapy. In: Mendelsohn J, Howley PM, Israle MA, Gray JW, Thompson CB, eds. *The Molecular Basis of Cancer*. 3rd ed. Philadelphia, PA: Saunders/Elsevier; 2008:593–604.

10

BIOLOGY OF CANCER

KAILIN YANG AND JENNIFER S. YU

Question 1

What is a hallmark of cancer cells?

Question 2

What is a proto-oncogene?

Question 3

What is a tumor suppressor gene?

Question 4

What is a DNA stability gene?

Turn page to see the answers. **133**

Question 1 *What is a hallmark of cancer cells?*

Answer 1

The hallmark of cancer cells is deregulated control of cell division and failure for self-elimination. It is like a Darwinian-like process in which the fittest cells replicate to become the dominant population of a tumor.

Hall EJ, Giaccia AJ. Cancer biology. In: Hall EJ, Giaccia AJ, eds. *Radiobiology for the Radiologists*. 7th ed. Philadelphia, PA: Lippincott Williams & Wilkins; 2012:274–303.

Question 2 *What is a proto-oncogene?*

Answer 2

A proto-oncogene is a component of signaling networks that positively regulates cellular growth in response to mitogens, cytokines, and cell-to-cell contact. Gain-of-function mutation in only one copy of a proto-oncogene is sufficient to produce an active oncogene in a dominant manner that often fails to be regulated by extracellular signals.

Hall EJ, Giaccia AJ. Cancer biology. In: Hall EJ, Giaccia AJ, eds. *Radiobiology for the Radiologists*. 7th ed. Philadelphia, PA: Lippincott Williams & Wilkins; 2012:274–303.

Question 3 *What is a tumor suppressor gene?*

Answer 3

A tumor suppressor gene is a negative growth regulator. It modulates cellular proliferation and survival by antagonizing the functions of proto-oncogenes or responding to unchecked growth signals. In most cases, loss-of-function mutations of both copies of tumor suppressor are needed for tumor progression.

Hall EJ, Giaccia AJ. Cancer biology. In: Hall EJ, Giaccia AJ, eds. *Radiobiology for the Radiologists*. 7th ed. Philadelphia, PA: Lippincott Williams & Wilkins; 2012:274–303.

Question 4 *What is a DNA stability gene?*

Answer 4

DNA stability genes are a group of genes involved in monitoring and maintaining genomic integrity. Loss of DNA stability genes causes defects in proper sensing of DNA lesions and error-prone repair of a damaged DNA template.

Hall EJ, Giaccia AJ. Cancer biology. In: Hall EJ, Giaccia AJ, eds. *Radiobiology for the Radiologists*. 7th ed. Philadelphia, PA: Lippincott Williams & Wilkins; 2012:274–303.

Question 5
What causes normal tissues to transform into tumors and metastasize?

Question 6
What are the steps of malignant progression?

Question 7
Are tumors composed of a homogenous or heterogeneous group of neoplastic cells?

Question 8
In classic experiments performed in the 1970s, why could Rous sarcoma virus (RSV), but not the similar avian leukosis virus (ALV), cause cellular transformation and induce sarcoma?

Question 5 *What causes normal tissues to transform into tumors and metastasize?*

Answer 5

Malignant progression occurs in a series of steps over a period of time. Malignant progression is typically caused by gain-of-function mutations that activate oncogenes, loss-of-function mutations that inactivate tumor suppressor genes, and loss of activity of DNA stability genes that increases the probability of genomic instability. These gene changes result from random errors or exposure to various agents including chemical mutagen, ionizing radiation, ultraviolet light, and viral infection. Malignant progression gradually alters the regulatory mechanisms of a single cell in proliferation, self-elimination, immortalization, and genetic stability, creating the clonal origin of a tumor. Tumors also evade immune mechanisms.

Hall EJ, Giaccia AJ. Cancer biology. In: Hall EJ, Giaccia AJ, eds. *Radiobiology for the Radiologists*. 7th ed. Philadelphia, PA: Lippincott Williams & Wilkins; 2012:274–303.

Question 6 *What are the steps of malignant progression?*

Answer 6

Cancers seem to develop progressively. Between the two extremes of fully normal and highly metastatic tissues, there are a spectrum of steps, including hyperplasia, metaplasia, dysplasia, and neoplasia.

Weinberg RA. *The Biology of Cancer*. New York, NY: Garland Science; 2007.

Question 7 *Are tumors composed of a homogenous or heterogeneous group of neoplastic cells?*

Answer 7

Although tumor cells are considered clonal in origin, most tumor types contain heterogeneous populations of cells that differ in their ability to repopulate the tumor or form metastases. In many cancers, only a small percentage of tumor cells possess the ability to form a tumor, leading to the concept that tumors possess "stem-like cells" and that elimination of these stem-like cells is essential for controlling tumor growth.

Hall EJ, Giaccia AJ. Cancer biology. In: Hall EJ, Giaccia AJ, eds. *Radiobiology for the Radiologists*. 7th ed. Philadelphia, PA: Lippincott Williams & Wilkins; 2012:274–303.

Question 8 *In classic experiments performed in the 1970s, why could Rous sarcoma virus (RSV), but not the similar avian leukosis virus (ALV), cause cellular transformation and induce sarcoma?*

Answer 8

RSV, an RNA retrovirus, contains approximately 1,500 more base pairs (bp) of sequence than ALV. This unique piece of sequence was later found to contain genetic information to encode the *v-src* gene, which drives cellular transformation. The *v-src* gene is the malignant form of the cellular proto-oncogene *c-src*.

Hall EJ, Giaccia AJ. Cancer biology. In: Hall EJ, Giaccia AJ, eds. *Radiobiology for the Radiologists*. 7th ed. Philadelphia, PA: Lippincott Williams & Wilkins; 2012:274–303.

Question 9
What are four mechanisms for oncogene activation in human neoplasms?

Question 10
What is the Philadelphia chromosome seen in chronic myeloid leukemia (CML) patients?

Question 11
Which gene is mutated in familial retinoblastoma (Rb)? What is the epidemiological inheritance pattern of this mutation?

Question 12
What is the key paradigm shift in the "two-hit hypothesis" proposed by Knudson?

Question 9 *What are four mechanisms for oncogene activation in human neoplasms?*

Answer 9

Four mechanisms are retroviral integration through recombination, DNA mutation of regulatory sites, gene amplification, and chromosome translocation.

Hall EJ, Giaccia AJ. Cancer biology. In: Hall EJ, Giaccia AJ, eds. *Radiobiology for the Radiologists*. 7th ed. Philadelphia, PA: Lippincott Williams & Wilkins; 2012:274–303.

Question 10 *What is the Philadelphia chromosome seen in chronic myeloid leukemia (CML) patients?*

Answer 10

The Philadelphia chromosome, the shortened version of chromosome 22, is caused by symmetric translocation between chromosomes 9 and 22 that creates a novel fusion transcript encoding bcr-abl whose aberrant expression drives the development of CML.

Hall EJ, Giaccia AJ. Cancer biology. In: Hall EJ, Giaccia AJ, eds. *Radiobiology for the Radiologists*. 7th ed. Philadelphia, PA: Lippincott Williams & Wilkins; 2012:274–303.

Question 11 *Which gene is mutated in familial retinoblastoma (Rb)? What is the epidemiological inheritance pattern of this mutation?*

Answer 11

In familial *Rb*, patients possess a germline mutation of the *Rb* gene, a tumor suppressor gene, in all the cells of the body. Epidemiologically, mutation in one allele of *Rb* gene seems to be inherited in an autosomal dominant manner. Patients carrying *Rb* mutation develop bilateral or multifocal disease at an earlier age than those with sporadic *Rb*.

Hall EJ, Giaccia AJ. Cancer biology. In: Hall EJ, Giaccia AJ, eds. *Radiobiology for the Radiologists*. 7th ed. Philadelphia, PA: Lippincott Williams & Wilkins; 2012:274–303.

Question 12 *What is the key paradigm shift in the "two-hit hypothesis" proposed by Knudson?*

Answer 12

Inactivation of one allele of the retinoblastoma (*Rb*) gene does not give rise to retinoblastoma, but a mutation in the other allele is required for retinoblastoma development. The "two-hit hypothesis" underlines the significance that mutations in both alleles of a tumor suppressor gene are needed for tumor progression. Germline mutation of one allele of a tumor suppressor gene increases the susceptibility of cancer development. Frequently, loss of heterozygosity (LOH) is seen whereby one allele is mutated and the other allele is deleted, often in the setting of loss of the entire chromosome arm.

Knudson AG. Mutation and cancer: statistical study of retinoblastoma. *Proc Natl Acad Sci USA*. 1971;68:820–823.

Question 13

What is Li-Fraumeni syndrome (LFS)? What is the unique gene mutation in this syndrome?

Question 14

What are the unique clinical characteristics of familial breast cancer compared to sporadic breast cancer?

Question 15

What genes are mutated in familial breast cancer?

Question 16

What cancer predisposition syndrome is associated with germline mutation in *NF1, NF2, APC, VHL, E-CAD, PTCH, PTEN,* or *MEN1*, respectively?

Question 13 *What is Li-Fraumeni syndrome (LFS)? What is the unique gene mutation in this syndrome?*

Answer 13

LFS is a rare autosomal dominant disease, and affected patients are predisposed to develop osteosarcoma, soft-tissue sarcoma, rhabdomyosarcoma, leukemia, brain tumor, and lung and breast carcinoma. Patients have germline mutations in one allele of a *p53* gene that either inactivates its tumor suppressive functions or causes gain of function. Often, mutant *p53* is stabilized and overexpressed in tumors. Inactivation of the second allele of a wild-type *p53* gene (second hit) is required for tumor development in affected patients.

Li FP, Fraumeni JF. Prospective study of a family cancer syndrome. *J Amer Med Assoc*. 1982;247:2692–2694.

Question 14 *What are the unique clinical characteristics of familial breast cancer compared to sporadic breast cancer?*

Answer 14

Familial breast cancer accounts for 5% to 10% of all breast cancer cases. It is characterized by earlier age of onset, increased frequency of bilateral breast tumors, association with familial ovarian and prostate cancer, and overall higher incidence of cancer within an affected family. However, familial breast cancer is indistinguishable from sporadic breast cancer regarding histology and anatomy.

Hall EJ, Giaccia AJ. Cancer biology. In: Hall EJ, Giaccia AJ, eds. *Radiobiology for the Radiologists*. 7th ed. Philadelphia, PA: Lippincott Williams & Wilkins; 2012:274–303.

Question 15 *What genes are mutated in familial breast cancer?*

Answer 15

The breast cancer susceptibility genes (*BRCA1* and *BRCA2*) are mutated in familial breast cancer patients. *BRCA1* and *BRCA2* function in DNA damage and repair, cell cycle progression, gene transcription, protein ubiquitination, apoptosis, and stem cell regulation.

Hall EJ, Giaccia AJ. Cancer biology. In: Hall EJ, Giaccia AJ, eds. *Radiobiology for the Radiologists*. 7th ed. Philadelphia, PA: Lippincott Williams & Wilkins; 2012:274–303.

Question 16 *What cancer predisposition syndrome is associated with germline mutation in NF1, NF2, APC, VHL, E-CAD, PTCH, PTEN, or MEN1, respectively?*

Answer 16

NF1, neurofibromatosis type 1 (neurofibroma, sarcoma).
NF2, neurofibromatosis type 2 (schwannoma, meningioma).
APC, familial adenomatous polyposis (colon and stomach cancer).
VHL, von Hippel-Lindau disease (kidney and adrenal cancer).
E-CAD (E-cadherin), familial gastric cancer (stomach and breast cancer).
PTCH (Patched), Gorlin syndrome (basal cell carcinoma).
PTEN, Cowden syndrome (hamartoma).
MEN1, multiple endocrine neoplasia (pituitary, pancreas, and parathyroid cancer).

Hall EJ, Giaccia AJ. Cancer biology. In: Hall EJ Giaccia AJ, eds. *Radiobiology for the Radiologists*. 7th ed. Philadelphia, PA: Lippincott Williams & Wilkins; 2012:274–303.

Question 17
How are tumor suppressor genes lost in sporadic cancers?

Question 18
What is the significance of cellular transformation on proliferation?

Question 19
What is the most important determinant of G1/S transition in proliferating cells?

Question 20
What are the two major pathways mediating programmed cell death (apoptosis)?

Question 17 *How are tumor suppressor genes lost in sporadic cancers?*

Answer 17

In reality, the loss of both alleles of a tumor suppressor gene seems to occur more commonly through the somatic homozygosity process: a single inactivation of the tumor suppressor gene occurs in one chromosome while the other chromosome is lost completely; the chromosome with the inactive tumor suppressor gene then replicates to generate a homozygous chromosome pair.

Hall EJ, Giaccia AJ. Cancer biology. In: Hall EJ, Giaccia AJ, eds. *Radiobiology for the Radiologists*. 7th ed. Philadelphia, PA: Lippincott Williams & Wilkins; 2012:274–303.

Question 18 *What is the significance of cellular transformation on proliferation?*

Answer 18

Untransformed cells use cell surface receptors to transduce extracellular growth signals into intracellular circuits and promote growth. In contrast, transformed cells are able to maintain cellular growth in an autonomous manner, through secreting autocrine growth factors, overexpression or activation of growth factor receptors, or downstream signaling molecules.

Hall EJ, Giaccia AJ. Cancer biology. In: Hall EJ, Giaccia AJ, eds. *Radiobiology for the Radiologists*. 7th ed. Philadelphia, PA: Lippincott Williams & Wilkins; 2012:274–303.

Question 19 *What is the most important determinant of G1/S transition in proliferating cells?*

Answer 19

The G1/S transition is regulated by the retinoblastoma (*RB*) family of proteins. In the hypophosphorylated state, *RB* sequesters the E2 factor (*E2F*) transcription factor, which is essential for the transcription of genes necessary for G1/S transition, and therefore inhibits the progression into the S phase. When *RB* is phosphorylated by cyclin-dependent kinases (CDKs), the inhibition on E2F is released, leading to the transcription of E2F target genes and progression into the S phase. Antiproliferative signals, such as transforming growth factor beta (*TGF-β*), inhibit the hyperphosphorylation of *RB*.

Hall EJ, Giaccia AJ. Cancer biology. In: Hall EJ, Giaccia AJ, eds. *Radiobiology for the Radiologists*. 7th ed. Philadelphia, PA: Lippincott Williams & Wilkins; 2012:274–303.

Question 20 *What are the two major pathways mediating programmed cell death (apoptosis)?*

Answer 20

The two major pathways mediating apoptosis start either from the cell membrane (Fas ligand binding to Fas receptor) or release of cytochrome c from mitochondria, which is regulated by proapoptotic regulators such as BCL-2-associated X protein (*BAX*), BCL-2 antagonist/Killer (*BAK*), BH3 interacting-domain death agonist (*BID*), and BCL-2-like protein 11 (*BIM*), and antiapoptotic regulators such as B-cell lymphoma 2 (*BCL-2*), B-cell lymphoma-extra large (*BCL-XL*), and myeloid cell leukemia 1 (*MCL-1*). The signaling from either pathway leads to the activation of intracellular cysteine proteases, called caspases, which in turn start the apoptotic cascade.

Hall EJ, Giaccia AJ. Cancer biology. In: Hall EJ, Giaccia AJ, eds. *Radiobiology for the Radiologists*. 7th ed. Philadelphia, PA: Lippincott Williams & Wilkins; 2012:274–303.

Question 21
How does the *p53* tumor suppressor gene regulate apoptosis?

Question 22
What is the paradoxical role of the *MYC* oncogene on cell proliferation and apoptosis?

Question 23
What determines the cellular fate (transformation vs. senescence) of untransformed primary cells upon overexpressing the oncogene *RAS*?

Question 24
How does a cancer cell maintain its telomeres?

Question 21 *How does the* p53 *tumor suppressor gene regulate apoptosis?*

Answer 21

Tumor suppressor gene *p53* is a key modulator of apoptosis. In an unstressed condition, *p53* is downregulated by its binding partner, murine double minute (MDM2), which through its E3-ligase activity degrades *p53* via ubiquitin-mediated proteasome degradation. Cellular stresses, such as ionizing radiation, serum starvation, and hypoxia, lead to an elevated p53 protein level through protein stabilization and increased protein synthesis. Stabilized *p53* then acts as a transcriptional factor to stimulate apoptosis through upregulating the expression of proapoptotic genes including *BAX, PUMA, NOXA,* and *PERP*.

Hall EJ, Giaccia AJ. Cancer biology. In: Hall EJ, Giaccia AJ, eds. *Radiobiology for the Radiologists*. 7th ed. Philadelphia, PA: Lippincott Williams & Wilkins; 2012:274–303.

Question 22 *What is the paradoxical role of the* MYC *oncogene on cell proliferation and apoptosis?*

Answer 22

Overexpression of the *MYC* oncogene can lead to a cellular state of oncogenic transformation or programmed cell death, depending on the microenvironment and *p53* mutation status. In cells with an intact *p53* gene, *MYC* deregulation stabilizes p53 proteins through the cell cycle inhibitor p19[ARF] and sensitizes cells to apoptosis under growth-restrictive conditions caused by nutrient deprivation or hypoxia. Inactivation of a *p53* tumor suppressor gene would significantly attenuate the sensitivity of *MYC*-overexpressing cells to stress-induced apoptosis and therefore promote cellular transformation.

Hall EJ, Giaccia AJ. Cancer biology. In: Hall EJ, Giaccia AJ, eds. *Radiobiology for the Radiologists*. 7th ed. Philadelphia, PA: Lippincott Williams & Wilkins; 2012:274–303.

Question 23 *What determines the cellular fate (transformation vs. senescence) of untransformed primary cells upon overexpressing the oncogene* RAS?

Answer 23

The differential effect of the oncogene *RAS* on the cellular fate of untransformed primary cells depends on the presence of a p53 tumor suppressor and p16 cell cycle inhibitor. When both proteins are intact, overexpression of *RAS* causes elevated p53 and p16 protein levels, leading to permanent cell cycle arrest or senescence. In primary cells lacking p53 or p16, overexpressing *RAS* alone is sufficient to cause transformation and cellular immortalization.

Hall EJ, Giaccia AJ. Cancer biology. In: Hall EJ, Giaccia AJ, eds. *Radiobiology for the Radiologists*. 7th ed. Philadelphia, PA: Lippincott Williams & Wilkins; 2012:274–303.

Question 24 *How does a cancer cell maintain its telomeres?*

Answer 24

Telomeres, also referred to as the "molecular clock," are long arrays of a repeated TTAGGG sequence of 1.5 to 150 kb present on both ends of mammalian chromosomes. In normal somatic cells, successive cell divisions will lead to progressive shortening of telomeres. When protective telomeres are depleted from the chromosome ends, cells will undergo senescence, a process mediated by a *p53* tumor suppressor gene, and therefore enter permanent cell cycle arrest. Cancer cells activate the enzyme telomerase, a reverse transcriptase that polymerizes TTAGGG repeat sequences on both ends of the chromosome to compensate for the telomere loss during cell division. As a result, the biochemical activity of telomerase enables unlimited replicative potential in cancer cells.

Hall EJ, Giaccia AJ. Cancer biology. In: Hall EJ, Giaccia AJ, eds. *Radiobiology for the Radiologists*. 7th ed. Philadelphia, PA: Lippincott Williams & Wilkins; 2012:274–303.

Question 25
What is angiogenesis? How do tumor cells stimulate angiogenesis?

Question 26
How do tumor cells invade locally?

Question 27
What are the key steps in a successful metastatic process?

Question 25 *What is angiogenesis? How do tumor cells stimulate angiogenesis?*

Answer 25

Angiogenesis refers to the formation of new blood vessels to regions of chronically low blood and oxygen supply. Angiogenesis is essential for tumor growth in order to provide a sustained supply of oxygen and nutrients. Tumor cells stimulate angiogenesis through secreting proangiogenetic factors, such as vascular endothelial growth factor (VEGF), and downregulating antiangiogenetic factors, such as thrombospondins (TSPs). Secreted VEGF then binds to VEGF receptor, a transmembrane receptor tyrosine kinase, on the cell surface of endothelial cells and initiates endothelial proliferation and migration.

Hall EJ, Giaccia AJ. Cancer biology. In: Hall EJ, Giaccia AJ, eds. *Radiobiology for the Radiologists*. 7th ed. Philadelphia, PA: Lippincott Williams & Wilkins; 2012:274–303.

Question 26 *How do tumor cells invade locally?*

Answer 26

In order to become locally invasive, tumor cells need to break down epithelial integrity through decreasing cell-cell and cell-extracellular matrix (ECM) interactions, and undergo a significant alteration—the epithelial-mesenchymal transition (EMT). This process is mediated by the decreased expression or impaired function of cell adhesion molecules, such as E-cadherin (E-CAD) and neural cell adhesion molecule (N-CAM), and by the change of cell surface repertoire of integrin molecules, which relay signals from ECM into intracellular networks.

Hall EJ, Giaccia AJ. Cancer biology. In: Hall EJ, Giaccia AJ, eds. *Radiobiology for the Radiologists*. 7th ed. Philadelphia, PA: Lippincott Williams & Wilkins; 2012:274–303.

Question 27 *What are the key steps in a successful metastatic process?*

Answer 27

Metastatic cascade includes localized invasion, intravasation, transport through circulation, extravasation, formation of a micrometastasis, and colonization (formation of a macrometastasis).

Weinberg RA. *The Biology of Cancer*. New York, NY: Garland Science; 2007.

11

MODEL TUMOR SYSTEMS AND PREDICTIVE ASSAYS

C. MARC LEYRER, CAMILLE BERRIOCHOA, AND EHSAN H. BALAGAMWALA

Question 1

What are the five techniques to assay the response of solid tumors to treatment?

Question 2

How many cells are required for effective transmission to a recipient animal?

Question 3

What are the two methods used to measure tumor growth?

Turn page to see the answers.

Question 1 *What are the five techniques to assay the response of solid tumors to treatment?*

Answer 1

a. Tumor growth measurements.

b. Tumor cure assay.

c. In vivo dilution assay technique to determine tumor cell survival.

d. Lung colony assay to determine tumor cell survival.

e. In vivo treatment followed by in vitro assay for tumor cell survival.

Hall EJ, Giaccia AJ. Model tumor systems. In: Hall EJ, Giaccia AJ, eds. *Radiobiology for the Radiologist*. 7th ed. Philadelphia, PA: Lippincott Williams & Wilkins; 2012:356–371.

Question 2 *How many cells are required for effective transmission to a recipient animal?*

Answer 2

The number of cells required for effective transmission to a recipient animal is 10^4 to 10^6 cells.

Hall EJ, Giaccia AJ. Model tumor systems. In: Hall EJ, Giaccia AJ, eds. *Radiobiology for the Radiologist*. 7th ed. Philadelphia, PA: Lippincott Williams & Wilkins; 2012:356–371.

Question 3 *What are the two methods used to measure tumor growth?*

Answer 3

a. Using growth delay, which follows the time required for a tumor to return to the original size prior to radiation.

b. Evaluating the time required for a tumor to grow to a specified size after radiation therapy (RT), which is better utilized in tumors that do not respond to radiation.

Hall EJ, Giaccia AJ. Model tumor systems. In: Hall EJ, Giaccia AJ, eds. *Radiobiology for the Radiologist*. 7th ed. Philadelphia, PA: Lippincott Williams & Wilkins; 2012:356–371.

Question 4
What are the different types of programmed cell death?

Question 5
In which cell line does apoptosis play an important role?

Question 6
How long does it take for cells to show signs of death by apoptosis?

Question 4 *What are the different types of programmed cell death?*

Answer 4

a. Apoptosis—regulated cell death, which can occur in multicellular organisms and leads to characteristic morphological changes in the cell. This includes rounding up of the cell, plasma membrane blebbing, cell shrinkage, nuclear/chromosomal fragmentation, and chromatin condensation.

b. Autophagy—regulated cell death without chromatin condensation but instead by autophagic vacuolization of the cytoplasm containing degenerating organelles or cytosol.

c. Cornification—a specific type of programmed cell death occurring exclusively in the epidermis that is responsible for producing the dead keratinocytes necessary for the cornified skin layer. This process is often called keratinization.

d. Necrosis—cell death due to external factors and/or unfavorable conditions such as trauma, infection, and/or environmental changes.

e. Mitotic death—occurs during or shortly after a dysregulated/failed mitosis.

Kroemer G, Galluzzi L, Vandenabeele P, et al. Classification of cell death: recommendations of the Nomenclature Committee on Cell Death 2009. *Cell Death Differ.* 2009;16(1):3–11.

Question 5 *In which cell line does apoptosis play an important role?*

Answer 5

Apoptosis plays an important role in lymphomas.

Hall EJ, Giaccia AJ. Model tumor systems. In: Hall EJ, Giaccia AJ, eds. *Radiobiology for the Radiologist.* 7th ed. Philadelphia, PA: Lippincott Williams & Wilkins; 2012:356–371.

Question 6 *How long does it take for cells to show signs of death by apoptosis?*

Answer 6

Signs of cell death by apoptosis can occur as soon as 3 to 5 hours after irradiation.

Hall EJ, Giaccia AJ. Model tumor systems. In: Hall EJ, Giaccia AJ, eds. *Radiobiology for the Radiologist.* 7th ed. Philadelphia, PA: Lippincott Williams & Wilkins; 2012:356–371.

Question 7
What is cellular senescence?

Question 8
What are the downsides to using cell lines highly susceptible to apoptosis?

Question 9
What is a tumor control/cure assay?

Question 10
What does TCD_{50} represent?

Question 7 *What is cellular senescence?*

Answer 7

Cellular senescence is a cellular state where the cell remains metabolically active but has permanently lost the ability to divide. This state can be initiated by many factors including telomere shortening, DNA damage, chromatin changes, and activation of cellular oncogenes.

Campis J, d'Adda di Fagagna F. Cellular senescence: when bad things happen to good cells. *Nat Rev Mol Cell Biol.* 2007;8(9):729–740.

Question 8 *What are the downsides to using cell lines highly susceptible to apoptosis?*

Answer 8

a. As the cells die off and cells more resistant to apoptosis remain, the population can self-select for more resistant variants over time. This can change your ability to accurately measure tumor response to treatment.

b. Tumors sensitive to apoptosis are also more susceptible to changes in the microenvironment such as oxygenation, pH, and nutrients.

Hall EJ, Giaccia AJ. Model tumor systems. In: Hall EJ, Giaccia AJ, eds. *Radiobiology for the Radiologist.* 7th ed. Philadelphia, PA: Lippincott Williams & Wilkins; 2012:356–371.

Question 9 *What is a tumor control/cure assay?*

Answer 9

A tumor control/cure assay is an experiment where animals with similar tumors are divided. They then receive gradually increasing doses of radiation and are then observed for local control/recurrence. The control/recurrence can then be plotted as a function of dose.

Hall EJ, Giaccia AJ. Model tumor systems. In: Hall EJ, Giaccia AJ, eds. *Radiobiology for the Radiologist.* 7th ed. Philadelphia, PA: Lippincott Williams & Wilkins; 2012:356–371.

Question 10 *What does* TCD_{50} *represent?*

Answer 10

It is the dose at which 50% of the tumors are controlled.

Hall EJ, Giaccia AJ. Model tumor systems. In: Hall EJ, Giaccia AJ, eds. *Radiobiology for the Radiologist.* 7th ed. Philadelphia, PA: Lippincott Williams & Wilkins; 2012:356–371.

Question 11
What is a dilution assay?

Question 12
What does TD_{50} represent?

Question 13
How are the cell survival curves modeled with radiotherapy?

Question 14
How does a spleen colony assay differ from a dilution assay?

Question 11 *What is a dilution assay?*

Answer 11

A suspension of a known tumor (usually leukemia) is quantified, diluted, and transplanted into a number of recipient animals. They are then observed and the amount of cells required to produce a tumor are recorded.

Hall EJ, Giaccia AJ. Model tumor systems. In: Hall EJ, Giaccia AJ, eds. *Radiobiology for the Radiologist.* 7th ed. Philadelphia, PA: Lippincott Williams & Wilkins; 2012:356–371.

Question 12 *What does TD_{50} represent?*

Answer 12

The number of cells required to produce a tumor in 50% of the animals in a dilution assay. Note that this acronym differs from the commonly discussed "TD 5/5," which is a term used to describe the tolerance dose that within 5 years will cause a minimal 5% complication rate. This latter term sounds similar to TD_{50} but has a very different meaning.

Hall EJ, Giaccia AJ. Model tumor systems. In: Hall EJ, Giaccia AJ, eds. *Radiobiology for the Radiologist.* 7th ed. Philadelphia, PA: Lippincott Williams & Wilkins; 2012:356–371.

Question 13 *How are the cell survival curves modeled with radiotherapy?*

Answer 13

Cell survival curves are modeled with radiotherapy using a dilution assay as a control. The process is then repeated where the animal containing the known tumor receives a given dose of radiation. The tumor cells are harvested and transplanted into known groups and the TD_{50} is calculated at a specific dose. The surviving fraction is then calculated by comparing the TD_{50} of the nonirradiated group to the TD_{50} of the specific radiation dose group (TD_{50} control/TD_{50} irradiated). This is repeated for a various number of doses and the surviving fraction is plotted in relation to dose to create a survival curve.

Hall EJ, Giaccia AJ. Model tumor systems. In: Hall EJ, Giaccia AJ, eds. *Radiobiology for the Radiologist.* 7th ed. Philadelphia, PA: Lippincott Williams & Wilkins; 2012:356–371.

Question 14 *How does a spleen colony assay differ from a dilution assay?*

Answer 14

Spleen colony assay uses normal bone marrow cells rather than tumor cells and evaluates colony formation in the spleen of sterilized mice.

Hall EJ, Giaccia AJ. Model tumor systems. In: Hall EJ, Giaccia AJ, eds. *Radiobiology for the Radiologist.* 7th ed. Philadelphia, PA: Lippincott Williams & Wilkins; 2012:356–371.

Question 15

What is used to quantify surviving clonogenic cells in a lung colony assay?

Question 16

What is an in vivo/in vitro assay and how is it used to quantify tumor response? How is tumor response quantified in an in vivo/in vitro assay?

Question 17

What are the three commonly used systems for an in vivo/in vitro assay?

Question 18

What is the main drawback of the in vivo/in vitro assay?

Question 15 *What is used to quantify surviving clonogenic cells in a lung colony assay?*

Answer 15

The number of lung nodules created ~18 to 21 days after injection of tumor cells into a recipient animal is used to quantify the surviving clonogenic cells in a lung colony assay.

Hall EJ, Giaccia AJ. Model tumor systems. In: Hall EJ, Giaccia AJ, eds. *Radiobiology for the Radiologist.* 7th ed. Philadelphia, PA: Lippincott Williams & Wilkins; 2012:356–371.

Question 16 *What is an in vivo/in vitro assay and how is it used to quantify tumor response? How is tumor response quantified in an in vivo/in vitro assay?*

Answer 16

A known number of cells of tumor taken from an irradiated animal (in vivo) is transferred to a growth medium (in vitro). The number of colonies created from clonogenic cells after ~10 days (depending on growth kinetics) is then quantified.

Hall EJ, Giaccia AJ. Model tumor systems. In: Hall EJ, Giaccia AJ, eds. *Radiobiology for the Radiologist.* 7th ed. Philadelphia, PA: Lippincott Williams & Wilkins; 2012:356–371.
Rasey JS. In vitro assays for tumors grown in vivo: a review of kinetic techniques. In: Gray JW, Darzynkiewicz Z, eds. *Techniques in Cell Cycle Analysis.* Clifton, NJ: Humana Press; 1987:73–92.

Question 17 *What are the three commonly used systems for an in vivo/in vitro assay?*

Answer 17

The three most commonly used systems for in vivo/in in vitro assay are rhabdomyosarcoma in rats, fibrosarcoma in mice, and EMT6 mammary tumor in mice.

Hall EJ, Giaccia AJ. Model tumor systems. In: Hall EJ, Giaccia AJ, eds. *Radiobiology for the Radiologist.* 7th ed. Philadelphia, PA: Lippincott Williams & Wilkins; 2012:356–371.
Rasey JS. In vitro assays for tumors grown in vivo: a review of kinetic techniques. In: Gray JW, Darzynkiewicz Z, eds. *Techniques in Cell Cycle Analysis.* Clifton, NJ: Humana Press; 1987:73–92.

Question 18 *What is the main drawback of the in vivo/in vitro assay?*

Answer 18

It can be difficult to equate the tumor models used in the assay with those in humans as these cells must survive in an animal model and transfer to a growth medium in the lab.

Hall EJ, Giaccia AJ. Model tumor systems. In: Hall EJ, Giaccia AJ, eds. *Radiobiology for the Radiologist.* 7th ed. Philadelphia, PA: Lippincott Williams & Wilkins; 2012:356–371.
Rasey JS. In vitro assays for tumors grown in vivo: a review of kinetic techniques. In: Gray JW, Darzynkiewicz Z, eds. *Techniques in Cell Cycle Analysis.* Clifton, NJ: Humana Press; 1987:73–92.

Question 19
What do a dilution assay, lung colony assay, and in vivo/in vitro assay have in common?

Question 20
What is a common site of tumor transplantation?

Question 21
What is a xenograft?

Question 22
What techniques are used to overcome normal immune response to a xenograft?

Question 19 *What do a dilution assay, lung colony assay, and in vivo/in vitro assay have in common?*

Answer 19

They are clonogenic assays, which measure the cell surviving fraction. This is created from a single-cell suspension taken from a tumor.

Hall EJ, Giaccia AJ. Model tumor systems. In: Hall EJ, Giaccia AJ, eds. *Radiobiology for the Radiologist.* 7th ed. Philadelphia, PA: Lippincott Williams & Wilkins; 2012:356–371.

Question 20 *What is a common site of tumor transplantation?*

Answer 20

The most common site of tumor transplantation is the flank or back.

Hall EJ, Giaccia AJ. Model tumor systems. In: Hall EJ, Giaccia AJ, eds. *Radiobiology for the Radiologist.* 7th ed. Philadelphia, PA: Lippincott Williams & Wilkins; 2012:356–371.

Question 21 *What is a xenograft?*

Answer 21

A xenograft is a transplant from one species to another such as a human tumor into an animal model. This requires suppression of the animal immune system to allow tumor growth. These tumors maintain human karyotypes along with some of the growth mechanisms present in the initial human tumor.

Hall EJ, Giaccia AJ. Model tumor systems. In: Hall EJ, Giaccia AJ, eds. *Radiobiology for the Radiologist.* 7th ed. Philadelphia, PA: Lippincott Williams & Wilkins; 2012:356–371.
Jin K, Teng L, Shen Y, He K, Xu Z, Li G. Patient-derived human tumour tissue xenografts in immunodeficient mice: a systematic review. *Clin Transl Oncol.* 2010;12(7):473–480.

Question 22 *What techniques are used to overcome normal immune response to a xenograft?*

Answer 22

Immune suppression with medications/RT or creation of animal models that lack an immune system are techniques used to overcome normal immune response/rejection. Nude mice are an example of an immunodeficient animal model. These mice have a spontaneous deletion in FOXN1, which causes them to be athymic.

Hall EJ, Giaccia AJ. Model tumor systems. In: Hall EJ, Giaccia AJ, eds. *Radiobiology for the Radiologist.* 7th ed. Philadelphia, PA: Lippincott Williams & Wilkins; 2012:356–371.
Jin K, Teng L, Shen Y, He K, Xu Z, Li G. Patient-derived human tumour tissue xenografts in immunodeficient mice: a systematic review. *Clin Transl Oncol.* 2010;12(7):473–480.

Question 23
What are the drawbacks of a xenograft in modeling tumors?

Question 24
What are autochthonous tumors?

Question 25
What is the challenge to irradiation of spontaneous tumor models?

Question 23 *What are the drawbacks of a xenograft in modeling tumors?*

Answer 23

a. It can be difficult to accurately model control due to rejection of the xenograft.

b. There is an inherent change in cell selection and kinetics with the transplantation process.

c. Even though xenografts retain the human karyotypes and histology, the stromal tissue is different. This makes it difficult to use in studies where vasculature and immune system response is important.

Hall EJ, Giaccia AJ. Model tumor systems. In: Hall EJ, Giaccia AJ, eds. *Radiobiology for the Radiologist*. 7th ed. Philadelphia, PA: Lippincott Williams & Wilkins; 2012:356–371.

Question 24 *What are autochthonous tumors?*

Answer 24

Autochthonous tumors are spontaneous primary tumors in animal models usually due to chemical, viral, or physical carcinogenesis. Tumors of this type are usually due to the mouse mammary tumor virus (MMTV) that can be transmitted in mouse milk. These tumor models can be advantageous since, in contrast to transplanted tumors, these develop organically and are naturally influenced by the host environment (stroma/immune system). As a result, they metastasize via typical lymphatic and vascular vessels and are also devoid of transplantation-induced changes. Though these tumors have obvious advantages, they exhibit variability in the time required to develop and the number of animals necessary to provide representative biological conclusions. Thus, these tumor models are typically utilized for confirmation of studies rather than providing primary biological data.

Hall EJ, Giaccia AJ. Model tumor systems. In: Hall EJ, Giaccia AJ, eds. *Radiobiology for the Radiologist*. 7th ed. Philadelphia, PA: Lippincott Williams & Wilkins; 2012:356–371.
Talmadge JE, Singh RK, Fidler IJ, Raz A. Murine models to evaluate novel and conventional therapeutic strategies for cancer. *Am J Pathol*. 2007;170(3):793–804.

Question 25 *What is the challenge to irradiation of spontaneous tumor models?*

Answer 25

They remain within the tissue of the animal and not superficial as in transplanted tumors. These require more complex radiation plans to achieve similar results.

Hall EJ, Giaccia AJ. Model tumor systems. In: Hall EJ, Giaccia AJ, eds. *Radiobiology for the Radiologist*. 7th ed. Philadelphia, PA: Lippincott Williams & Wilkins; 2012:356–371.

Question 26

What is a spheroid tumor model?

Question 27

What is the advantage of spheroids in tumor modeling?

Question 28

What are the three cell populations that make up a mature spheroid?

Question 26 *What is a spheroid tumor model?*

Answer 26

A spheroid tumor model is an in vitro method of growing multicellular tumors, which allows the tumor to grow in three dimensions; this is usually accomplished through attachment to a glass/plastic surface, suspension in a spinning flask, or growth on nonadherent surfaces.

Hall EJ, Giaccia AJ. Model tumor systems. In: Hall EJ, Giaccia AJ, eds. *Radiobiology for the Radiologist*. 7th ed. Philadelphia, PA: Lippincott Williams & Wilkins; 2012:356–371.
Sutherland R, Carlsson J, Durand R, et al. Spheroids in cancer research. *Cancer Res*. 1981;41:2980–2984.

Question 27 *What is the advantage of spheroids in tumor modeling?*

Answer 27

Mature spheroids better mimic in vivo tumor models due to the heterogenous exposure caused by variable diffusion of oxygen and nutrients to the central portion of the spheroid. They are simpler, easier to reproduce/manipulate, and less expensive to maintain than standard animal models.

Hall EJ, Giaccia AJ. Model tumor systems. In: Hall EJ, Giaccia AJ, eds. *Radiobiology for the Radiologist*. 7th ed. Philadelphia, PA: Lippincott Williams & Wilkins; 2012:356–371.
Sutherland R, Carlsson J, Durand R, Yuhas J. Spheroids in cancer research. *Cancer Res*. 1981;41:2980–2984.

Question 28 *What are the three cell populations that make up a mature spheroid?*

Answer 28

The three cell populations from the outside to the inside: asynchronous aerobic cycling cells, aerated noncycling G1-like cells, and noncycling G1-like hypoxic cells in the center.

Hall EJ, Giaccia AJ. Model tumor systems. In: Hall EJ, Giaccia AJ, eds. *Radiobiology for the Radiologist*. 7th ed. Philadelphia, PA: Lippincott Williams & Wilkins; 2012:356–371.

12

CELL KINETICS

MATTHEW C. WARD AND RICHARD BLAKE ROSS

Question 1
What are cyclin-dependent kinases (Cdks)? How are they related to cyclins?

Question 2
What are the names of the three most important checkpoints a cell encounters during the cell cycle?

Question 3
At which checkpoint are p53 and Rb most relevant?

Question 4
What is the mitotic index (MI) and how is it calculated?

Turn page to see the answers.

Question 1 *What are cyclin-dependent kinases (Cdks)? How are they related to cyclins?*

Answer 1

Cdks are enzymes that regulate the cell cycle. Cdks complex with cyclins (labeled A–H), which are proteins. The activation of a cyclin protein by a Cdk will allow the cell to progress through the cell cycle. While Cdk levels are constant throughout the cell cycle, cyclin levels vary based on the cell cycle phase.

Hall EJ, Giaccia AJ. Cell, tissue and tumor kinetics. In: Hall EJ, Giaccia AJ, eds. *Radiobiology for the Radiologist.* 7th ed. Philadelphia, PA: Lippincott Williams & Wilkins; 2012:372–390.

Question 2 *What are the names of the three most important checkpoints a cell encounters during the cell cycle?*

Answer 2

The cell encounters the G1/S checkpoint, S phase checkpoint, and G2/M checkpoint.

Hall EJ, Giaccia AJ. Cell, tissue and tumor kinetics. In: Hall EJ, Giaccia AJ, eds. *Radiobiology for the Radiologist.* 7th ed. Philadelphia, PA: Lippincott Williams & Wilkins; 2012:372–390.

Question 3 *At which checkpoint are p53 and Rb most relevant?*

Answer 3

The purpose of a cell's checkpoint is to check for errors prior to initiating the next step of the cell cycle. The proteins p53 and Rb are keys within the G1 checkpoint whose purpose is to detect DNA damage prior to initiating DNA synthesis. p53 also mediates the G2/M checkpoint.

Hall EJ, Giaccia AJ. Cell, tissue and tumor kinetics. In: Hall EJ, Giaccia AJ, eds. *Radiobiology for the Radiologist.* 7th ed. Philadelphia, PA: Lippincott Williams & Wilkins; 2012:372–390.

Question 4 *What is the mitotic index (MI) and how is it calculated?*

Answer 4

The MI is the fraction of cells undergoing mitosis. The MI can be observed by counting the number of cells undergoing mitosis or calculated using the formula:

$$MI = \frac{\lambda T_M}{T_C}$$

where T_M is the time required for a cell to undergo mitosis and T_C is the time required for a cell to undergo the entire cell cycle. λ is a correction factor accounting for the uneven distribution of cells throughout the cell cycle.

Hall EJ, Giaccia AJ. Cell, tissue and tumor kinetics. In: Hall EJ, Giaccia AJ, eds. *Radiobiology for the Radiologist.* 7th ed. Philadelphia, PA: Lippincott Williams & Wilkins; 2012:372–390.

Question 5
What is the labeling index (LI) and how is it calculated?

Question 6
What technique, beyond the mitotic index (MI) and labeling index (LI), is required to determine the length of all phases in the cell cycle?

Question 7
Which phase of the cell cycle is the most variable and accounts for the majority of variation in cycle times between malignant and benign cell lines?

Question 8
What are the general principles of flow cytometry?

Question 5 *What is the labeling index (LI) and how is it calculated?*

Answer 5

The LI is used to determine the length of time required for a cell to pass through the S phase of the cell cycle. It is calculated by "flash labeling" cells with 5-bromodeoxyuridine and counting the proportion of cells that are labeled. The formula:

$$LI = \frac{\lambda T_S}{T_C}$$

can be used to calculate the duration of the S phase (T_s) of the cell cycle.

Hall EJ, Giaccia AJ. Cell, tissue and tumor kinetics. In: Hall EJ, Giaccia AJ, eds. *Radiobiology for the Radiologist.* 7th ed. Philadelphia, PA: Lippincott Williams & Wilkins; 2012:372–390.

Question 6 *What technique, beyond the mitotic index (MI) and labeling index (LI), is required to determine the length of all phases in the cell cycle?*

Answer 6

Although the MI and LI can be used to quickly and simply determine the length of the M and S phase of the cell cycle, the percent-labeled mitoses technique is necessary to determine the time required for cells to pass through the additional phases (G1 and G2). This technique involves labeling a cohort of cells and serially sampling the cells, each time counting the fraction undergoing mitosis. It is a time and labor-intensive process and is difficult to perform in vivo due to the large number of samples required.

Hall EJ, Giaccia AJ. Cell, tissue and tumor kinetics. In: Hall EJ, Giaccia AJ, eds. *Radiobiology for the Radiologist.* 7th ed. Philadelphia, PA: Lippincott Williams & Wilkins; 2012:372–390.

Question 7 *Which phase of the cell cycle is the most variable and accounts for the majority of variation in cycle times between malignant and benign cell lines?*

Answer 7

The G1 phase is highly variable whereas S, G2, and M are fairly consistent across cell lines.

Hall EJ, Giaccia AJ. Cell, tissue and tumor kinetics. In: Hall EJ, Giaccia AJ, eds. *Radiobiology for the Radiologist.* 7th ed. Philadelphia, PA: Lippincott Williams & Wilkins; 2012:372–390.

Question 8 *What are the general principles of flow cytometry?*

Answer 8

Flow cytometry is a method by which single cells (usually fluorescently labeled) are passed through a light beam (usually a laser matched to the fluorescent dye) in order to count the fraction of cells labeled with the dye.

Hall EJ, Giaccia AJ. Cell, tissue and tumor kinetics. In: Hall EJ, Giaccia AJ, eds. *Radiobiology for the Radiologist.* 7th ed. Philadelphia, PA: Lippincott Williams & Wilkins; 2012:372–390.

Question 9
What is the growth fraction (GF)?

Question 10
Why do tumors typically grow more slowly than is predicted by the calculated cell cycle time?

Question 11
How is the cell loss factor defined?

Question 12
How does the tumor diameter doubling time relate to the cell doubling time?

Question 9 *What is the growth fraction (GF)?*

Answer 9

The GF is defined as the fraction of cells proliferating. Although highly variable, the typical GF for cancerous cell lines is between 30% and 50%.

$$GF = \frac{\text{Proliferating}}{\text{Proliferating} + \text{Quiescent}}$$

Hall EJ, Giaccia AJ. Cell, tissue and tumor kinetics. In: Hall EJ, Giaccia AJ, eds. *Radiobiology for the Radiologist.* 7th ed. Philadelphia, PA: Lippincott Williams & Wilkins; 2012:372–390.

Question 10 *Why do tumors typically grow more slowly than is predicted by the calculated cell cycle time?*

Answer 10

A tumor's in situ behavior is often much different than the behavior of its cell line in vitro. Possible explanations for this include cell loss from hypoxia, tumor heterogeneity, nutritional deficits, the immune system, or exfoliation (skin or gastrointestinal tumors).

Hall EJ, Giaccia AJ. Cell, tissue and tumor kinetics. In: Hall EJ, Giaccia AJ, eds. *Radiobiology for the Radiologist.* 7th ed. Philadelphia, PA: Lippincott Williams & Wilkins; 2012:372–390.

Question 11 *How is the cell loss factor defined?*

Answer 11

The cell loss factor is a measure of the difference between the predicted and observed doubling time. It is defined mathematically as:

$$\phi = 1 - \frac{T_{pot}}{T_d}$$

where T_{pot} = the potential doubling time and T_d = the actual doubling time.

Hall EJ, Giaccia AJ. Cell, tissue and tumor kinetics. In: Hall EJ, Giaccia AJ, eds. *Radiobiology for the Radiologist.* 7th ed. Philadelphia, PA: Lippincott Williams & Wilkins; 2012:372–390.

Question 12 *How does the tumor diameter doubling time relate to the cell doubling time?*

Answer 12

Considering that a volume of a sphere is:

$$V = \frac{4\pi}{3} r^3$$

And diameter = $2r$, then:

$$V = \frac{\pi}{6} d^3$$

$$V_2 = \frac{\pi}{6}(2d_0)^3$$

$$V_1 = \frac{\pi}{6} d_0^3$$

$$V_2 = 8 \cdot V_1$$

Therefore, a doubling in the diameter implies at least an 8-fold increase in the number of cells.

Hall EJ, Giaccia AJ. Cell, tissue and tumor kinetics. In: Hall EJ, Giaccia AJ, eds. *Radiobiology for the Radiologist.* 7th ed. Philadelphia, PA: Lippincott Williams & Wilkins; 2012:372–390.

Question 13
What is the typical cell-loss factor for solid tumors?

Question 14
What are typical doubling times for human solid tumors?

Question 15
What is the most radiosensitive phase of the cell cycle?

Question 16
What is the most radioresistant phase of the cell cycle?

Question 13 *What is the typical cell-loss factor for solid tumors?*

Answer 13

The cell loss factor varies dramatically from nearly 0% to nearly 100% for solid tumors. Sarcomas tend toward a cell loss factor less than 50% and carcinomas tend to have a cell loss factor greater than 70%, but this is highly variable.

Hall EJ, Giaccia AJ. Cell, tissue and tumor kinetics. In: Hall EJ, Giaccia AJ, eds. *Radiobiology for the Radiologist.* 7th ed. Philadelphia, PA: Lippincott Williams & Wilkins; 2012:372–390.

Question 14 *What are typical doubling times for human solid tumors?*

Answer 14

Again, this is highly variable, but as a general rule they range from approximately 30 days to 90 days. Listing from short doubling times to long doubling times: lymphomas, sarcomas, squamous carcinomas, then adenocarcinoma.

Hall EJ, Giaccia AJ. Cell, tissue and tumor kinetics. In: Hall EJ, Giaccia AJ, eds. *Radiobiology for the Radiologist.* 7th ed. Philadelphia, PA: Lippincott Williams & Wilkins; 2012:372–390.

Question 15 *What is the most radiosensitive phase of the cell cycle?*

Answer 15

Cells are most radiosensitive in the G_2/M phase of the cell cycle.

Pawlik TM, Keyomarsi K. Role of cell cycle in mediating sensitivity to radiotherapy. *Int J Radiat Oncol Biol Phys.* 2004;59(4):928–942.

Question 16 *What is the most radioresistant phase of the cell cycle?*

Answer 16

Cells in the late S phase of the cell cycle are generally considered the most radioresistant.

Pawlik TM, Keyomarsi K. Role of cell cycle in mediating sensitivity to radiotherapy. *Int J Radiat Oncol Biol Phys.* 2004;59(4):928–942.

Question 17

At what phase in the cell cycle are cyclins A, B, D, and E active?

Question 18

What molecule is responsible for detection of DNA damage prior to the activation of p53, Chk2, Nijmegen breakage syndrome (Nbs), or any of the other downstream regulators?

Question 19

How does the growth rate of a tumor change with increasing size?

Question 20

If the labeling index (LI) of a tumor is noted to be 0.1, the cells are known to cycle every 20 hours, and the cells are evenly distributed along the cell cycle, what is the estimated length of the S phase of the cell cycle?

Question 17 *At what phase in the cell cycle are cyclins A, B, D, and E active?*

Answer 17

Cyclin levels vary throughout the cell cycle and bind to the Cdks to create complexes allowing for progression through the cell cycle. Cyclin D is most active during G1, cyclin E is active from late G1 to early S, cyclin A is active from late S through G2 to early M, and cyclin B is active from G2 to M.

Hall EJ, Giaccia AJ. Cell, tissue and tumor kinetics. In: Hall EJ, Giaccia AJ, eds. *Radiobiology for the Radiologist.* 7th ed. Philadelphia, PA: Lippincott Williams & Wilkins; 2012:372–390.

Question 18 *What molecule is responsible for detection of DNA damage prior to the activation of p53, Chk2, Nijmegen breakage syndrome (Nbs), or any of the other downstream regulators?*

Answer 18

ATM (ataxia-telangiectasia mutated) senses DNA damage and activates repair pathways.

Hall EJ, Giaccia AJ. Cell, tissue and tumor kinetics. In: Hall EJ, Giaccia AJ, eds. *Radiobiology for the Radiologist.* 7th ed. Philadelphia, PA: Lippincott Williams & Wilkins; 2012:372–390.

Question 19 *How does the growth rate of a tumor change with increasing size?*

Answer 19

Typically, the growth rate of a tumor decreases as its size increases due to increased hypoxia and necrosis within the tumor, which increases cell loss.

Hall EJ, Giaccia AJ. Cell, tissue and tumor kinetics. In: Hall EJ, Giaccia AJ, eds. *Radiobiology for the Radiologist.* 7th ed. Philadelphia, PA: Lippincott Williams & Wilkins; 2012:372–390.

Question 20 *If the labeling index (LI) of a tumor is noted to be 0.1, the cells are known to cycle every 20 hours, and the cells are evenly distributed along the cell cycle, what is the estimated length of the S phase of the cell cycle?*

Answer 20

$$LI = \frac{\lambda T_S}{T_C}$$

$$0.1 = \frac{1 \times T_S}{20 \ \text{hours}}$$

$$T_S = 2 \ \text{hours}$$

Hall EJ, Giaccia AJ. Cell, tissue and tumor kinetics. In: Hall EJ, Giaccia AJ, eds. *Radiobiology for the Radiologist.* 7th ed. Philadelphia, PA: Lippincott Williams & Wilkins; 2012:372–390.

Question 21

If a cell line under ideal in vitro conditions doubles every 3 days but is observed in situ to double every 30 days, what is the estimated cell loss factor?

Question 22

The potential doubling time for a tumor with a cell loss factor of 66% is known to be 10 days. What is the actual doubling time after accounting for cell loss?

Question 23

Which two tumors (adenocarcinomas) are most likely to have the same doubling time: a lung and liver metastases in the same patient or two lung metastases in different patients?

Question 21 *If a cell line under ideal in vitro conditions doubles every 3 days but is observed in situ to double every 30 days, what is the estimated cell loss factor?*

Answer 21

$$\phi = 1 - \frac{T_{pot}}{T_d}$$

$$\phi = 1 - \frac{3 \text{ days}}{30 \text{ days}}$$

$$\phi = 90\%$$

Hall EJ, Giaccia AJ. Cell, tissue and tumor kinetics. In: Hall EJ, Giaccia AJ, eds. *Radiobiology for the Radiologist*. 7th ed. Philadelphia, PA: Lippincott Williams & Wilkins; 2012:372–390.

Question 22 *The potential doubling time for a tumor with a cell loss factor of 66% is known to be 10 days. What is the actual doubling time after accounting for cell loss?*

Answer 22

$$\phi = 1 - \frac{T_{pot}}{T_d}$$

$$0.66 = 1 - \frac{10 \text{ days}}{T_d}$$

Therefore, the actual doubling time is closer to 30 days.

Hall EJ, Giaccia AJ. Cell, tissue and tumor kinetics. In: Hall EJ, Giaccia AJ, eds. *Radiobiology for the Radiologist*. 7th ed. Philadelphia, PA: Lippincott Williams & Wilkins; 2012:372–390.

Question 23 *Which two tumors (adenocarcinomas) are most likely to have the same doubling time: a lung and liver metastases in the same patient or two lung metastases in different patients?*

Answer 23

Although heterogeneity exists between metastases, the two lesions in the same patient are more likely to have the same doubling time than two metastases in different patients with the same histology. Doubling times across metastatic lesions are typically relatively similar.

Hall EJ, Giaccia AJ. Cell, tissue and tumor kinetics. In: Hall EJ, Giaccia AJ, eds. *Radiobiology for the Radiologist*. 7th ed. Philadelphia, PA: Lippincott Williams & Wilkins; 2012:372–390.

Question 24

Cells are known not to be evenly distributed through the cell cycle as evidenced by the correction factor λ necessary when calculating the mitotic index (MI) and labeling index (LI). Which phase of the cell cycle is most prevalent under the simplest assumptions?

Question 25

Which cell cycle checkpoint is key to preventing damaged cells from entering mitosis?

Question 26

Using the percent-labeled mitosis technique, how is the length of mitosis (T_M) calculated?

Question 24 *Cells are known not to be evenly distributed through the cell cycle as evidenced by the correction factor λ necessary when calculating the mitotic index (MI) and labeling index (LI). Which phase of the cell cycle is most prevalent under the simplest assumptions?*

Answer 24

Cells double after passing through the M phase, so the simplest assumption for λ when calculating the MI and LI is that the G1 phase is most prevalent and is exponentially distributed throughout the cell cycle, leading to an assumed value of $λ = \ln(2) = 0.693$.

Hall EJ, Giaccia AJ. Cell, tissue and tumor kinetics. In: Hall EJ, Giaccia AJ, eds. *Radiobiology for the Radiologist.* 7th ed. Philadelphia, PA: Lippincott Williams & Wilkins; 2012:372–390.

Question 25 *Which cell cycle checkpoint is key to preventing damaged cells from entering mitosis?*

Answer 25

The G_2/M checkpoint is the most regulated checkpoint and is the critical checkpoint for the prevention of damaged cells from progressing to mitosis. Cells that are lacking this checkpoint are radiosensitive; thus, the inhibition of regulators of this checkpoint can potentially increase radiosensitivity.

Hall EJ, Giaccia AJ. Cell, tissue and tumor kinetics. In: Hall EJ, Giaccia AJ, eds. *Radiobiology for the Radiologist.* 7th ed. Philadelphia, PA: Lippincott Williams & Wilkins; 2012:372–390.

Question 26 *Using the percent-labeled mitosis technique, how is the length of mitosis (T_M) calculated?*

Answer 26

A percent-labeled mitosis curve can be generated by plotting the percentage of labeled mitoses versus time. The length of mitosis can be calculated by measuring the time it takes for the percentage of labeled mitoses to reach 100%. This measurement coincides with the time it takes for the leading edge (the first cells in the sample) of the labeled sample to undergo mitosis (time between *b* and *c* in the following figure).

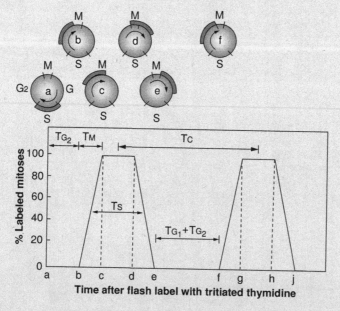

Source: Figure from Hall EJ, Giaccia AJ. Cell, tissue and tumor kinetics. In: Hall EJ, Giaccia AJ, eds. *Radiobiology for the Radiologist.* 7th ed. Philadelphia, PA: Lippincott Williams & Wilkins; 2012:372–390. Reprinted with permission.

Question 27

Using the percent-labeled mitosis technique, how is the duration of the DNA synthetic period or S period (T_s) calculated?

Question 28

Generally, how does the cell loss factor (ϕ) differ between sarcomas and carcinomas? How does this difference affect radiotherapy?

Question 29

Generally, how does the cell cycle time of malignant cells compare to normal tissue? How does radiotherapy affect the cell cycle times?

Question 30

What is the correlation between cell growth fraction (GF), cell turnover rate, and radiosensitivity in humans?

Question 27 *Using the percent-labeled mitosis technique, how is the duration of the DNA synthetic period or S period (T_s) calculated?*

Answer 27

A percent-labeled mitosis curve can be generated by plotting the percentage of labeled mitoses versus time. The S period can be approximated by measuring the time span of the first peak from the 50% level of the ascending portion to the 50% level of the descending portion (see figure for Question 26).

Hall EJ, Giaccia AJ. Cell, tissue and tumor kinetics. In: Hall EJ, Giaccia AJ, eds. *Radiobiology for the Radiologist.* 7th ed. Philadelphia, PA: Lippincott Williams & Wilkins; 2012:372–390.

Question 28 *Generally, how does the cell loss factor (ϕ) differ between sarcomas and carcinomas? How does this difference affect radiotherapy?*

Answer 28

Generally, carcinomas have large cell loss factors, while sarcomas have smaller cell loss factors. This is due to apoptosis being a common occurrence in carcinoma processes. Because of the higher cell loss, there is a quicker reduction of tumor volume in carcinomas than sarcomas. Thus, carcinomas are typically more radioresponsive and have a shorter response time to radiotherapy.

Hall EJ, Giaccia AJ. Cell, tissue and tumor kinetics. In: Hall EJ, Giaccia AJ, eds. *Radiobiology for the Radiologist.* 7th ed. Philadelphia, PA: Lippincott Williams & Wilkins; 2012:372–390.

Question 29 *Generally, how does the cell cycle time of malignant cells compare to normal tissue? How does radiotherapy affect the cell cycle times?*

Answer 29

Typically, malignant cell cycle times are shorter than those of normal tissue. Irradiated malignant cells generally have an increase in cell cycle time, while this effect is the opposite in normal tissue.

Hall EJ, Giaccia AJ. Cell, tissue and tumor kinetics. In: Hall EJ, Giaccia AJ, eds. *Radiobiology for the Radiologist.* 7th ed. Philadelphia, PA: Lippincott Williams & Wilkins; 2012:372–390.

Question 30 *What is the correlation between cell growth fraction (GF), cell turnover rate, and radiosensitivity in humans?*

Answer 30

Similar to the response to chemotherapy, human tumors with the fastest GFs and turnover rates also tend to be the most radiosensitive.

Hall EJ, Giaccia AJ. Cell, tissue and tumor kinetics. In: Hall EJ, Giaccia AJ, eds. *Radiobiology for the Radiologist.* 7th ed. Philadelphia, PA: Lippincott Williams & Wilkins; 2012:372–390.

13

FACTORS INFLUENCING TUMOR CONTROL AND COMPLICATIONS

DAESUNG LEE

Question 1

Quantitative radiobiology is based on a target model. What is the major target in cells for radiation-induced cell killing?

Question 2

Suppose we have 10,000 clonogenic cells. After receiving 2 Gy, 9,000 cells stopped reproducing and we now have 1,000 clonogenic cells. Would another 2 Gy eradicate the remaining 1,000 cells?

Question 3

If we have a small tumor measuring 1 cm in diameter with 10^9 cells and if a radiation dose of 6 Gy will kill 90% of cells, how many fractions of 6 Gy are necessary for a 90% chance of tumor control if there is no repopulation of cells between each dose?

Turn page to see the answers.

Question 1 *Quantitative radiobiology is based on a target model. What is the major target in cells for radiation-induced cell killing?*

Answer 1

A target theory is based on modeling that radiation induces cell killing by hitting specific targets in the cell. The major target is nuclear DNA. DNA double-strand breaks are the most important damage, leading to possible cell killing at the time of reproduction (mitotic cell death). However, other molecular events such as clustered single-strand breaks, DNA base damage, DNA–DNA crosslinks, and DNA–protein cross links can also possibly lead to mitotic cell death or trigger p53-mediated or p53-independent pathways to apoptosis.

Prise KM, Schettino G, Folkard M, Held KD. New insights of cell death from radiation exposure. *Lancet Oncol.* 2005;6:520–528.
Zhoa L, Mi D, Hu B, Sun Y. A generalized target theory and its applications. *Sci Rep.* 2015;5:14568.

Question 2 *Suppose we have 10,000 clonogenic cells. After receiving 2 Gy, 9,000 cells stopped reproducing and we now have 1,000 clonogenic cells. Would another 2 Gy eradicate the remaining 1,000 cells?*

Answer 2

No. Radiation-induced cell kill is logarithmic. It is proportional to the existing cell population that is observed in studies with bacteria and then with mammalian cells. As "hits" (lethal lesions) on the "targets" (DNA) are distributed randomly, the probability that a certain cell will have "hits" can be described by Poisson statistics. For example, if there are 100 cells and a given radiation dose resulting in 100 hits, about 37 cells (100 cells $\times$ e^{-1}) can be expected to survive. If the dose is doubled, about 14 cells (100 cells $\times$ e^{-2}) will survive. If the dose is tripled, about 5 cells (100 cells $\times$ e^{-3}) will survive, and so on. So for our question, another 2 Gy will result in 100 surviving cells.

McBride WH, Withers HR. Biologic basis of radiation therapy. In: Halperin EC, Wazer DE, Perez CA, Brady LW, eds. *Perez and Brady's Principles and Practice of Radiation Oncology.* 6th ed. Philadelphia, PA: Lippincott Williams & Wilkins; 2013:61–88.

Question 3 *If we have a small tumor measuring 1 cm in diameter with 10^9 cells and if a radiation dose of 6 Gy will kill 90% of cells, how many fractions of 6 Gy are necessary for a 90% chance of tumor control if there is no repopulation of cells between each dose?*

Answer 3

The proportion of surviving cells is 10% after each fraction. So after the first fraction, $10^9 \times 0.1 = 10^8$ cells survive. After the second fraction, $10^8 \times 0.1 = 10^7$ cells, do. After the third, 10^6 cells, and so on. If we continue, after nine fractions, one cell will survive and another fraction of 6 Gy will give a 90% chance of that cell being killed. Therefore, 10 fractions of 6 Gy will give a 90% chance of tumor control.

Halperin EC, Wazer DE, Perez CA. The discipline of radiation oncology. In: Halperin EC, Wazer DE, Perez CA, Brady LW, eds. *Perez and Brady's Principles and Practice of Radiation Oncology.* 6th ed. Philadelphia, PA: Lippincott Williams & Wilkins; 2013:2–60.

Question 4

The total radiation dose necessary to control a tumor depends on the initial number of tumor cells (volume) and radiosensitivity of tumor cells (proportion of cells killed for a given dose of radiation). Why might a large gross tumor require a higher dose than predicted?

Question 5

Subclinical disease is defined as a deposit of tumor cells too small to be detected clinically and microscopically but with the capacity to grow into a clinically apparent tumor if untreated. If 50 Gy in 25 fractions is required to control subclinical disease in preoperative patients, how much dose is usually used in postoperative patients suspected to have subclinical disease in the operative bed?

Question 6

How much dose would be necessary to treat a patient with positive surgical margins for the same type of cancer as in question 5?

Question 4 *The total radiation dose necessary to control a tumor depends on the initial number of tumor cells (volume) and radiosensitivity of tumor cells (proportion of cells killed for a given dose of radiation). Why might a large gross tumor require a higher dose than predicted?*

Answer 4

One possible reason is the proportion of hypoxic cells. There is an inverse relationship between the size of the tumor and oxygen pressure. Higher proportions of hypoxic cells in large tumors will require higher doses as the radiosensitivity decreases by a factor of two to three in hypoxic cells. Another possible reason is repopulation. In some tumors, accelerated repopulation is triggered after a certain time. Larger tumors will require more prolonged treatment time if the same dose per fraction is used. Higher total dose may be required to account for additional cells generated by accelerated repopulation.

Steel GG, Peacock JH. Why are some human tumours more radiosensitive than others? *Radiother Oncol.* 1989;15:63–72.
Vaupel P, Kelleher DK, Hockel M. Oxygen status of malignant tumors: pathogenesis of hypoxia and significance for tumor therapy. Treatment resistance of solid tumors: role of hypoxia and anemia. *Semin Oncol.* 2001;28:29–35.

Question 5 *Subclinical disease is defined as a deposit of tumor cells too small to be detected clinically and microscopically but with the capacity to grow into a clinically apparent tumor if untreated. If 50 Gy in 25 fractions is required to control subclinical disease in preoperative patients, how much dose is usually used in postoperative patients suspected to have subclinical disease in the operative bed?*

Answer 5

Clinically, it has been shown that a higher radiation dose is necessary in an operative bed because the dissected surgical field is thought to be less oxygenated. Therefore, 56 to 60 Gy in 28 to 30 fractions is necessary in postoperative settings, which is considered equivalent to 50 Gy in 25 fractions in preoperative settings.

Ang KK, Adam GS. *Radiotherapy for Head and Neck Cancers.* 2nd ed. Philadelphia, PA: Lippincott Williams & Wilkins; 2002:80–104.
Peters LJ, Goepfert H, Ang KK, et al. Evaluation of the dose for postoperative radiation therapy for head and neck cancer: first report of a prospective randomized trial. *Int J Radiat Oncol Biol Phys.* 1993;26(1):3–11.

Question 6 *How much dose would be necessary to treat a patient with positive surgical margins for the same type of cancer as in question 5?*

Answer 6

It is estimated that a pathologist can detect malignancy microscopically when cell aggregates are larger than 10^6 cells/cm^3 Therefore, a higher dose than used in subclinical disease is necessary for treating microscopic disease. In addition, when it is in the surgical bed, a higher dose is required for comparable control to a similar number of cells in the intact tumor bed. Therefore, a dose in the range of 60 to 66 Gy would be appropriate.

Ang KK, Adam GS. *Radiotherapy for Head and Neck Cancers.* 2nd ed. Philadelphia, PA: Lippincott Williams & Wilkins; 2002:80–104.
Halperin EC, Wazer DE, Perez CA. The discipline of radiation oncology. In: Halperin EC, Wazer DE, Perez CA, Brady LW, eds. *Perez and Brady's Principles and Practice of Radiation Oncology.* 6th ed. Philadelphia, PA: Lippincott Williams & Wilkins, 2013:2–60.

Question 7

Suppose your patient has a 1 cm tumor with an estimated number of cancer clonogens of 10^7 cells. Estimated tumor control probability (TCP) is 10% at 52 Gy, 50% at 58 Gy, and 90% at 64 Gy. You prescribed 66 Gy in 2 Gy per fraction for definitive treatment. About halfway through treatment at 32 Gy, the patient has decided to quit treatments. He is asking you if his efforts for 3 weeks of treatment did anything good. What would be your answer?

Question 8

Suppose your patient had surgical resection of a tumor without any remaining gross or microscopic disease. He has a 40% chance of harboring subclinical disease and you decide to offer adjuvant radiation treatment. You prescribed 60 Gy with 2 Gy per fraction. About halfway through treatment at 30 Gy, the patient has decided to quit treatment. He is asking you if his efforts for 3 weeks of treatment did any good. What would be your answer?

Question 9

When tumor control probability (TCP) is plotted against dose, we see a sigmoid curve. TCP curves from experimental animal data are steep; however, those for human tumor control are much shallower and a given dose of radiation can produce a wide range of responses. What are some possible sources of such heterogeneity in actual tumor characteristics?

Question 7 *Suppose your patient has a 1 cm tumor with an estimated number of cancer clonogens of 10^7 cells. Estimated tumor control probability (TCP) is 10% at 52 Gy, 50% at 58 Gy, and 90% at 64 Gy. You prescribed 66 Gy in 2 Gy per fraction for definitive treatment. About halfway through treatment at 32 Gy, the patient has decided to quit treatments. He is asking you if his efforts for 3 weeks of treatment did anything good. What would be your answer?*

Answer 7

Unfortunately, with 32 Gy, his gross tumor may regress in size, but the chance for cure is close to 0%. For gross disease with a certain number of clonogens, there is a minimum threshold dose above which you start to have a chance of killing the last standing clonogen cell. Because cell killing is a random process, you need to combine the probability of getting to that last standing cell and probability of killing that last standing cell with an additional radiation dose to generate TCP at a given dose. For the aforementioned example, you're not likely to see tumor control at doses lower than 50 Gy.

McBride WH, Withers HR. Biologic basis of radiation therapy. In: Halperin EC, Wazer DE, Perez CA, Brady LW, eds. *Perez and Brady's Principles and Practice of Radiation Oncology.* 6th ed. Philadelphia, PA: Lippincott Williams & Wilkins; 2013:61–88.

Question 8 *Suppose your patient had surgical resection of a tumor without any remaining gross or microscopic disease. He has a 40% chance of harboring subclinical disease and you decide to offer adjuvant radiation treatment. You prescribed 60 Gy with 2 Gy per fraction. About halfway through treatment at 30 Gy, the patient has decided to quit treatment. He is asking you if his efforts for 3 weeks of treatment did any good. What would be your answer?*

Answer 8

His treatment, even at 32 Gy, did improve his chance for cure. Because he has subclinical disease, the number of remaining cancer clonogens can be anywhere between 0 and 10^6 cells/cm^3. If he had a lower number of remaining cells, let's say less than 10^3 cells/cm^3, then 32 Gy has a significant chance to eradicate them.

McBride WH, Withers HR. Biologic basis of radiation therapy. In: Halperin EC, Wazer DE, Perez CA, Brady LW, eds. *Perez and Brady's Principles and Practice of Radiation Oncology.* 6th ed. Philadelphia, PA: Lippincott Williams & Wilkins; 2013:61–88.

Question 9 *When tumor control probability (TCP) is plotted against dose, we see a sigmoid curve. TCP curves from experimental animal data are steep; however, those for human tumor control are much shallower and a given dose of radiation can produce a wide range of responses. What are some possible sources of such heterogeneity in actual tumor characteristics?*

Answer 9

The heterogeneity in actual tumor characteristics may be a result of molecular differences in cancer and proportion of cancer stem cells. This will lead to differences in intrinsic radiosensitivity, redistribution and repopulation kinetics, and reoxygenation rates, as well as the overall response to radiation treatment.

McBride WH, Withers HR. Biologic basis of radiation therapy. In: Halperin EC, Wazer DE, Perez CA, Brady LW, eds. *Perez and Brady's Principles and Practice of Radiation Oncology.* 6th ed. Philadelphia, PA: Lippincott Williams & Wilkins, 2013:61–88.

Question 10

Similar to tumor control probability (TCP) curves, normal tissue complication probability (NTCP) curves can be drawn against dose and they are sigmoid curves as well. Do you expect the curves to be steeper or shallower compared to TCP curves?

Question 11

What is LD_{50} or TD_{50}?

Question 12

What is the definition of functional subunits (FSUs) and how is FSU important in normal tissue tolerance to radiation?

Question 13

Some functional subunits (FSUs) are arranged serially and others in parallel. Suppose organ A has FSUs arranged serially with free movement of stem cells among FSUs and organ B has FSUs arranged in parallel with strict compartmentalization and no movement of stem cells among FSUs. Which organ will tend to have a higher dose tolerance to uniform radiation dose to the entire organ?

Question 10 *Similar to tumor control probability (TCP) curves, normal tissue complication probability (NTCP) curves can be drawn against dose and they are sigmoid curves as well. Do you expect the curves to be steeper or shallower compared to TCP curves?*

Answer 10

They tend to be steeper because normal tissues are more homogenous with respect to their composition, response, and repair to radiation.

McBride WH, Withers HR. Biologic basis of radiation therapy. In: Halperin EC, Wazer DE, Perez CA, Brady LW, eds. *Perez and Brady's Principles and Practice of Radiation Oncology.* 6th ed. Philadelphia, PA: Lippincott Williams & Wilkins; 2013:61–88.

Question 11 *What is LD_{50} or TD_{50}?*

Answer 11

It is a dose that can cause lethality in 50% of a population or a dose that can cause intolerance (or specific undesirable organ effects) in 50% of a population. For example, TD_{50} for an ear can be either 30 Gy or 55 Gy if intolerance is defined as acute serous otitis (30 Gy) or as chronic serous otitis (55 Gy).

Emami B, Lyman J, Brown A, et al. Tolerance of normal tissue to therapeutic irradiation. *Int J Radiat Oncol Biol Phys.* May 1991;21(1):109–122.

Question 12 *What is the definition of functional subunits (FSUs) and how is FSU important in normal tissue tolerance to radiation?*

Answer 12

It is "the minimum clonogenic entity required for regeneration of a structure." Normal tissue tolerance depends on the intrinsic radiosensitivity of normal tissue and the number of stem cells similar to the lethal tumor dose. In addition, how FSUs are composed and organized is an important factor in determining tolerance at a given dose.

McBride WH, Withers HR. Biologic basis of radiation therapy. In: Halperin EC, Wazer DE, Perez CA, Brady LW, eds. *Perez and Brady's Principles and Practice of Radiation Oncology.* 6th ed. Philadelphia, PA: Lippincott Williams & Wilkins; 2013:61–88.

Question 13 *Some functional subunits (FSUs) are arranged serially and others in parallel. Suppose organ A has FSUs arranged serially with free movement of stem cells among FSUs and organ B has FSUs arranged in parallel with strict compartmentalization and no movement of stem cells among FSUs. Which organ will tend to have a higher dose tolerance to uniform radiation dose to the entire organ?*

Answer 13

Organ A. Suppose there are 10 stem cells in each organ and 10 FSUs. As a result, there is one stem cell in each FSUs. For organ B with parallel FSUs, a radiation dose high enough to kill one stem cell is required to disable its function. However, for organ A, all 10 stem cells need to be killed because even one remaining stem cell can migrate and regenerate other FSUs. Although it is not a perfect example because of differences in radiosensitivity and incomplete stem cell mobility, the spinal cord (serial organ) has a higher dose tolerance than the kidneys (parallel organ).

McBride WH, Withers HR. Biologic basis of radiation therapy. In: Halperin EC, Wazer DE, Perez CA, Brady LW, eds. *Perez and Brady's Principles and Practice of Radiation Oncology.* 6th ed. Philadelphia, PA: Lippincott Williams & Wilkins; 2013:61–88.

Question 14

Suppose organ A has functional subunits (FSUs) arranged serially with free movement of stem cells among FSUs and organ B has FSUs arranged in parallel with strict compartmentalization and no movement of stem cells among FSUs. Which organ can tolerate a higher dose if only a small part of each organ receives radiation?

Question 15

Even in serial organs such as the spinal cord, there may be a volume effect on the tolerance dose. What is a "bath and shower" effect observed in the rat spinal cord?

Question 16

Regarding the "bath and shower" effect in question 15, what happens if there is a significant interval between administration of a low-dose bath and high-dose shower?

Question 17

The "bath and shower" effect is also observed in rat parotid glands. When 50% of the parotid gland received a high shower dose of 30 Gy, the functional loss was greater if the other 50% of the parotid gland had a low bath dose as low as 1 Gy. What does it suggest about the parallel functional subunits (FSUs) concept?

Question 14 *Suppose organ A has functional subunits (FSUs) arranged serially with free movement of stem cells among FSUs and organ B has FSUs arranged in parallel with strict compartmentalization and no movement of stem cells among FSUs. Which organ can tolerate a higher dose if only a small part of each organ receives radiation?*

Answer 14

Organ B. For a parallel organ, a small number of disabled FSUs may not disrupt overall function of the organ as long as it is below the organ's spare capacity. But for a serial organ, totally disabled FSUs will render the entire organ dysfunctional. For example, a small volume of the kidneys can tolerate a high dose of 60 Gy as long as the majority volume of the kidney receives a dose below 18 Gy. However, the spinal cord has high risks of dysfunction even if a small part of it receives 60 Gy.

McBride WH, Withers HR. Biologic basis of radiation therapy. In: Halperin EC, Wazer DE, Perez CA, Brady LW, eds. *Perez and Brady's Principles and Practice of Radiation Oncology*. 6th ed. Philadelphia, PA: Lippincott Williams & Wilkins; 2013:61–88.

Question 15 *Even in serial organs such as the spinal cord, there may be a volume effect on the tolerance dose. What is a "bath and shower" effect observed in the rat spinal cord?*

Answer 15

It was observed that right after a modest dose of 4 Gy was given to a large segment of the spinal cord (low-dose "bath"), the dose to the smaller volume of the spinal cord (high-dose "shower") required to cause paralysis decreased substantially from 88 Gy to 61 Gy. The exact mechanism is not known but inhibition of cell migration can be a possible cause. It may play an important role in understanding spinal cord toxicity in stereotactic radiotherapy where a large dose to smaller volume is accompanied with a low dose to large volume.

McBride WH, Withers HR. Biologic basis of radiation therapy. In: Halperin EC, Wazer DE, Perez CA, Brady LW, eds. *Perez and Brady's Principles and Practice of Radiation Oncology*. 6th ed. Philadelphia, PA: Lippincott Williams & Wilkins; 2013:61–88.

Question 16 *Regarding the "bath and shower" effect in question 15, what happens if there is a significant interval between administration of a low-dose bath and high-dose shower?*

Answer 16

It is observed that the effect gradually disappears over 24 hours. The repair kinetics are different from those of fractionated radiation repair of sublethal damage, suggesting different molecular events.

Philippens ME, Pop LA, Viser AG, Peeters WJ, van der Kogel AJ. The bath and shower effect in spinal cord: the effect of time interval. *Int J Radiat Oncol Biol Phys*. February 2009;73(2):514–522.

Question 17 *The "bath and shower" effect is also observed in rat parotid glands. When 50% of the parotid gland received a high shower dose of 30 Gy, the functional loss was greater if the other 50% of the parotid gland had a low bath dose as low as 1 Gy. What does it suggest about the parallel functional subunits (FSUs) concept?*

Answer 17

It suggests that each FSU may not be completely independent even in some parallel organ. The organ function may be arranged in parallel subunits but stem cells or progenitor cells may not be strictly compartmentalized. Therefore, low dose volume may also play an important role in predicting long-term dysfunction.

Van Luijk, P, Faber H, Schippers JM, et al. Bath and shower effects in the rat parotid gland explain increased relative risk of parotid gland dysfunction after intensity-modulated radiotherapy. *Int J Radiat Oncol Biol Phys*. July 2009;74(4):1002–1005.

Question 18
What is a cancer stem cell model for human tumor growth?

Question 19
How does a cancer stem cell model give uncertainties in predicting the total radiation dose required for tumor control based on tumor size?

Question 20
How does the cancer stem cell model give uncertainties in predicting curability based on the response of a tumor undergoing radiation treatment?

Question 21
Which two inherent factors in tumor cell lines are important in determining radiocurability in fractionated radiation treatment?

Question 18 *What is a cancer stem cell model for human tumor growth?*

Answer 18

It is a model based on the observation that the target cell density is much less than the cell density in a given tumor and that the dose required to control the tumor clinically is far less than the prediction based on radiosensitivity and a tumor cell density. Therefore, only a small fraction of tumor cells may have the capacity to regrow and they behave like stem cells in normal tissue. The estimated fraction of stem cells differs widely among tumors and can range from 10^{-2} to 10^{-10}.

Brenner DJ. Dose, volume, and tumor-control predictions in radiotherapy. *Int J Radiat Oncol Biol Phys.* April 1993;26(1):171–179.

Question 19 *How does a cancer stem cell model give uncertainties in predicting the total radiation dose required for tumor control based on tumor size?*

Answer 19

It is not clear if the proportion of stem cells remains the same when the tumor size changes. If a tumor with 1 cm^3 volume has stem cells consisting of 1% of the tumor volume and another 10 cm^3 tumor with stem cells consisting of 0.1%, the number of target cells are the same despite a big difference in volume. This is an extreme example, but it illustrates a point that the number of stem cells may not be accurately estimated by the size of the tumor.

Brenner DJ. Dose, volume, and tumor-control predictions in radiotherapy. *Int J Radiat Oncol Biol Phys.* April 1993;26(1):171–179.

Question 20 *How does the cancer stem cell model give uncertainties in predicting curability based on the response of a tumor undergoing radiation treatment?*

Answer 20

The decrease in the size of a tumor while undergoing radiation treatment depends on the amount of dead cancer cells and the speed of clearing those dead cells. In sarcomas and in some carcinomas with low turnover of cells, it is observed that the efficiency of removing dead cells either by phagocytosis or autolysis is low. Therefore, changes in gross tumor volume in those tumors do not necessarily reflect the amount of dead cancer cells. In addition, the amount of dead cancer cells may not necessarily correlate with the amount of dead cancer stem cells. Some stem cells may reside in more hypoxic regions and may be more resistant than other cancer cells.

Brenner DJ. Dose, volume, and tumor-control predictions in radiotherapy. *Int J Radiat Oncol Biol Phys.* April 1993;26(1):171–179.

Question 21 *Which two inherent factors in tumor cell lines are important in determining radiocurability in fractionated radiation treatment?*

Answer 21

One factor is the ability to repair potentially lethal radiation damage. It has been shown that there is considerable variation of repair capacity between melanoma cell lines and breast cancer cell lines, partly explaining their difference in radiocurability. The other factor is the difference in accelerated repopulation if the duration of the radiation treatment course is sufficiently long enough.

Steel GG, Peacock JH. Why are some human tumours more radiosensitive than others? *Radiother Oncol.* 1989;15:63–72.
Weichselbaum RR, Little JB. Radioresistance in some human tumor cells conferred in vitro by repair of potentially lethal x-ray damage. *Radiology.* 1982;145:511–513.

Question 22

One factor influencing complications is a history of previous radiation treatment to the same region. Which tissue tends to tolerate retreatment better, early-responding tissue or late-responding tissue?

Question 23

There are two possible mechanisms for detrimental complications of retreatment. One is irreversible vascular damage and the other is depletion of stem/progenitor cells that can maintain and regenerate functional cells. What three factors help assess if retreatment is feasible if the dominant mechanism is stem/progenitor cell depletion?

Question 24

Preclinical data using monkeys and clinical data suggest the partial recovery of the spinal cord after initial radiation treatment. How much recovery is estimated at least 6 months after the initial radiation treatment to the full circumference of the spinal cord?

Question 25

In preclinical data using rats, what other factors were witnessed to increase the spinal cord tolerance dose?

Question 22 *One factor influencing complications is a history of previous radiation treatment to the same region. Which tissue tends to tolerate retreatment better, early-responding tissue or late-responding tissue?*

Answer 22

Early-responding tissue tolerates retreatment better; it has a rapidly proliferating stem cell compartment; if stem cells can migrate to the irradiated area, restoring the tissue architecture, it can possibly tolerate retreatment almost to the full dose. However, late-responding tissue tends to have a slowly proliferating stem cell compartment with incomplete functional recovery and also incomplete proliferative capacity recovery. Therefore, late-responding tissue has more difficulties with retreatment.

Hall EJ, Giaccia AJ. Retreatment after radiotherapy: the possibilities and the perils. In: Hall EJ, Giaccia AJ, eds. *Radiobiology for the Radiologist*. 7th ed. Philadelphia, PA: Lippincott Williams & Wilkins; 2012:412–418.

Question 23 *There are two possible mechanisms for detrimental complications of retreatment. One is irreversible vascular damage and the other is depletion of stem/progenitor cells that can maintain and regenerate functional cells. What three factors help assess if retreatment is feasible if the dominant mechanism is stem/progenitor cell depletion?*

Answer 23

a. Initial radiation dose to assess cell depletion.
b. Time elapsed.
c. Regeneration speed of the target tissue to assess tissue restoration.

McBride WH, Withers HR. Biologic basis of radiation therapy. In: Halperin EC, Wazer DE, Perez CA, Brady LW, eds. *Perez and Brady's Principles and Practice of Radiation Oncology*. 6th ed. Philadelphia, PA: Lippincott Williams & Wilkins; 2013:61–88.

Question 24 *Preclinical data using monkeys and clinical data suggest the partial recovery of the spinal cord after initial radiation treatment. How much recovery is estimated at least 6 months after the initial radiation treatment to the full circumference of the spinal cord?*

Answer 24

When an α/β ratio of 3 is used, it is estimated that a cumulative biologically effective dose (BED) can be 130% to 135% of the acceptable BED in a single course of therapy. More recent study suggests an α/β ratio of 0.87; using that value, it is estimated that at least 125% of the cumulative BED can be tolerated with standard fractionation.

Hall EJ, Giaccia AJ. Retreatment after radiotherapy: the possibilities and the perils. In: Hall EJ Giaccia AJ, eds. *Radiobiology for the Radiologist*. 7th ed. Philadelphia, PA: Lippincott Williams & Wilkins; 2012:412–418.
Kirckpatrick JP, van der Kogel AJ, Schultheiss TE. Radiation dose-volume effects in the spinal cord. *Int J Radiat Oncol Biol Phys*. March 2010;76(suppl 3):S42–49.

Question 25 *In preclinical data using rats, what other factors were witnessed to increase the spinal cord tolerance dose?*

Answer 25

An immature spinal cord in rats has a modestly lower tolerance dose compared to adult rats (ED50 19.5 Gy vs. 21.5 Gy), suggesting more care is needed with the pediatric population. Chemotherapy such as intrathecal Ara-C and intraperitoneal fludarabine also had a dose-modifying factor of 1.2 to 1.3 in rats. However, clinical data have not been conclusive.

Kirckpatrick JP, van der Kogel AJ, Schultheiss TE. Radiation dose-volume effects in the spinal cord. *Int J Radiat Oncol Biol Phys*. March 2010;76(Suppl 3):S42–49.

Question 26
Based on mouse studies, which organs do not recover from late functional damage?

Question 27
Ethyol (amifostine) is one radioprotector that is approved by the Food and Drug Administration (FDA) to reduce the incidence of moderate to severe xerostomia in patients undergoing postoperative treatment for head and neck cancer. How does it work to decrease complications in the normal tissue?

Question 28
Hyperthermia can be combined with radiation treatment to improve cancer control. Some clinical trials proved its efficacy in the treatment of superficial breast cancer and chest wall recurrence. How does hyperthermia complement radiation treatment?

Question 26 *Based on mouse studies, which organs do not recover from late functional damage?*

Answer 26

Unlike the spinal cord, the kidney and bladder may not recover their tolerance to radiation. In mouse studies, tolerance decreased significantly with increasing the interval between treatments up to 26 weeks, suggesting progression rather than recovery from the initial damage.

Hall EJ, Giaccia AJ. Retreatment after radiotherapy: the possibilities and the perils. In: Hall EJ, Giaccia AJ, eds. *Radiobiology for the Radiologist*. 7th ed. Philadelphia, PA: Lippincott Williams & Wilkins; 2006:412–418.
Stewart FA, Oussoren Y, Van Tinteren H, Bentzen SM. Loss of reirradiation tolerance in the kidney with increasing time after single or fractionated partial tolerance doses. *Int J Radiat Oncol Biol Phys*. August 1994;66(2):169–179.

Question 27 *Ethyol (amifostine) is one radioprotector that is approved by the Food and Drug Administration (FDA) to reduce the incidence of moderate to severe xerostomia in patients undergoing postoperative treatment for head and neck cancer. How does it work to decrease complications in the normal tissue?*

Answer 27

It is believed that the active metabolites of amifostine, WR-1065, eliminate free radicals, thus reducing the effects of radiation. To produce the active metabolites, it needs to be dephosphorylated by cellular-bound alkaline phosphatase. Alkaline phosphatase is in higher concentration in normal tissues and amifostine may selectively protect normal tissues. However, the FDA has warnings that amifostine should not be used in patients receiving definitive radiation treatment except in clinical trials because there is insufficient data excluding a tumor-protective effect. There are also reports of serious cutaneous reactions with fatalities with the administration of amifostine.

Halperin EC, Wazer DE, Perez CA. The discipline of radiation oncology. In: Halperin EC, Wazer DE, Perez CA, Brady LW, eds. *Perez and Brady's Principles and Practice of Radiation Oncology*. 6th ed. Philadelphia, PA: Lippincott Williams & Wilkins; 2013:2–60.

Question 28 *Hyperthermia can be combined with radiation treatment to improve cancer control. Some clinical trials proved its efficacy in the treatment of superficial breast cancer and chest wall recurrence. How does hyperthermia complement radiation treatment?*

Answer 28

Unlike radiation treatment, heat is more effective in killing hypoxic cells. Cells in S phase of the proliferative cycle are resistant to radiation but more sensitive to heat.

Halperin EC, Wazer DE, Perez CA. The discipline of radiation oncology. In: Halperin EC, Wazer DE, Perez CA, Brady LW, eds. *Perez and Brady's Principles and Practice of Radiation Oncology*. 6th ed. Philadelphia, PA: Lippincott Williams & Wilkins; 2013:2–60.
Zagar TM, Oleson JR, Vujaskovic Z, et al. Hyperthermia combined with radiation therapy for superficial breast cancer and chest wall recurrence: a review of the randomized data. *Int J Hyperthermia*. 2010;26(7):612–617.

Question 29

Cetuximab, an epidermal growth factor receptor (EGFR) inhibitor, increases the tumor control rate in locally advanced squamous cell carcinoma of the head and neck. How does it work synergistically with radiation?

Question 30

Suppose you have a tumor with a large portion of cancer cells in a hypoxic environment and most cells in the late S phase of the mitotic cell cycle. What type of radiation can overcome these radiation-resistant factors?

Question 29 *Cetuximab, an epidermal growth factor receptor (EGFR) inhibitor, increases the tumor control rate in locally advanced squamous cell carcinoma of the head and neck. How does it work synergistically with radiation?*

Answer 29

Expression of EGFR in cancer cells increases with radiation. EGFR inhibition increases cellular sensitivity to radiation by improving the tumor cell response to radiation through changes in the cell cycle distribution, decreasing DNA damage response, inhibiting accelerated repopulation, and triggering radiation-induced apoptosis.

Halperin EC, Wazer DE, Perez CA. The discipline of radiation oncology. In: Halperin EC, Wazer DE, Perez CA, Brady LW, eds. *Perez and Brady's Principles and Practice of Radiation Oncology*. 6th ed. Philadelphia, PA: Lippincott Williams & Wilkins; 2013:2–60.

Morris ZS, Harari PM. Interaction of radiation therapy with molecular targeted agents. *J Clin Oncol*. September 2014;32(26):2886–2893.

Question 30 *Suppose you have a tumor with a large portion of cancer cells in a hypoxic environment and most cells in the late S phase of the mitotic cell cycle. What type of radiation can overcome these radiation-resistant factors?*

Answer 30

High-linear energy transfer (LET) radiation such as neutrons, pi mesons, and heavy ions can overcome these radiation-resistant factors. High-LET radiation has a lower oxygen enhancement ratio (OER) and is less dependent on oxygen because of more dense ionization events along its path. One possible mechanism of radiation resistance in S phase is that low-LET radiation slows cells in the S phase, allowing more time for repair. However, in high-LET radiation, this is not observed. One caveat is high-LET radiation such as a neutron irradiation may also have increased effects on normal tissue and complications.

Blakely E, Change P, Lommel L, et al. Cell-cycle radiation response: role of intracellular factors. *Adv Space Res*. 1989;9(10): 177–186.

Todd P. Biological aspects of high LET radiation therapy. *Radiology*. November 1977;125:493–496.

14

IMPACT OF TIME, DOSE, AND FRACTIONATION IN RADIATION ONCOLOGY

DAESUNG LEE

Question 1

Biological effects of radiation on tissues depend on total dose, number of fractions, fraction size, and total time. However, not all tissues respond in the same way to changes in fraction size and overall treatment time, even if the total dose remains the same. When was it first realized that fractionation can be utilized to spare normal tissue better while achieving the desired effect of radiation?

Question 2

What are the 4 R's of radiobiology to explain advantages of fractionated radiation treatment?

Question 3

How does fractionation affect oxygenation in normal tissue and a tumor?

Turn page to see the answers.

Question 1 *Biological effects of radiation on tissues depend on total dose, number of fractions, fraction size, and total time. However, not all tissues respond in the same way to changes in fraction size and overall treatment time, even if the total dose remains the same. When was it first realized that fractionation can be utilized to spare normal tissue better while achieving the desired effect of radiation?*

Answer 1

In the 1920s and 1930s, in France, radiation was thought to be a candidate for sterilization of rams to replace surgical castration, which had high morbidity rates. However, a single dose of radiation to sterilize rams also caused significant irritation of scrotum skin. When smaller fractionated doses were given over several days, sterilization was achieved while sparing scrotum skin, showing that biological effects can be differentially modulated among tissue types by varying dose, fractionation, and time.

Hall EJ, Giaccia AJ. Time, dose, and fractionation in radiotherapy. In: Hall EJ, Giaccia AJ, eds. *Radiobiology for the Radiologist.* 7th ed. Philadelphia, PA: Lippincott Williams & Wilkins, 2012:391–411.

Question 2 *What are the 4 R's of radiobiology to explain advantages of fractionated radiation treatment?*

Answer 2

    a. Repair of sublethal damage for better normal tissue sparing.

    b. Reassortment of cells within the cell cycle to improve tumor cell killing.

    c. Repopulation for better normal tissue recovery.

    d. Reoxygenation to improve cell killing.

Hall EJ, Giaccia AJ. Time, dose, and fractionation in radiotherapy. In: Hall EJ, Giaccia AJ, eds. *Radiobiology for the Radiologist.* 7th ed. Philadelphia, PA: Lippincott Williams & Wilkins; 2012:391–411.

Question 3 *How does fractionation affect oxygenation in normal tissue and a tumor?*

Answer 3

In normal tissue, oxygenation changes slightly, if any, between fractions. The tumor consists of aerated cells and hypoxic cells. A dose of radiation kills more aerated cells than hypoxic cells because aerated cells are more sensitive. Therefore, immediately after radiation treatment, the proportion of hypoxic cells increases because of a decrease in aerated cells killed by radiation. Then, there is reoxygenation of the remaining cells and the proportion of aerated cells return to the pretreatment level. Fractionation is one method to overcome hypoxia.

Halperin EC, Wazer DE, Perez CA. The discipline of radiation oncology. In: Halperin EC, Wazer DE, Perez CA, Brady LW, eds. *Perez and Brady's Principles and Practice of Radiation Oncology.* 6th ed. Philadelphia, PA: Lippincott Williams & Wilkins; 2013:2–60.

Question 4

How does tumor cell killing improve oxygenation in the remaining cells?

Question 5

In stereotactic body radiation therapy (SBRT), a single fraction or only limited number of fractions up to five are given. This means that most hypoxic cells need to be killed in the hypoxic state and a higher biological effective dose will be required compared to the standard fractionation regimen. However, a clinically effective SBRT dose is lower than what is predicted to be necessary to kill hypoxic cells. It suggests that there are other possible ways SBRT can improve cell killing not seen in a conventional radiation treatment regimen. What are two proposed mechanisms?

Question 6

Redistribution means that cells in resistant phases of the cell cycle can move to a more sensitive phase at the next fraction. Does this improve the therapeutic ratio?

Question 4 *How does tumor cell killing improve oxygenation in the remaining cells?*

Answer 4

If there is a constant supply of oxygen, fewer surviving cells means better access to that amount of oxygen per each cell. Another possible mechanism is that blood vessels can be compressed by a rapidly growing cancer and they can be decompressed with tumor regression, resulting in better vascular and oxygen flow.

Halperin EC, Wazer DE, Perez CA. The discipline of radiation oncology. In: Halperin EC, Wazer DE, Perez CA, Brady LW, eds. *Perez and Brady's Principles and Practice of Radiation Oncology.* 6th ed. Philadelphia, PA: Lippincott Williams & Wilkins; 2013:20.

Question 5 *In stereotactic body radiation therapy (SBRT), a single fraction or only limited number of fractions up to five are given. This means that most hypoxic cells need to be killed in the hypoxic state and a higher biological effective dose will be required compared to the standard fractionation regimen. However, a clinically effective SBRT dose is lower than what is predicted to be necessary to kill hypoxic cells. It suggests that there are other possible ways SBRT can improve cell killing not seen in a conventional radiation treatment regimen. What are two proposed mechanisms?*

Answer 5

SBRT with a large dose per fraction can cause heterogeneous tumor vascular damage at doses higher than 10 Gy/fraction. It can also trigger active immune responses against tumor cells.

Brown JM, Diehn M, Loo BW Jr. Stereotactic ablative radiotherapy should be combined with a hypoxic cell radiosensitizer. *Int J Radiat Oncol Biol Phys.* 2010;78(2):323–327.
Garcia-Barros M, Paris F, Cordon-Cardo C, et al. Tumor response to radiotherapy regulated by endothelial cell apoptosis. *Science.* May 2003;300(5622):1155–1159.

Question 6 *Redistribution means that cells in resistant phases of the cell cycle can move to a more sensitive phase at the next fraction. Does this improve the therapeutic ratio?*

Answer 6

It would improve the therapeutic ratio if redistribution occurs in tumor cells and not in normal tissue stem cells. Tumor cells proliferate rapidly enough to move to different phases of the cell cycle between radiation fractions, but the normal tissue stem cells cycle slowly and stay mostly in the G_0 phase of the cell cycle. However, in the cancer stem cell hypothesis, unlike cancer progenitor cells, cancer stem cells cycle slowly and it is not clear if redistribution gives a particularly strong advantage in cancer cure.

Pajonk F, Vlashi E, McBride WH. Radiation resistance of cancer stem cells: the 4 R's of radiobiology revisited. *Stem Cells.* April 2010;28(4):639–648.

Question 7

Among the 4 R's of radiobiology, which 2 R's improve sparing of the normal tissues?

Question 8

Repopulation can occur in tumor cells. Does repopulation increase the therapeutic ratio in fractionated radiation treatment?

Question 9

What is accelerated repopulation?

Question 10

In head and neck cancer, neoadjuvant chemotherapy failed to improve the final outcome despite initial tumor regression. What is a possible explanation?

Question 7 *Among the 4 R's of radiobiology, which 2 R's improve sparing of the normal tissues?*

Answer 7

Repair of sublethal damage between dose fractions and repopulation of normal tissue cells for sufficiently prolonged overall treatment time help improve sparing of normal tissues.

Hall EJ, Giaccia AJ. Time, dose, and fractionation in radiotherapy. In: Hall EJ, Giaccia AJ, eds. *Radiobiology for the Radiologist*. 7th ed. Philadelphia, PA: Lippincott Williams & Wilkins; 2012:391–411.

Question 8 *Repopulation can occur in tumor cells. Does repopulation increase the therapeutic ratio in fractionated radiation treatment?*

Answer 8

Meaningful repopulation can start at different time points for normal tissues and tumor cells. Estimating from the extra dose required to counteract proliferation after starting daily irradiation, the mouse small intestine mucosa tissue (early reaction tissue) starts repopulation at day 1 or 2, the mouse skin starts at day 14, and rat spinal cord (late reaction tissue) starts at around day 42. In humans, it is estimated that repopulation of human skin starts at around 4 weeks. For human oropharyngeal cancers, meaningful repopulation starts at about 30 days. Therefore, repopulation may offer a modest advantage in tumor control with respect to early reaction tissue toxicities. For late reaction tissue toxicities, repopulation may work against the therapeutic ratio if treatment time is prolonged over a month in tumors such as oropharyngeal cancers. Although repopulation may not be an important factor in improving therapeutic ratio, it improves radiation treatment tolerance and compliance by mitigating acute normal tissue reaction.

Hall EJ, Giaccia AJ. Time, dose, and fractionation in radiotherapy. In: Hall EJ, Giaccia AJ, eds. *Radiobiology for the Radiologist*. 7th ed. Philadelphia, PA: Lippincott Williams & Wilkins; 2012:391–411.
Kim JJ, Tannock IF. Repopulation of cancer cells during therapy: an important cause of treatment failure. *Nat Rev Cancer*. 2005; 5:516–525.
Withers HR. Biologic basis for altered fractionation schemed. *Cancer*. 1985;55:2086–2095.

Question 9 *What is accelerated repopulation?*

Answer 9

Tumor growth and doubling time decrease with the growth of the tumor. With reduction of tumor cells by any cytotoxic agent such as radiation treatment and chemotherapy, surviving tumor clonogens are triggered to grow faster than the growth rate at the time of treatment initiation. This is called accelerated repopulation. It has a various lag time depending on tumor type. For human oropharygeal cancers, accelerated repopulation starts after about 1 month. This is when you start to see clinically significant repopulation, requiring an additional radiation dose to counter repopulation.

Hall EJ, Giaccia AJ. Time, dose, and fractionation in radiotherapy. In: Hall EJ, Giaccia AJ, eds. *Radiobiology for the Radiologist*. 7th ed. Philadelphia, PA: Lippincott Williams & Wilkins; 2012:391–411.
Kim JJ, Tannock IF. Repopulation of cancer cells during therapy: an important cause of treatment failure. *Nat. Rev. Cancer*. 2005;5:516–525.

Question 10 *In head and neck cancer, neoadjuvant chemotherapy failed to improve the final outcome despite initial tumor regression. What is a possible explanation?*

Answer 10

Accelerated repopulation is triggered by chemotherapy as well as radiation therapy. When radiation treatment starts after chemotherapy, the tumor is already at an accelerated repopulation stage, using up about 0.61 Gy/day to kill repopulated cells from day 1 of radiation treatment.

Hall EJ, Giaccia AJ. Time, dose, and fractionation in radiotherapy. In: Hall EJ, Giaccia AJ, eds. *Radiobiology for the Radiologist*. 7th ed. Philadelphia, PA: Lippincott Williams & Wilkins; 2012:391–411.

Question 11

Repair of sublethal damage occurs in tumor cells as well as in normal cells. Does repair increase the therapeutic ratio in fractionated radiation treatment?

Question 12

The Strandquist plot is isoeffect curves relating the total dose to the overall treatment time for a given biological effect such as skin necrosis, cure of skin carcinoma, moist desquamation of skin, dry desquamation of skin, and skin erythema. What shape is the curve in logarithmic scales?

Question 13

Ellis improved on the Strandquist plot by separating overall treatment time and number of fractions and introduced the nominal standard dose (NSD) system with the following formula.

Total dose = $(NSD)T^{0.11}N^{0.24}$

where T is overall treatment time, N is the number of fractions, and NSD is a constant to adjust the unit to dose.

What are two major criticisms of this formula?

Question 14

The linear-quadratic model was developed to describe cell survival curves and assumes two components of cell killing. Barendsen suggested the biologically effective dose (BED) by describing the biological effect (E) of a single dose (D) by those two components.

$E = \alpha D + \beta D^2$

And for n fractions of dose d,

$E = n(\alpha d + \beta d^2)$

It can be rearranged to calculate E/α, BED. What is the equation?

Question 11 *Repair of sublethal damage occurs in tumor cells as well as in normal cells. Does repair increase the therapeutic ratio in fractionated radiation treatment?*

Answer 11

Yes. Cancer cells were shown to have lower repair capacity of sublethal damage compared to normal cell lines in split-dose experiments where a single-dose radiation treatment to various cancer cell lines was compared to two split-dose radiation treatments administered 6 hours apart. Among normal tissues, late-responding tissue cells have more capacity for repair than early-responding tissue cells.

Schwachofer JH, Crooijmans RP, Hoogenhout J, et al. Sublethal damage repair in two radioresistant human tumor cell lines irradiated as multicellular spheroids. *Tumour Biol.* 1991;12(4):207–216.
Withers HR. Biologic basis for altered fractionation schemed. *Cancer.* 1985;55:2086–2095.

Question 12 *The Strandquist plot is isoeffect curves relating the total dose to the overall treatment time for a given biological effect such as skin necrosis, cure of skin carcinoma, moist desquamation of skin, dry desquamation of skin, and skin erythema. What shape is the curve in logarithmic scales?*

Answer 12

They are straight lines with a slope of about 0.33. Because they are plotted in logarithmic scales, the total dose is proportional to $T^{0.33}$ where T is overall treatment time. The data is derived from fractionated treatment of 280 cases of carcinoma of the skin and lips; treatments were given in 3 or 5 fractions/week.

Hall EJ, Giaccia AJ. Time, dose, and fractionation in radiotherapy. In: Hall EJ, Giaccia AJ, eds. *Radiobiology for the Radiologist.* 7th ed. Philadelphia, PA: Lippincott Williams & Wilkins; 2012:391–411.

Question 13 *Ellis improved on the Strandquist plot by separating overall treatment time and number of fractions and introduced the nominal standard dose (NSD) system with the following formula.*

Total dose = (NSD)$T^{0.11}N^{0.24}$

where T is overall treatment time, N is the number of fractions, and NSD is a constant to adjust the unit to dose.

What are two major criticisms of this formula?

Answer 13

It is derived from acute skin reaction data and does not predict late effects. When the number of fractions remains the same, total dose is proportional to $T^{0.11}$ from the very start of irradiation. But meaningful repopulation requiring an extra dose starts with a lag of a few days to weeks in experimental data.

Hall EJ, Giaccia AJ. Time, dose, and fractionation in radiotherapy. In: Hall EJ, Giaccia AJ, eds. *Radiobiology for the Radiologist.* 7th ed. Philadelphia, PA: Lippincott Williams & Wilkins; 2006:391–411.

Question 14 *The linear-quadratic model was developed to describe cell survival curves and assumes two components of cell killing. Barendsen suggested the biologically effective dose (BED) by describing the biological effect (E) of a single dose (D) by those two components.*

$E = \alpha D + \beta D^2$

And for n fractions of dose d,

$E = n(\alpha d + \beta d^2)$

It can be rearranged to calculate E/α, BED. What is the equation?

Answer 14

BED = total dose $\times$ relative effectiveness = $E/\alpha = (nd) \times (1 + d/(\alpha/\beta))$

Hall EJ, Giaccia AJ. Time, dose, and fractionation in radiotherapy. In: Hall EJ, Giaccia AJ, eds. *Radiobiology for the Radiologist.* 7th ed. Philadelphia, PA: Lippincott Williams & Wilkins; 2012:391–411.

Question 15

Isoeffect curves are plotted with the total dose necessary for a given radiation effect versus the dose/fraction. It is observed that isoeffect curves for late effects are steeper than those for acute effects. What does it tell us about the magnitude of impact of changes in the dose/fraction in late-responding tissues?

Question 16

Early-responding tissues and late-responding tissues react differently to changes in dose per fraction. The biologically effective dose (BED) formula allows that difference by using different α/β values for different tissues. Late-responding tissue is much more sensitive to changes in dose per fraction. Which tissue has a higher α/β ratio?

Question 17

Suppose you plan to give 70 Gy in 35 fractions with 2 Gy/fraction. What is the biologically effective dose (BED) for tumor control and BED for osteoradionecrosis of the mandible (late tissue effects)? Assume α/β is 3 Gy for osteoradionecrosis and 10 Gy for tumor cells.

Question 18

Please see question 17. Now, you want to change the fraction size to 1.2 Gy. For the same biological effects as 70 Gy with 2 Gy/fraction, what should your total dose be?

Question 15 *Isoeffect curves are plotted with the total dose necessary for a given radiation effect versus the dose/fraction. It is observed that isoeffect curves for late effects are steeper than those for acute effects. What does it tell us about the magnitude of impact of changes in the dose/fraction in late-responding tissues?*

Answer 15

Late effects are more sensitive to changes in fraction size than acute effects. If the fraction size gets larger, late complications may increase more than the gains in tumor control for a given total dose.

Hall EJ, Giaccia AJ. Time, dose, and fractionation in radiotherapy. In: Hall EJ, Giaccia AJ, eds. *Radiobiology for the Radiologist*. 7th ed. Philadelphia, PA: Lippincott Williams & Wilkins; 2012:391–411.

Question 16 *Early-responding tissues and late-responding tissues react differently to changes in dose per fraction. The biologically effective dose (BED) formula allows that difference by using different α/β values for different tissues. Late-responding tissue is much more sensitive to changes in dose per fraction. Which tissue has a higher α/β ratio?*

Answer 16

BED = (total dose) × (relative effectiveness). Relative effectiveness is $(1 + d/(\alpha/\beta))$. Effectiveness of a single dose d is divided by α/β. If α/β is large, the impact of a single dose gets smaller. Therefore, α/β is large for early-responding tissues and is small for late-responding tissues.

Hall EJ, Giaccia AJ. Time, dose, and fractionation in radiotherapy. In: Hall EJ, Giaccia AJ, eds. *Radiobiology for the Radiologist*. 7th ed. Philadelphia, PA: Lippincott Williams & Wilkins; 2012:391–411.

Question 17 *Suppose you plan to give 70 Gy in 35 fractions with 2 Gy/fraction. What is the biologically effective dose (BED) for tumor control and BED for osteoradionecrosis of the mandible (late tissue effects)? Assume α/β is 3 Gy for osteoradionecrosis and 10 Gy for tumor cells.*

Answer 17

BED = $(nd) \times (1 + d/(\alpha/\beta))$, where nd is total dose and d is dose per fraction. For tumor control, 70 Gy × $(1 + 2$ Gy/10 Gy$) = 84$ Gy$_{10}$, and for osteoradionecrosis, 70 Gy × $(1 + 2$ Gy/3 Gy$) = 116.67$ Gy$_3$. Subscript of Gy$_3$ denotes α/β used for BED calculation.

Hall EJ, Giaccia AJ. Time, dose, and fractionation in radiotherapy. In: Hall EJ, Giaccia AJ, eds. *Radiobiology for the Radiologist*. 7th ed. Philadelphia, PA: Lippincott Williams & Wilkins; 2012:391–411.

Question 18 *Please see question 17. Now, you want to change the fraction size to 1.2 Gy. For the same biological effects as 70 Gy with 2 Gy/fraction, what should your total dose be?*

Answer 18

First, you need to define which biological effects are needed. For tumor control using an α/β ratio of 10 Gy, the biologically effective dose (BED) is 84 Gy$_{10}$ from the aforementioned calculation and BED = $(nd) \times (1 + d/(\alpha/\beta))$, where nd is total dose and d is dose/fraction. Therefore, 84 Gy$_{10}$ = total dose × $(1 + 1.2$ Gy/10 Gy$)$. Solving for total dose = 84 Gy$_{10}$/$(1 + 1.2$ Gy/10 Gy$) = 75$ Gy.
For osteoradionecrosis, 116.67 Gy$_3$ = total dose × $(1 + 1.2$ Gy/3 Gy$)$. Total dose = 83.33 Gy.
When the fraction size gets smaller, you need a smaller amount of extra dose to achieve the same biological early effects (in this case 5 Gy) than to have the same late effects (in this case 13.33 Gy).

Hall EJ, Giaccia AJ. Time, dose, and fractionation in radiotherapy. In: Hall EJ, Giaccia AJ, eds. *Radiobiology for the Radiologist*. 7th ed. Philadelphia, PA: Lippincott Williams & Wilkins; 2012:391–411.

Question 19

What is hyperfractionation and how can it improve the therapeutic ratio?

Question 20

The Radiation Therapy Oncology Group (RTOG) 9003 trial proved that hyperfractionation treatment can indeed improve therapeutic ratio over the standard treatment. What fractionation regimen was used for this trial?

Question 21

What is accelerated treatment and how does it improve therapeutic ratio?

Question 22

EORTC (European Organisation for Research and Treatment of Cancer) 22851 was a randomized trial testing accelerated treatment in head and neck cancer. It compared 72 Gy with 1.6 Gy/fraction three fractions per day (minimum 4 hours apart between fractions) with a 2-week break in the middle (overall treatment time of 5 weeks) to the standard treatment of 70 Gy in 35 fractions over 7 weeks. What were the unexpected findings?

Question 19 *What is hyperfractionation and how can it improve the therapeutic ratio?*

Answer 19

Hyperfractionation is using a lower fraction size multiple times a day while keeping the overall treatment time and total dose about the same. It can improve the therapeutic ratio because late effect complications are more sensitive to fraction size than early effects such as tumor cell death. For tumor control, 75 Gy in a 1.2 Gy/fraction has a similar chance of tumor control as 70 Gy in a 2 Gy/fraction. But the risk of late complications is lower at 75 Gy in a 1.2 Gy/fraction compared to 70 Gy in a 2 Gy/fraction.

Or you can improve the chance for tumor control by increasing the dose to 83.33 Gy in 1.2 Gy/fraction while keeping late complication risks similar.

(Note: It actually will be 75.6 Gy and 84 Gy if the numbers of fractions are integers.)

Hall EJ, Giaccia AJ. Time, dose, and fractionation in radiotherapy. In: Hall EJ, Giaccia AJ, eds. *Radiobiology for the Radiologist.* 7th ed. Philadelphia, PA: Lippincott Williams & Wilkins; 2012:391–411.

Question 20 *The Radiation Therapy Oncology Group (RTOG) 9003 trial proved that hyperfractionation treatment can indeed improve therapeutic ratio over the standard treatment. What fractionation regimen was used for this trial?*

Answer 20

The hyperfractionation regimen was one of the three experimental arms. It used 81.6 Gy total dose in 1.2 Gy/fraction twice daily at least 6 hours apart between fractions over 7 weeks. It was compared to 70 Gy total dose in 2 Gy/fraction once daily over 7 weeks in treatment of locally advanced head and neck cancer. As you can see in question 19, 81.6 Gy is higher than the biologically equivalent dose of 75 Gy with respect to tumor control but slightly lower than the biologically equivalent dose for late effects. The study showed improvement in local-regional control and increased acute effects but similar late complications.

Fu KK, Pajak TF, Trotti A, et al. A Radiation Therapy Oncology Group (RTOG) phase III randomized study to compare hyperfractionation and two variants of accelerated fractionation to standard fractionation radiotherapy for head and neck squamous cell carcinoma: first report of RTOG 9003. *Int J Radiat Oncol Biol Phys.* 2000;48(1):7–16.

Question 21 *What is accelerated treatment and how does it improve therapeutic ratio?*

Answer 21

Accelerated treatment shortens overall treatment time by giving multiple fractions a day but keeps the fraction size and total dose similar. It can potentially improve therapeutic ratio by reducing repopulation with shortening of overall treatment time. As fraction size and total dose are similar, late complications are not expected to increase.

Hall EJ, Giaccia AJ. Time, dose, and fractionation in radiotherapy. In: Hall EJ, Giaccia AJ, eds. *Radiobiology for the Radiologist.* 7th ed. Philadelphia, PA: Lippincott Williams & Wilkins; 2012:391–411.

Question 22 *EORTC (European Organisation for Research and Treatment of Cancer) 22851 was a randomized trial testing accelerated treatment in head and neck cancer. It compared 72 Gy with 1.6 Gy/fraction 3 fractions/day (minimum 4 hours apart between fractions) with a 2-week break in the middle (overall treatment time of 5 weeks) to the standard treatment of 70 Gy in 35 fractions over 7 weeks. What were the unexpected findings?*

Answer 22

As expected, local-regional control improved and acute effects increased. Unexpectedly, severe late complications increased significantly, such as severe fibrosis, radiation myelitis (spinal cord dose at 42 Gy and 48 Gy), peripheral neuropathy, and severe mucosa sequelae including necrosis.

Horiot JC, Bontemps P, van den Bogaert W, et al. Accelerated fractionation compared to conventional fractionation improves loco-regional control in the radiotherapy of advanced head and neck cancers: results of the EORTC 22851 randomized trial. *Radiother Oncol.* 1997;44(2):111–121.

Question 23

Which variant of accelerated treatment was shown to improve local-regional control without an increase in late complications?

Question 24

What is continuous hyperfractionated accelerated radiation therapy (CHART) and how does it improve therapeutic ratio?

Question 25

An initial continuous hyperfractionated accelerated radiation therapy (CHART) trial had a few episodes of spinal cord myelitis reported. At least 4 hours of break was required between fractions given on the same day. One patient had myelitis with total dose of 42.5 Gy to the spinal cord. Another patient developed myelitis with total dose of 46 Gy to the spinal cord. Those doses are close to the tolerance dose for conventional radiation treatment with once-a-day treatment. What does it tell about repair in the spinal cord?

Question 26

One randomized trial comparing continuous hyperfractionated accelerated radiation therapy (CHART) 54 Gy to conventional treatment of 66 Gy in 33 fractions over 6.5 weeks in head and neck cancer showed similar local control. How were late complication rates different between two treatment arms?

Question 23 *Which variant of accelerated treatment was shown to improve local-regional control without an increase in late complications?*

Answer 23

Concomitant boost was one experimental arm of Radiation Therapy Oncology Group (RTOG) 9003. The accelerated fractionation with concomitant boost regimen was 1.8 Gy/fraction/day, 5 days/week and 1.5 Gy/fraction/day to a boost field as a second daily treatment for the last 12 treatment days to 72 Gy/42 fractions/6 weeks. It decreased overall treatment time by 1 week and local-regional control improved without an increase in late complications.

Fu KK, Pajak TF, Trotti A, et al. A Radiation Therapy Oncology Group (RTOG) phase III randomized study to compare hyperfractionation and two variants of accelerated fractionation to standard fractionation radiotherapy for head and neck squamous cell carcinoma: first report of RTOG 9003. *Int J Radiat Oncol Biol Phys.* August 2000;48(1):7–16.

Question 24 *What is continuous hyperfractionated accelerated radiation therapy (CHART) and how does it improve therapeutic ratio?*

Answer 24

CHART is an extreme form of accelerated treatment. It stands for continuous hyperfractionated accelerated radiation therapy and started at the Mount Vernon Hospital in the United Kingdom in 1985. It consists of 36 fractions of 1.4 to 1.5 Gy over 12 consecutive days without weekend breaks and three fractions daily at least 6 hours apart between fractions to the total dose of 50 to 54 Gy. It improves therapeutic ration by reducing overall treatment time drastically, countering repopulation. It also decreases late complication rates by using lower dose per fraction and lower total dose. An accelerated treatment regimen in the EORTC 22851 trial used a higher total dose than conventional treatment and only 4 hours apart between fractions.

Hall EJ, Giaccia AJ. Time, dose, and fractionation in radiotherapy. In: Hall EJ, Giaccia AJ, eds. *Radiobiology for the Radiologist.* 7th ed. Philadelphia, PA: Lippincott Williams & Wilkins; 2012:391–411.

Question 25 *An initial continuous hyperfractionated accelerated radiation therapy (CHART) trial had a few episodes of spinal cord myelitis reported. At least 4 hours of break was required between fractions given on the same day. One patient had myelitis with total dose of 42.5 Gy to the spinal cord. Another patient developed myelitis with total dose of 46 Gy to the spinal cord. Those doses are close to the tolerance dose for conventional radiation treatment with once-a-day treatment. What does it tell about repair in the spinal cord?*

Answer 25

Six hours may not be long enough for maximum repair of tissues pertaining to cord myelitis. Therefore, to account for incomplete repair, the spinal cord dose was reduced in subsequent CHART trials. When the spinal cord dose was limited to 40 Gy generally and 44 Gy as an absolute maximum in CHART treatment arms, no case of spinal cord myelitis was reported.

Dische S, Saunders MI. Continuous, hyperfractionated, accelerated radiotherapy (CHART): an interim report upon late morbidity. *Radiother Oncol.* 1989;16:67–74.
Saunders MI, Dische S, Barrett A, et al. Randomised multicenter trials of CHART vs. conventional radiotherapy in head and neck cancer and non-small cell lung cancer: an interim report. *Br J Cancer.* 1996;73:1455–1462.

Question 26 *One randomized trial comparing continuous hyperfractionated accelerated radiation therapy (CHART) 54 Gy to conventional treatment of 66 Gy in 33 fractions over 6.5 weeks in head and neck cancer showed similar local control. How were late complication rates different between two treatment arms?*

Answer 26

Some late effects such as skin telangiectasia, laryngeal edema, and mucosa ulceration occurred in lower rates in the CHART arm compared to the standard arm.

Dische S, Saunders M, Barret A, et al. A randomized multicenter trial of CHART versus conventional radiotherapy in head and neck cancer. *Radiother Oncol.* August 1997;44(2):132–136.

Question 27

Another randomized trial comparing continuous hyperfractionated accelerated radiation therapy (CHART) 54 Gy to standard radiation treatment 60 Gy in 30 fractions over 6 weeks in locally advanced non–small cell lung cancer showed similar late complications. (Please note that total dose in the conventional arm is lower than the trial mentioned in question 26.) How were local control and overall survival rates different between the two treatment arms?

Question 28

Overall treatment time is shown to be important in tumor control in head and neck cancer and non–small cell lung cancer as shown in continuous hyperfractionated accelerated radiation therapy (CHART) trials mentioned in the aforementioned questions. Acute complications were also higher with shorter overall treatment time. What impact does overall treatment time have on late complications?

Question 29

The initial formula for biologically effective dose (BED) does not have a variable for overall treatment time, which has significant impact on certain tumors or early effects. Fowler suggested modification by adding a time component.

$$BED = E/\alpha = (\text{Total dose})[1 + d/(\alpha/\beta)] - (0.693/\alpha)(t/T_{pot})$$

Rapid repopulation starts with a lag of 21 to 28 days. Therefore, 21 or 28 days are subtracted from overall treatment time and $t = T$ (overall time) $- T_k$ (kick-off time, typically 21–28 days). T_{pot} is potential doubling time. α is estimated to be 0.3. What is time-corrected BED of 70 Gy in 35 fractions over 7 weeks (46 α) assuming $\alpha/\beta = 10$ Gy, $T_k = 21$ days, and $T_{pot} = 5$ days?

Question 27 *Another randomized trial comparing continuous hyperfractionated accelerated radiation therapy (CHART) 54 Gy to standard radiation treatment 60 Gy in 30 fractions over 6 weeks in locally advanced non–small cell lung cancer showed similar late complications. (Please note that total dose in the conventional arm is lower than the trial mentioned in question 26.) How were local control and overall survival rates different between the two treatment arms?*

Answer 27

Local control and overall survival rate were significantly higher in the CHART arm. It proved that repopulation is an important factor in locally advanced non–small lung cancer that needs to be overcome by shortening overall treatment time. This may be one factor regarding why we see better outcomes with concurrent chemoradiation treatment compared to sequential chemotherapy and then radiation treatment in non–small cell lung cancer.

Saunders M, Dische S, Barrett A, et al. Continuous, hyperfractionated, accelerated radiotherapy (CHART) versus conventional radiotherapy in non-small cell lung cancer: mature data from the randomized multicenter trial. CHART Steering Committee. *Radiother Oncol.* August 1999;52(2):137–148.

Question 28 *Overall treatment time is shown to be important in tumor control in head and neck cancer and non–small cell lung cancer as shown in continuous hyperfractionated accelerated radiation therapy (CHART) trials mentioned in the aforementioned questions. Acute complications were also higher with shorter overall treatment time. What impact does overall treatment time have on late complications?*

Answer 28

As shown in the aforementioned trials, fraction size and total dose are important factors in late complication. However, overall treatment time has little impact on late complication because accelerated repopulation starts at a much later time (later than the typical length of radiation treatment) for most late-responding tissues.

Hall EJ, Giaccia AJ. Time, dose, and fractionation in radiotherapy. In: Hall EJ, Giaccia AJ, eds. *Radiobiology for the Radiologist.* 7th ed. Philadelphia, PA: Lippincott Williams & Wilkins; 2012:391–411.

Question 29 *The initial formula for biologically effective dose (BED) does not have a variable for overall treatment time, which has significant impact on certain tumors or early effects. Fowler suggested modification by adding a time component.*

$$BED = E/\alpha = (Total\ dose)[1 + d/(\alpha/\beta)] - (0.693/\alpha)(t/T_{pot})$$

Rapid repopulation starts with a lag of 21 to 28 days. Therefore, 21 or 28 days are subtracted from overall treatment time and $t = T$ (overall time) $- T_k$ (kick-off time, typically 21–28 days). T_{pot} is potential doubling time. α is estimated to be 0.3. What is time-corrected BED of 70 Gy in 35 fractions over 7 weeks (46 days) assuming $\alpha/\beta = 10$ Gy, $T_k = 21$ days, and $T_{pot} = 5$ days?

Answer 29

$BED = 70\ Gy \times [1 + (2/10)] - (0.693/0.3)(46\ days - 21\ days)/5\ days = 84\ Gy_{10} - 11.55\ Gy_{10} = 72.45\ Gy_{10}$

Hall EJ, Giaccia AJ. Time, dose, and fractionation in radiotherapy. In: Hall EJ, Giaccia AJ, eds. *Radiobiology for the Radiologist.* 7th ed. Philadelphia, PA: Lippincott Williams & Wilkins; 2012:391–411.

Question 30

Please see question 29. To calculate correction for time, many values such as α, T_{pot}, and T_k are estimated. As those values are multiplied and divided, even small differences in estimates can be magnified; thus, the calculated number is only a rough estimate. Instead of using estimates of constants to calculate estimated dose, Dr. Lester Peters uses estimates of time correcting dose. He adds 3 Gy/week to account for accelerated repopulation for head and neck cancer between overall treatment of 5 and 7 weeks.

Suppose you plan to treat head and neck cancer with intensity modulated radiation therapy (IMRT) using simultaneous integrated boost over 7 weeks. How much dose do you need to prescribe to the subclinical disease region where 50 Gy in 5 weeks were sufficient traditionally?

Question 31

For tumors with rapid repopulation such as head and neck cancer, local control decreases with prolonged overall treatment time. It is estimated that local control is reduced by 1.4% (0.4%–2.5%) for each extra day added to overall treatment time. What other cancer has overall treatment time as an important predictive factor for local control?

Question 32

In some tumors with longer potential tumor doubling time (T_{pot}) such as prostate cancer and breast cancer, overall treatment time was not found to be critical. T_{pot} is 40 days for prostate cancer and 14 days for breast cancer compared to 4 days in head and neck cancer. What is the estimated α/β ratio of prostate and breast cancer?

Question 30 *Please see question 29. To calculate correction for time, many values such as α, T_{pot}, and T_k are estimated. As those values are multiplied and divided, even small differences in estimates can be magnified; thus, the calculated number is only a rough estimate. Instead of using estimates of constants to calculate estimated dose, Dr. Lester Peters uses estimates of time correcting dose. He adds 3 Gy/week to account for accelerated repopulation for head and neck cancer between overall treatment of 5 and 7 weeks.*

Suppose you plan to treat head and neck cancer with intensity modulated radiation therapy (IMRT) using simultaneous integrated boost over 7 weeks. How much dose do you need to prescribe to the subclinical disease region where 50 Gy in 5 weeks were sufficient traditionally?

Answer 30

Previously, we treated 50 Gy in 5 weeks to a large field and then gave a boost to a smaller field. Simultaneous integrated boost let us keep the overall treatment field the same over the entire treatment course but give a different total dose. Using Dr. Lester Peters' rule, 6 Gy needs to be added to the total dose as overall treatment time is extended by 2 weeks and 3 Gy per each week is necessary to counter repopulation. Therefore, 56 Gy in 35 fractions over 7 weeks is considered to be equivalent to 50 Gy in 25 fractions over 5 weeks.

Hall EJ, Giaccia AJ. Time, dose, and fractionation in radiotherapy. In: Hall EJ, Giaccia AJ, eds. *Radiobiology for the Radiologist*. 7th ed. Philadelphia, PA: Lippincott Williams & Wilkins; 2012:391–411.

Question 31 *For tumors with rapid repopulation such as head and neck cancer, local control decreases with prolonged overall treatment time. It is estimated that local control is reduced by 1.4% (0.4%–2.5%) for each extra day added to overall treatment time. What other cancer has overall treatment time as an important predictive factor for local control?*

Answer 31

Cervical carcinoma. Local control may be reduced by 0.5% (0.3%–1.1%) for each extra day of radiation treatment time.

Hall EJ, Giaccia AJ. Time, dose, and fractionation in radiotherapy. In: Hall EJ, Giaccia AJ, eds. *Radiobiology for the Radiologist*. 7th ed. Philadelphia, PA: Lippincott Williams & Wilkins; 2012:391–411.

Question 32 *In some tumors with longer potential tumor doubling time (T_{pot}) such as prostate cancer and breast cancer, overall treatment time was not found to be critical. T_{pot} is 40 days for prostate cancer and 14 days for breast cancer compared to 4 days in head and neck cancer. What is the estimated α/β ratio of prostate and breast cancer?*

Answer 32

The estimated α/β ratio of prostate cancer is low. Brenner estimated it to be 1.5 Gy (0.8 Gy–2.2 Gy). The estimated α/β ratio of breast cancer is 3.5 Gy (1.2 Gy–5.7 Gy) based on results in the UK Standardisation of Breast Radiotherapy (START) trials. Breast cancer and prostate cancer may behave more like late-responding tissues than early-responding tissues, unlike head and neck squamous cell carcinoma.

Brenner DJ, Hall EJ. Fractionation and protraction for radiotherapy of prostate carcinoma. *Int J Radiat Oncol Biol Phys*. March 1999;43(5):1095–1101.

Haviland JS, Owen JR, Dewar JA, et al. The UK standardisation of breast radiotherapy (START) trials of radiotherapy hypofractionation for treatment of early breast cancer: 10-year follow-up results of two randomized controlled trials. *Lancet Oncol*. 2013;14:1086–1094.

Question 33

What is hypofractionation treatment and why is there renewed interest in its application?

Question 33 *What is hypofractionation treatment and why is there renewed interest in its application?*

Answer 33

The standard fraction is 1.8 to 2 Gy/fraction. Fraction size larger than 2 Gy is called hypofractionation. Hypofractionation was traditionally used for palliative radiation treatment when the total dose is low. For definitive or adjuvant treatment requiring a high dose, it fell out of favor when earlier experience showed high rates of late complications. In the 1950s and 1960s, when postoperative radiation treatments were delivered with 4.35 to 4.58 Gy/fraction to a total dose of 43.5 to 55 Gy, brachial plexopathy was reported in 10% to 73% of patients. Recently, with recognition of a low α/β ratio of breast cancer and prostate cancer, moderate hypofractionation regimens are explored and used for patient convenience and cost savings. In START trials done in the United Kingdom, no case of brachial plexopathy was reported when 39 to 41.6 Gy were delivered with 2.67 to 3.2 Gy/fraction. Improved dose control using intensity modulated radiation therapy (IMRT) and Image-Guided Radiation Therapy (IGRT) also decreases the volume of normal tissue exposed to hypofractionated radiation.

Hall EJ, Giaccia AJ. Time, dose, and fractionation in radiotherapy. In: Hall EJ, Giaccia AJ, eds. *Radiobiology for the Radiologist.* 7th ed. Philadelphia, PA: Lippincott Williams & Wilkins; 2012:391–411.
Stoll BA, Andrews JT. Radiation-induced peripheral neuropathy. *Br Med J.* 1966;1:834–837.

15

EFFECTS OF TOTAL BODY IRRADIATION

SUDHA AMARNATH

Question 1
What is acute radiation syndrome (ARS)?

Question 2
What are the various forms of acute radiation syndrome (ARS)?

Question 3
At what dose level exposures would you expect the following syndromes to occur: cerebrovascular, hematopoietic, and gastrointestinal (GI)?

Question 4
What typically follows the prodromal syndrome?

Turn page to see the answers.

Question 1 *What is acute radiation syndrome (ARS)?*

Answer 1

ARS is defined as the biological changes and symptoms, including death, that can occur within weeks after a high-intensity total body irradiation exposure. The various forms of ARS arise based on the level of radiation exposure and at various time points after the exposure.

Hall EJ, Giaccia AJ. Acute radiation syndrome. In: Hall EJ, Giaccia AJ, eds. *Radiobiology for the Radiologist*. 7th ed. Philadelphia, PA: Lippincott Williams & Wilkins; 2012:114–128.

Question 2 *What are the various forms of acute radiation syndrome (ARS)?*

Answer 2

The four major recognized forms of ARS are the prodromal radiation syndrome, the cerebrovascular syndrome, the gastrointestinal (GI) syndrome, and the hematopoietic syndrome.

Hall EJ, Giaccia AJ. Acute radiation syndrome. In: Hall EJ, Giaccia AJ, eds. *Radiobiology for the Radiologist*. 7th ed. Philadelphia, PA: Lippincott Williams & Wilkins; 2012:114–128.

Question 3 *At what dose level exposures would you expect the following syndromes to occur: cerebrovascular, hematopoietic, and gastrointestinal (GI)?*

Answer 3

The cerebrovascular syndrome is associated with total body exposures in excess of 100 Gy and death typically occurs within 24 to 48 hours after the exposure. The GI syndrome is associated with more intermediate total body dose exposures (5–12 Gy) and death typically occurs within 9 to 10 days after exposure. The hematopoietic syndrome can occur after lower dose exposures (2.5–5 Gy) and if death occurs, it typically happens several weeks to 2 months after exposure.

Hall EJ, Giaccia AJ. Acute radiation syndrome. In: Hall EJ, Giaccia AJ, eds. *Radiobiology for the Radiologist*. 7th ed. Philadelphia, PA: Lippincott Williams & Wilkins; 2012:114–128.

Question 4 *What typically follows the prodromal syndrome?*

Answer 4

The prodromal syndrome is typically followed by a *latent period*, in which the symptoms from the initial prodromal syndrome subside and the exposed person will feel well again, only to be followed by the development of one of the life-threatening syndromes (cerebrovascular, GI, or hematopoietic) within hours to weeks, depending on the level of dose exposure. The higher the dose exposure, the shorter the latent period is expected to be (inverse relationship). The most important consequences of radiation exposure, namely tissue damage that can lead to death, occur during the "latent" period.

Hall EJ, Giaccia AJ. Acute radiation syndrome. In: Hall EJ, Giaccia AJ, eds. *Radiobiology for the Radiologist*. 7th ed. Philadelphia, PA: Lippincott Williams & Wilkins; 2012:114–128.

Question 5

What factor(s) determine the time to onset, maximum severity, and duration of symptoms an exposed person will develop during the prodromal syndrome?

Question 6

What are the expected signs and symptoms of the prodromal syndrome? How do they vary by dose?

Question 7

What laboratory test can diagnose the acute radiation syndrome (ARS)?

Question 8

What is the mechanism of tissue damage and subsequent death with the cerebrovascular syndrome?

Question 5 *What factor(s) determine the time to onset, maximum severity, and duration of symptoms an exposed person will develop during the prodromal syndrome?*

Answer 5

Depending on the *dose level* at the time of exposure, the time to onset, maximum severity, and duration of the symptoms that develop can vary. For example, at higher dose level exposures (10+ Gy), all exposed individuals will develop all prodromal symptoms within 5 to 15 minutes and these symptoms will peak at about 30 minutes and persist for a few days. This is then followed by a latent period and then the development of either the cerebrovascular syndrome or the GI syndrome (depending on the dose exposure). At lower doses, it becomes harder to predict the timing and severity of symptoms, but typically a presentation of more severe prodromal symptoms equals a poorer prognosis.

Hall EJ, Giaccia AJ. Acute radiation syndrome. In: Hall EJ, Giaccia AJ, eds. *Radiobiology for the Radiologist.* 7th ed. Philadelphia, PA: Lippincott Williams & Wilkins; 2012:114–128.

Question 6 *What are the expected signs and symptoms of the prodromal syndrome? How do they vary by dose?*

Answer 6

The prodromal syndrome typically has signs and symptoms related to the neuromuscular and gastrointestinal (GI) systems. The most common symptoms at sublethal doses (or LD_{50}) are nausea, vomiting, anorexia, and easy fatigability. At higher doses, symptoms can also include fever, hypotension, sweating, headache, listlessness, and immediate diarrhea.

Hall EJ, Giaccia AJ. Acute radiation syndrome. In: Hall EJ, Giaccia AJ, eds. *Radiobiology for the Radiologist.* 7th ed. Philadelphia, PA: Lippincott Williams & Wilkins; 2012:114–128.

Question 7 *What laboratory test can diagnose the acute radiation syndrome (ARS)?*

Answer 7

The *absolute lymphocyte count* is the best and most useful lab test to diagnose ARS and determine the level of exposure. Circulating lymphocytes are one of the most radiosensitive cell lines and count levels can drop with exposures as low as 0.5 Gy. Chromosomal aberration analysis from cultured lymphocytes is the most widely used and accepted method of biological dosimetry and can detect dose exposures as low as 0.2 Gy of gamma- or x-rays.

Hall EJ, Giaccia AJ. Acute radiation syndrome. In: Hall EJ, Giaccia AJ, eds. *Radiobiology for the Radiologist.* 7th ed. Philadelphia, PA: Lippincott Williams & Wilkins; 2012:114–128.

Question 8 *What is the mechanism of tissue damage and subsequent death with the cerebrovascular syndrome?*

Answer 8

The exact cause of death and mechanism of tissue damage is not fully understood. It has been hypothesized that with very high exposures (>40 Gy), there is immediate damage to the microvasculature in the body. This causes small vessels in the brain to leak, leading to cerebral edema, increased intracranial pressure, and perhaps eventual death.

Hall EJ, Giaccia AJ. Acute radiation syndrome. In: Hall EJ, Giaccia AJ, eds. *Radiobiology for the Radiologist.* 7th ed. Philadelphia, PA: Lippincott Williams & Wilkins; 2012:114–128.

Question 9
What are the symptoms associated with the cerebrovascular syndrome?

Question 10
What are the symptoms associated with the gastrointestinal (GI) syndrome?

Question 11
What is the mechanism of tissue damage in the gastrointestinal (GI) syndrome?

Question 12
What is the mechanism of tissue damage and potential death in the hematopoietic syndrome?

Question 9 *What are the symptoms associated with the cerebrovascular syndrome?*

Answer 9

At doses high enough to cause the cerebrovascular syndrome (>40 Gy), all organ systems are seriously damaged and the exposed individual succumbs to death within 24 to 48 hours. Typically, an exposed individual develops severe nausea, vomiting, and abdominal cramping within minutes and then subsequently develops disorientation, loss of muscular coordination, difficulty breathing, hypotension, bloody diarrhea, seizures, coma, and ultimately death.

Hall EJ, Giaccia AJ. Acute radiation syndrome. In: Hall EJ, Giaccia AJ, eds. *Radiobiology for the Radiologist.* 7th ed. Philadelphia, PA: Lippincott Williams & Wilkins; 2012:114–128.

Question 10 *What are the symptoms associated with the gastrointestinal (GI) syndrome?*

Answer 10

GI syndrome is typically caused by a total body exposure of 10+ Gy and usually ends in death about 3 to 10 days after onset. The most common symptoms are nausea, vomiting, prolonged diarrhea (a poor prognostic sign if lasting several days), poor appetite, and lethargy. It typically results in dehydration, weight loss, wasting, complete exhaustion, and, finally, death. No human in recorded history has survived a total body exposure in excess of 10 Gy.

Hall EJ, Giaccia AJ. Acute radiation syndrome. In: Hall EJ, Giaccia AJ, eds. *Radiobiology for the Radiologist.* 7th ed. Philadelphia, PA: Lippincott Williams & Wilkins; 2012:114–128.

Question 11 *What is the mechanism of tissue damage in the gastrointestinal (GI) syndrome?*

Answer 11

Radiation exposure in excess of 10 Gy sterilizes a large proportion of dividing cells in the crypts of the intestinal epithelium, but does not damage the differentiated/functioning cells of the intestinal villi. Over time, the differentiated cells slough off with normal use and would typically be replaced by the dividing cells in the crypt. However, due to the radiation exposure and sterilization of dividing cells, there are no new replacement cells; after a few days, the intestinal villi shrink and shorten. Eventually, the surface epithelium is completely denuded of villi and intestinal contents, including gut bacteria, can access the bloodstream, which can lead to sepsis and death. This process usually occurs over 7 to 10 days in humans.

Hall EJ, Giaccia AJ. Acute radiation syndrome. In: Hall EJ, Giaccia AJ, eds. *Radiobiology for the Radiologist.* 7th ed. Philadelphia, PA: Lippincott Williams & Wilkins; 2012:114–128.

Question 12 *What is the mechanism of tissue damage and potential death in the hematopoietic syndrome?*

Answer 12

The hematopoietic syndrome results from dose exposures of about 2.5 to 5 Gy. Similar to the gastrointestinal (GI) syndrome, mitotically active (dividing) precursor cells of the hematological system are sterilized by radiation. As the mature circulating red blood cells (RBCs), white blood cells (WBCs), and platelets die off normally over a few weeks, there are no new cells to replace them, leading to a hematological crisis (primarily due to granulocyte and platelet depression, which have a shorter circulating life span than RBC). Without transplant and/or supportive care, exposed individuals die of infection and bleeding.

Hall EJ, Giaccia AJ. Acute radiation syndrome. In: Hall EJ, Giaccia AJ, eds. *Radiobiology for the Radiologist.* 7th ed. Philadelphia, PA: Lippincott Williams & Wilkins; 2012:114–128.

Question 13
What are the symptoms associated with the hematopoietic syndrome?

Question 14
What is the concept of LD_{50}?

Question 15
What is the LD_{50} for radiation exposure in humans?

Question 16
What is the time point for peak incidence of death from hematological damage in humans after radiation exposure?

Question 13 *What are the symptoms associated with the hematopoietic syndrome?*

Answer 13

After the initial prodromal syndrome, most exposed individuals have a latent period of about 3 weeks before symptoms start to appear. These include chills, fatigue, skin petechial hemorrhages, mouth ulcers, and hair loss. Due to granulocyte depression, patients can present with infections and fever; platelet depression leads to bleeding and possibly anemia from bleeding (anemia due to RBC depression is rare). Unless the bone marrow has started to regenerate at this point, death is inevitable. Antibiotics can be administered to decrease the chance of infection-related death.

Hall EJ, Giaccia AJ. Acute radiation syndrome. In: Hall EJ, Giaccia AJ, eds. *Radiobiology for the Radiologist.* 7th ed. Philadelphia, PA: Lippincott Williams & Wilkins; 2012:114–128.

Question 14 *What is the concept of LD_{50}?*

Answer 14

LD_{50} is the 50% lethal dose or, rather, the dose of any agent that causes a mortality rate of 50% in an experimental group within a specified period. This concept has been borrowed from pharmacology and applied to radiation exposure. In humans, the typical reported time range is 60 days, which is abbreviated as $LD_{50/60}$.

Hall EJ, Giaccia AJ. Acute radiation syndrome. In: Hall EJ, Giaccia AJ, eds. *Radiobiology for the Radiologist.* 7th ed. Philadelphia, PA: Lippincott Williams & Wilkins; 2012:114–128.

Question 15 *What is the LD_{50} for radiation exposure in humans?*

Answer 15

The sensitivity of individual humans to total body radiation exposure can vary based on a number of factors, but in general, it is estimated to be between 3 and 4 Gy for young adults without medical intervention. It may be raised to 7 Gy with the use of antibiotics, as seen in Chernobyl.

Hall EJ, Giaccia AJ. Acute radiation syndrome. In: Hall EJ, Giaccia AJ, eds. *Radiobiology for the Radiologist.* 7th ed. Philadelphia, PA: Lippincott Williams & Wilkins; 2012:114–128.

Question 16 *What is the time point for peak incidence of death from hematological damage in humans after radiation exposure?*

Answer 16

The peak incidence of death in humans due to the hematopoietic syndrome is 30 days after exposure, but deaths can continue for up to 60 days depending on individual factors.

Hall EJ, Giaccia AJ. Acute radiation syndrome. In: Hall EJ, Giaccia AJ, eds. *Radiobiology for the Radiologist.* 7th ed. Philadelphia, PA: Lippincott Williams & Wilkins; 2012:114–128.

Question 17

What is the life span of the following mature circulating blood elements: red blood cells (RBCs), white blood cells (WBCs), and platelets?

Question 18

What is cutaneous radiation injury (CRI)?

Question 19

What are the signs and symptoms of cutaneous radiation injury (CRI)?

Question 20

How do radiation burns to the skin differ from thermal or chemical burns?

Question 17 *What is the life span of the following mature circulating blood elements: RBCs, WBCs, and platelets?*

Answer 17

RBCs typically have a life span of 100 to 120 days (which is why anemia from RBC depression is rarely seen). WBCs typically have a life span of a few hours to a few weeks (depending on the type of WBC). Platelets typically last for 8 to 9 days in the circulating bloodstream.

Daniels VG, Wheater PR, Burkitt HG. *Functional Histology: A Text and Colour Atlas*. Edinburgh: Churchill Livingstone; 1979.

Leekshma CHW, Cohen JA. Determination of the life span of human blood platelets using labelled diisopropylfluoro-phosphonate. *J Clin Invest*. 1956;35(9):964–969

Mock DM, Matthews NI, Zhu S, et al. Red blood cell (RBC) survival determined in humans using RBCs labeled at multiple biotin densities. *Transfusion*. 2011;51:1047–1057.

Question 18 *What is cutaneous radiation injury (CRI)?*

Answer 18

CRI is radiation damage to the skin and superficial microvasculature. It can occur both in the presence or absence of acute radiation syndrome (ARS) because nonpenetrating beta particles and low-energy photons may only deposit excess doses superficially. Depending on the dose, the injury may be seen within a few hours or delayed by a few weeks.

Hall EJ, Giaccia AJ. Acute radiation syndrome. In: Hall EJ, Giaccia AJ, eds. *Radiobiology for the Radiologist*. 7th ed. Philadelphia, PA: Lippincott Williams & Wilkins; 2012:114–128.

Question 19 *What are the signs and symptoms of cutaneous radiation injury (CRI)?*

Answer 19

The symptoms of radiation damage to the skin can include itching and tingling, erythema (threshold dose 3 Sv), hair loss (threshold dose 6 Sv), and edema, with progression to dry desquamation, wet desquamation, and ultimately ulceration and necrosis (>10 Sv). It can be complicated by chronic skin infections and recurrent ulceration. These symptoms can be quite painful (similar to second degree thermal burns) for exposed individuals.

Hall EJ, Giaccia AJ. Acute radiation syndrome. In: Hall EJ, Giaccia AJ, eds. *Radiobiology for the Radiologist*. 7th ed. Philadelphia, PA: Lippincott Williams & Wilkins; 2012:114–128.

Question 20 *How do radiation burns to the skin differ from thermal or chemical burns?*

Answer 20

The biggest difference between radiation burns and thermal or chemical burns is the delay between the exposure and the effect (typically delayed with radiation exposures, as opposed to the immediate burns seen with thermal or chemical injury). Radiation burns also have a tendency to undergo recurrent breakdown, even after a scar has formed.

Hall EJ, Giaccia AJ. Acute radiation syndrome. In: Hall EJ, Giaccia AJ, eds. *Radiobiology for the Radiologist*. 7th ed. Philadelphia, PA: Lippincott Williams & Wilkins; 2012:114–128.

Question 21

What is the recommended supportive care for human exposures of less than 4 to 5 Gy?

Question 22

What is the dose exposure window for which bone marrow transplantation is considered a useful "rescue" method for humans exposed to radiation?

Question 23

What is the major challenge to determining who might benefit from bone marrow transplantation "rescue"?

Question 21 *What is the recommended supportive care for human exposures of less than 4 to 5 Gy?*

Answer 21

According to the International Atomic Energy Agency and World Health Organization joint report, *Diagnosis and Treatment of Radiation Injuries*, close observation is recommended with symptom-specific treatment only (i.e., antibiotics for infection, platelets for hemorrhage). Prophylactic blood transfusions are not recommended because they can delay marrow element regeneration.

Hall EJ, Giaccia AJ. Acute radiation syndrome. In: Hall EJ, Giaccia AJ, eds. *Radiobiology for the Radiologist*. 7th ed. Philadelphia, PA: Lippincott Williams & Wilkins; 2012:114–128.

International Atomic Energy Agency. *Diagnosis and Treatment of Radiation Injuries*. Safety Report Series No. 2, Vienna, Austria: IAEA; 1998.

Question 22 *What is the dose exposure window for which bone marrow transplantation is considered a useful "rescue" method for humans exposed to radiation?*

Answer 22

The dose window for which bone marrow transplantation is considered useful is between 8 and 10 Gy. At doses below 8 Gy, most individuals will recover with antibiotics and supportive measures, so transplantation is not necessary. At doses above 10 Gy, death from the GI syndrome is considered inevitable, and bone marrow transplantation is not considered useful.

Hall EJ, Giaccia AJ. Acute radiation syndrome. In: Hall EJ, Giaccia AJ, eds. *Radiobiology for the Radiologist*. 7th ed. Philadelphia, PA: Lippincott Williams & Wilkins; 2012:114–128.

Question 23 *What is the major challenge to determining who might benefit from bone marrow transplantation "rescue"?*

Answer 23

The major challenge is obtaining accurate in vivo biological dosimetry after an exposure. Although chromosomal aberration analysis of circulating lymphocytes is an accurate means of determining dose in vitro, after exposures close to or above the LD_{50}, peripheral lymphocytes disappear before 24 hours, making it difficult to obtain cells for analysis.

Hall EJ, Giaccia AJ. Acute radiation syndrome. In: Hall EJ, Giaccia AJ, eds. *Radiobiology for the Radiologist*. 7th ed. Philadelphia, PA: Lippincott Williams & Wilkins; 2012:114–128.

Question 24

What are some useful rules of thumb/tests to help triage the care of radiation-exposed individuals (who are not wearing a dosimeter, so their dose level of exposure is unknown)?

Question 25

What are some of the rough guidelines for dose exposure and time to emesis in acute radiation exposures?

Question 26

What are the long-term side effects of acute radiation exposures that have been seen in long-term survivors of nuclear accidents?

Question 24 *What are some useful rules of thumb/tests to help triage the care of radiation-exposed individuals (who are not wearing a dosimeter, so their dose level of exposure is unknown)?*

Answer 24

There are a few different methods to help assess dose exposure for the triage of exposed individuals. The most accurate method is chromosomal aberration analysis of circulating lymphocytes stimulated to divide in vitro. With this method, doses of 0.2 Gy or above can be accurately determined. This method requires access to a cytogenetic laboratory and dose exposures less than the LD_{50} (see question 23). If a cytogenetic lab is not available, the drop in lymphocyte count can be monitored with serial blood draws and correlated with radiation dose using an algorithm developed by Guskova and colleagues. The best estimate is made 48-hours postexposure. Lastly, the average time to emesis will decrease with increasing radiation dose. Data from Goans and colleagues has correlated the presence and time to vomiting with radiation dose exposure. This is the most crude estimate since this can vary significantly from individual to individual.

Hall EJ, Giaccia AJ. Acute radiation syndrome. In: Hall EJ, Giaccia AJ, eds. *Radiobiology for the Radiologist*. 7th ed. Philadelphia, PA: Lippincott Williams & Wilkins; 2012:114–128.

Question 25 *What are some of the rough guidelines for dose exposure and time to emesis in acute radiation exposures?*

Answer 25

According to data from the Oak Ridge Associated Universities, at doses less than 1 Gy, few individuals will vomit. If the dose is greater than 2 Gy, then almost all individuals will vomit. If the time to emesis is less than 2 hours after exposure, the effective total body dose is estimated to be at least 3 Gy. If, however, no vomiting occurs during the first 4 hours after exposure, it is unlikely that any severe clinical effects from radiation exposure will occur.

Hall EJ, Giaccia AJ. Acute radiation syndrome. In: Hall EJ, Giaccia AJ, eds. *Radiobiology for the Radiologist*. 7th ed. Philadelphia, PA: Lippincott Williams & Wilkins; 2012:114–128.

Question 26 *What are the long-term side effects of acute radiation exposures that have been seen in long-term survivors of nuclear accidents?*

Answer 26

Approximately 70 long-term survivors of acute radiation exposures (mostly individuals employed in nuclear programs) have been studied closely over the years. In this population, there have been no observed long-term side effects, including early malignancies, shortened life span, or early cataracts, over the expected numbers for unirradiated individuals of the same age. It is hypothesized that the excess cancer risk that would be expected is difficult to detect in such a small group of individuals and is likely masked by other biological and health factors.

Hall EJ, Giaccia AJ. Acute radiation syndrome. In: Hall EJ, Giaccia AJ, eds. *Radiobiology for the Radiologist*. 7th ed. Philadelphia, PA: Lippincott Williams & Wilkins; 2012:114–128.

Question 27

What resources are available in the event of radiation accidents?

Question 28

How do patients survive supralethal doses of radiation exposure with total body irradiation techniques for the treatment of cancer?

Question 27 *What resources are available in the event of radiation accidents?*

Answer 27

The Oak Ridge Institute for Science and Education operates a Radiation Emergency Assistance Center/Training Site (REAC/TS), which provides 24-hour assistance with medical and health physics problems related to radiation-related accidents. Their website is http://www.orau.gov/reacts.

Hall EJ, Giaccia AJ. Acute radiation syndrome. In: Hall EJ, Giaccia AJ, eds. *Radiobiology for the Radiologist.* 7th ed. Philadelphia, PA: Lippincott Williams & Wilkins; 2012:114–128.

Question 28 *How do patients survive supralethal doses of radiation exposure with total body irradiation techniques for the treatment of cancer?*

Answer 28

Total body irradiation is often used in the conditioning regimens to either suppress the immune system or diminish the bone marrow elements for new bone marrow grafting. Due to the availability of supportive care measures and growth factors, bone marrow transplantation techniques have greatly improved and are now used widely for multiple types of cancer, most commonly leukemias.

Hall EJ, Giaccia AJ. Acute radiation syndrome. In: Hall EJ, Giaccia AJ, eds. *Radiobiology for the Radiologist.* 7th ed. Philadelphia, PA: Lippincott Williams & Wilkins; 2012:114–128.

16

RADIATION SENSITIZERS, RADIOPROTECTORS, AND BIOREDUCTIVE DRUGS

ADITYA JULOORI AND MICHAEL A. WELLER

Question 1
What is the mechanism by which antiangiogenesis agents increase radiosensitivity?

Question 2
What is the only radioprotective drug approved by the Food and Drug Administration (FDA) and what is the mechanism of this drug?

Question 3
Gemcitabine is a chemotherapy drug that is a well-known radiosensitizer. What is the mechanism by which this occurs?

Question 4
What is nimorazole?

Turn page to see the answers.

Question 1 *What is the mechanism by which antiangiogenesis agents increase radiosensitivity?*

Answer 1

Tumor angiogenesis is characterized by abnormal blood vessels—with irregular shape and high permeability—thus impairing the ability for oxygen to be delivered to the tumor. It is well understood that oxygen is a radiosensitizer. Thus, use of antiangiogenesis agents normalizes the vasculature of the tumor environment, increasing oxygen delivery to the tumor and thereby improving radiosensitivity.

Jain RK. Antiangiogenic therapy for cancer: current and emerging concepts. *Oncology*. 2005;19(4 suppl 3):7–16.
Jain RK. Normalization of tumor vasculature: an emerging concept in antiangiogenic therapy. *Science*. 2005;307:58–62.

Question 2 *What is the only radioprotective drug approved by the Food and Drug Administration (FDA) and what is the mechanism of this drug?*

Answer 2

Amifostine is approved by the FDA and has been shown to prevent the development of xerostomia in patients undergoing radiation therapy (RT) for head and neck cancer, as demonstrated by a Radiation Therapy Oncology Group (RTOG) trial. Amifostine is a prodrug and its active metabolite travels intracellularly and scavenges free radicals produced by ionizing radiation.

Anne PR, Machtay M, Rosenthal D, et al. A phase II trial of subcutaneous amifostine and radiation therapy in patients with head-and-neck cancer. *Int J Radiat Oncol Biol Phys*. 2007;67:445–452.
Hall EJ, Giaccia AJ. Radiation carcinogenesis. In: Hall EJ, Giaccia AJ, eds. *Radiobiology for the Radiologist*. 7th ed. Philadelphia, PA: Lippincott Williams & Wilkins; 2006:135–153.

Question 3 *Gemcitabine is a chemotherapy drug that is a well-known radiosensitizer. What is the mechanism by which this occurs?*

Answer 3

Gemcitabine is a nucleoside analog that interferes with DNA replication. Ribonucleotide reductase is an enzyme that plays an important role in DNA synthesis and serves to catalyze the production of deoxyribonucleotides from ribonucleotides. Gemcitabine is metabolized to 5′-diphosphate (dFdCDP), which interferes with the normal function of ribonucleotide reductase; by this process, it is believed gemcitabine acts as a radiosensitizer.

Pereira S, Fernandes PA, Ramos MJ. Mechanism for ribonucleotide reductase inactivation by the anticancer drug gemcitabine. *J Comput Chem*. 2004;25(10):1286–1294.
Shewach DS, Lawrence TS. Antimetabolite radiosensitizers. *J Clin Oncol*. 2007;25:4043–4050.

Question 4 *What is nimorazole?*

Answer 4

Nimorazole is a nitroimidazole compound, similar to misonidazole and etanidazole, which works as a radiosensitizer in hypoxic environments—mimicking the role oxygen plays in increasing radiosensitivity in regions that are not well vascularized.

Hall EJ, Giaccia AJ. Radiation carcinogenesis. In: Hall EJ, Giaccia AJ, eds. *Radiobiology for the Radiologist*. 7th ed. Philadelphia, PA: Lippincott Williams & Wilkins; 2006:135–153.

Question 5
What are the common side effects of amifostine?

Question 6
How is amifostine administered and why is this important?

Question 7
What did the Danish Head and Neck Cancer Study (DAHANCA) trial of nimorazole demonstrate?

Question 8
How does the radiosensitization potential of nimorazole compare to that of misonidazole and etanidazole?

Question 5 *What are the common side effects of amifostine?*

Answer 5

Nausea, emesis, hypotension, and allergic reactions are the most common side effects.

Gu J, Zhu S, Li X, Wu H, Li Y, Hua F. Effect of amifostine in head and neck cancer patients treated with radiotherapy: a systematic review and meta-analysis based on randomized controlled trials. *PLoS One*. May 2014;9(5):e95968.

Question 6 *How is amifostine administered and why is this important?*

Answer 6

Amifostine is given 30 minutes prior to radiation, reflective of the fact that it penetrates tumor at a slower rate than it penetrates normal tissue. By administering the radiation soon after amifostine is given, you are taking advantage of this differential penetration so that tumor is more radiosensitive than normal tissue.

Hall EJ, Giaccia AJ. Radiation carcinogenesis. In: Hall EJ, Giaccia AJ, eds. *Radiobiology for the Radiologist*. 7th ed. Philadelphia, PA: Lippincott Williams & Wilkins; 2006:135–153.

Question 7 *What did the Danish Head and Neck Cancer Study (DAHANCA) trial of nimorazole demonstrate?*

Answer 7

This was a Danish randomized trial that showed that nimorazole can be used as a radiosensitizer in head and neck cancer patients without dose-limiting toxicity and use of this drug along with radiation was associated with improved locoregional control.

Overgaard J, Hansen HS, Overgaard M, et al. A randomized double-blind phase III study of nimorazole as a hypoxic radiosensitizer of primary radiotherapy in supraglottic larynx and pharynx carcinoma. Results of the Danish Head and Neck Cancer Study (DAHANCA) Protocol 5–85. *Radiother Oncol*. February 1998;46(2):135–146.
Rockwell S, Dobrucki IT, Kim EY, et al. Hypoxia and radiation therapy: past history, ongoing research, and future promise. *Current Mol Med*. 2009;9:441–459.

Question 8 *How does the radiosensitization potential of nimorazole compare to that of misonidazole and etanidazole?*

Answer 8

Nimorazole has an NO_2 group at the fifth position on the imidazole ring rather than the second position—such as with imidazole and etanidazole. Thus, it is a less effective radiosensitizer.

Hall EJ, Giaccia AJ. Radiation carcinogenesis. In: Hall EJ, Giaccia AJ, eds. *Radiobiology for the Radiologist*. 7th ed. Philadelphia, PA: Lippincott Williams & Wilkins; 2006:135–153.
Rockwell S, Dobrucki IT, Kim EY, et al. Hypoxia and radiation therapy: past history, ongoing research, and future promise. *Current Mol Med*. 2009;9:441–459.

Question 9

What is the role of palifermin?

Question 10

By what means does androgen deprivation therapy (ADT) impact DNA repair when administered with radiation therapy (RT) in patients undergoing RT for prostate cancer?

Question 11

What is the mechanism of radiosensitization by the HIV protease inhibitor nelfinavir?

Question 12

How do Hsp90 inhibitors cause radiosensitization?

Question 9 *What is the role of palifermin?*

Answer 9

Palifermin functions as a keratinocyte growth factor that can be used to induce proliferation of mucosal cells of the gastrointestinal (GI) tract and can thus decrease the incidence of mucositis after radiation. It has been shown to decrease the duration and severity of oral mucositis in patients undergoing chemoradiotherapy for hematological malignancies.

Hall EJ, Giaccia AJ. Radiation carcinogenesis. In: Hall EJ, Giaccia AJ, eds. *Radiobiology for the Radiologist*. 7th ed. Philadelphia, PA: Lippincott Williams & Wilkins; 2006:135–153.

Question 10 *By what means does androgen deprivation therapy (ADT) impact DNA repair when administered with radiation therapy (RT) in patients undergoing RT for prostate cancer?*

Answer 10

The androgen receptor signaling pathway has been shown to be involved in upregulation of transcription of DNA repair genes. By blocking these receptors with ADT, one can inhibit the repair capacity of these prostate cancer cells and reduce radioresistance.

Goodwin JF, Schiewer MJ, Dean JL, et al. A hormone-DNA repair circuit governs the response to genotoxic insult. *Cancer Discov*. November 2013;3(11):1254–1271.
Polkinghorn WR, Parker JS, Lee MX, et al. Androgen receptor signaling regulates DNA repair in prostate cancers. *Cancer Discov*. November 2013;3(11):1245–1253.

Question 11 *What is the mechanism of radiosensitization by the HIV protease inhibitor nelfinavir?*

Answer 11

Nelfinavir induces radiosensitization by radiosensitizing endothelial cells, downregulating VEGF expression in the tumor microenvironment, and inhibiting the PI3K-AKT-mTOR pathway.

Cuneo KC, Tu T, Geng L, Fu A, Hallahan DE, Willey CD. HIV protease inhibitors enhance the efficacy of irradiation. *Cancer Res*. May 2007;67(10):4886–4993.
Fischer D, Bachar O, Nussinov R, Wolfson H. An efficient automated computer vision based technique for detection of three dimensional structural motifs in proteins. *J Biomol Struct Dyn*. February 1992;9(4):769–789.
Gupta AK, Li B, Cerniglia GJ, Ahmed MS, Hahn SM, Maity A. The HIV protease inhibitor nelfinavir downregulates Akt phosphorylation by inhibiting proteasomal activity and inducing the unfolded protein response. *Neoplasia*. April 2007;9(4):271–278.
Pore N, Gupta AK, Cerniglia GJ, et al. Nelfinavir down-regulates hypoxia-inducible factor 1alpha and VEGF expression and increases tumor oxygenation: implications for radiotherapy. *Cancer Res*. September 2006;66(18):9252–9259.

Question 12 *How do Hsp90 inhibitors cause radiosensitization?*

Answer 12

Heat-shock proteins like HSP90 allow tumor cells to survive in toxic conditions that are often characterized by varying degrees of hypoxia and the presence of reactive oxygen molecules. Hsp90 inhibitors disrupt the normal DNA damage repair pathways.

Gomez-Casal R, Bhattacharya C, Epperly MW, et al. The HSP90 inhibitor ganetespib radiosensitizes human lung adenocarcinoma cells. *Cancers (Basel)*. May 2015;7(2):876–907.

Question 13
What is the most radioresistant phase of the cell cycle?

Question 14
What is a radiation mitigator?

Question 15
How does flagellin function as a radiation protectant?

Question 16
What is the major side effect of hypoxic cell sensitizers like nimorazole?

Question 13 *What is the most radioresistant phase of the cell cycle?*

Answer 13

The S phase, during which DNA synthesis occurs, is the phase of the cell cycle during which cells are the least sensitive to the effects of radiation therapy (RT).

Hall EJ, Giaccia AJ. Radiation carcinogenesis. In: Hall EJ, Giaccia AJ, eds. *Radiobiology for the Radiologist.* 7th ed. Philadelphia, PA: Lippincott Williams & Wilkins; 2006:135–153.

Question 14 *What is a radiation mitigator?*

Answer 14

Radiation mitigators can be given after radiation therapy (RT) has administered (as opposed to radioprotectants, which must be given before or during RT). Radiation mitigators are given to lessen the toxicity associated with radiation. One example is a transforming growth factor-β (TGF-β) inhibitor that can be used to reduce the incidence of late radiation fibrosis.

Citrin D, Cotrim AP, Hyodo F, Baum BJ, Krishna MC, Mitchell JB. Radioprotectors and mitigators of radiation-induced normal tissue injury. *Oncologist.* 2010;15(4):360–371.

Question 15 *How does flagellin function as a radiation protectant?*

Answer 15

Flagellin is an activator of the NF-kB pathway and thus upregulates transcription of antiapoptosis genes and also upregulates proliferation of stem cells. The pathway also upregulates reactive oxygen species scavengers.

Burdelya LG, Krivokrysenko VI, Tallant TC, et al. An agonist of Toll-like receptor 5 has radioprotective activity in mouse and primate models. *Science.* April 11, 2008;320(5873):226–230.
Shakhov AN, Singh VK, Bone F, et al. Prevention and mitigation of acute radiation syndrome in mice by synthetic lipopeptide agonists of Toll-like receptor 2 (TLR2). *PLoS One.* 2012;7(3):e33044.

Question 16 *What is the major side effect of hypoxic cell sensitizers like nimorazole?*

Answer 16

The major dose-limiting toxicity in trials of head and neck cancer patients undergoing chemoradiotherapy along with nimorazole was peripheral neuropathy.

Overgaard J, Hansen HS, Overgaard M, et al. A randomized double-blind phase III study of nimorazole as a hypoxic radiosensitizer of primary radiation therapy (RT) in supraglottic larynx and pharynx carcinoma. Results of the Danish Head and Neck Cancer Study (DAHANCA) Protocol 5–85. *Radiother Oncol.* 1998;46:135–146.
Overgaard J. Hypoxic radiosensitization: adored and ignored. *J Clin Oncol.* 2007;25:4066–4074.

Question 17

How do sulfhydryl radioprotectors work?

Question 18

What is the mechanism by which cisplatin works as a radiosensitizer?

Question 19

What are some examples of mammalian target of rapamycin (mTOR) inhibitors?

Question 20

Are there radioprotectors that also may protect against carcinogenesis?

Question 17 *How do sulfhydryl radioprotectors work?*

Answer 17
Sulfhydryl radioprotectors like cysteine and glutathione work by scavenging free radicals.

Nair CKK, Parida DK, Nomura T. Radioprotectors in radiotherapy. *J Radiat Res*. 2001;42:21–37.

Question 18 *What is the mechanism by which cisplatin works as a radiosensitizer?*

Answer 18
One proposed mechanism that this may occur is that cisplatin inhibits DNA double-stand repair.

Wilson GD, Bentzen SM, Harari PM. Biologic basis for combining drugs with radiation. *Semin Radiat Oncol*. 2006;16:2–9.

Question 19 *What are some examples of mammalian target of rapamycin (mTOR) inhibitors?*

Answer 19
Rapamycin, temsirolimus, and everolimus act as radiosensitizers and are mTOR inhibitors.

Murphy JD, Spalding AC, Somnay YR, et al. Inhibition of mTOR radiosensitizes soft tissue sarcoma and tumor vasculature. *Clin Cancer Res*. 2009;15(2):588–596.
Sabatini DM. mTOR and cancer: insights into a complex relationship. *Nat Rev Cancer*. 2006;6:729–734.

Question 20 *Are there radioprotectors that also may protect against carcinogenesis?*

Answer 20
Amifostine was developed to protect against normal tissue cell kill during radiation therapy (RT) but has also been shown to protect against oncogenic transformation in mouse models and cell cultures.

Hall EJ, Giaccia AJ. Radiation carcinogenesis. In: Hall EJ, Giaccia AJ, eds. *Radiobiology for the Radiologist*. 7th ed. Philadelphia, PA: Lippincott Williams & Wilkins; 2006:135–153.

17

RADIATION CARCINOGENESIS

BINDU V. MANYAM AND MICHAEL A. WELLER

Question 1
What is the threshold dose?

Question 2
What is a deterministic effect?

Question 3
What is a stochastic effect?

Question 4
What is the latent period and which type of cancer has the shortest median latent period?

Turn page to see the answers. **257**

Question 1 *What is the threshold dose?*

Answer 1

Ionizing radiation leads to DNA damage which, if not adequately repaired, can prevent a cell from surviving or can lead to a mutation, which is retained through subsequent divisions. The organs and tissues in the body can continue to function in the event of a loss of a few cells; however, if there is a substantial loss of cells, there can be loss of organ or tissue function. At small radiation doses, the probability of this occurring is zero. However, the *threshold dose* is the dose at which the probability of observable harm and loss of tissue function approaches 100%.

Hall EJ, Giaccia AJ. Radiation carcinogenesis. In: Hall EJ, Giaccia AJ, eds. *Radiobiology for the Radiologist*. 7th ed. Philadelphia, PA: Lippincott Williams & Wilkins; 2012:135–153.

Question 2 *What is a deterministic effect?*

Answer 2

Deterministic effects are dose related, in that the probability of harm and severity of harm increases with increasing dose above the threshold dose. Examples of deterministic effects include radiation cataractogenesis and radiation dermatitis.

Hall EJ, Giaccia AJ. Radiation carcinogenesis. In: Hall EJ, Giaccia AJ, eds. *Radiobiology for the Radiologist*. 7th ed. Philadelphia, PA: Lippincott Williams & Wilkins; 2012:135–153.

Question 3 *What is a stochastic effect?*

Answer 3

Stochastic effects have no threshold dose—harmful effects can occur at any dose and the severity of harm is independent of dose. Similar to deterministic effects, the probability of harm increases with dose. Carcinogenesis is an example of a stochastic effect. A radiation dose of 1 Gy and a radiation dose of 10 Gy can both induce carcinogenesis with no difference in the severity of cancer, but a dose of 10 Gy has a higher probability of inducing carcinogenesis.

Hall EJ, Giaccia AJ. Radiation carcinogenesis. In: Hall EJ, Giaccia AJ, eds. *Radiobiology for the Radiologist*. 7th ed. Philadelphia, PA: Lippincott Williams & Wilkins; 2012:135–153.

Question 4 *What is the latent period and which type of cancer has the shortest median latent period?*

Answer 4

The *latent period* is the interval of time between the exposure to radiation and the development of malignancy. Leukemia has the shortest latent period. Observation of survivors of Hiroshima and Nagasaki demonstrated that prevalence of leukemia peaked by 5 to 7 years, with the vast majority of cases occurring within 15 years. On the other hand, solid tumors have latency periods of 10 to 60 years.

Hall EJ, Giaccia AJ. Radiation carcinogenesis. In: Hall EJ, Giaccia AJ, eds. *Radiobiology for the Radiologist*. 7th ed. Philadelphia, PA: Lippincott Williams & Wilkins; 2012:135–153.
Nakachi K, Hayashi T, Hamatani K, Eguchi H, Kusunoki Y. Sixty years of follow-up of Hiroshima and Nagasaki survivors: current progress in molecular epidemiology studies. *Mutat Res*. 2008;659:109–117.

Question 5

Can cancers induced by radiation be distinguished from those cancers not associated with radiation exposure?

Question 6

What is the radiation weighting factor (W_T) and what is the weighting factor for the breast, bladder, brain, gonads, and kidney?

Question 7

What models are used to assess the risk of cancer from radiation exposure?

Question 5 *Can cancers induced by radiation be distinguished from those cancers not associated with radiation exposure?*

Answer 5

No molecular markers have been identified to date, which can distinguish radiation-induced cancers from those not associated with radiation. Cahan et al. proposed three criteria in 1948 for a malignancy to be considered radiation induced: the neoplasm must arise within a previously irradiated field, a latent period of several years (>5 years) must exist between radiation therapy (RT) and development of malignancy, and the second malignancy must be histologically distinct from the first tumor.

Cahan WG, Woodard HQ, Higinbotham NL, Stewart FW, Coley BL. Sarcoma arising in irradiated bone: report of eleven cases. *Cancer*. 1998;82:8–34.

Hall EJ, Giaccia AJ. Radiation carcinogenesis. In: Hall EJ, Giaccia AJ, eds. *Radiobiology for the Radiologist*. 7th ed. Philadelphia, PA: Lippincott Williams & Wilkins; 2006:135–153.

Question 6 *What is the radiation weighting factor (W_T) and what is the weighting factor for the breast, bladder, brain, gonads, and kidney?*

Answer 6

W_T is a constant used to account for varying tissue sensitivities to radiation carcinogenesis. It is primarily used for radiation protection purposes to estimate the hazard of radiation. It is used to convert the physical dose, represented by the unit Gy, to an equivalent absorbed dose, unit Sievert (Sv), to represent the biological effect on different tissues. The W_T of the breast is 0.12, the W_T of the bladder and gonads is 0.05, and the W_T of the brain and kidney is 0.01. W_T is distinct from relative biological effectiveness (RBE).

Palmans H, Rabus H, Belchior AL, et al. Future development of biologically relevant dosimetry. *Br J Radiol*. 2015; 88:1045–1064.

Question 7 *What models are used to assess the risk of cancer from radiation exposure?*

Answer 7

The absolute risk model, the relative risk model, and the time-dependent relative risk models are used to assess the risk of cancer from radiation exposure. The absolute risk model theorizes that the excess risk of cancer due to radiation exposure is not dependent on the baseline risk of cancer when there is no radiation exposure. On the other hand, the relative risk model theorizes that the excess risk of cancer due to radiation exposure is dependent on the baseline risk of cancer. For example, the natural incidence of cancer increases significantly with age, and the relative risk model predicts that the excess risk is also increased with age. The time-dependent relative risk model is preferred by the Biological Effects of Ionizing Radiation (BEIR) committee. It predicts that the excess risk of cancer is dependent on a number of variables, including dose, the square of the dose, age at exposure, and time since exposure.

Little MP, Muirhead CR, Charles MW. Describing time and age variations in the risk of radiation-induced solid tumour incidence in the Japanese atomic bomb survivors using generalized relative and absolute risk models. *Stat Med*. 1999;15:17–33.

Question 8

How does the risk of radiation-induced cancer differ with age of exposure?

Question 9

What is the Childhood Cancer Survivor study? In this study, an increased incidence of which types of cancers were observed in children who received radiation therapy (RT)?

Question 10

What organ has the highest sensitivity for radiation carcinogenesis in children?

Question 11

What is the most common type of cancer found in children who were exposed to radiation after the Chernobyl nuclear power plant accident in 1986?

Question 8 *How does the risk of radiation-induced cancer differ with age of exposure?*

Answer 8

The risk of radiation-induced cancer decreases with increasing age at the time of exposure. Individuals exposed to radiation as adults demonstrate a decreasing dose–response relationship. There is a clear dose–response relationship for individuals who were exposed as children. Excessive relative risk (ERR) per Seivert was shown to be 9.5 for children exposed under the age of 10 years old, and 3.0 for individuals exposed at ages 10 to 19 years old. This phenomenon is likely secondary to the increased number of years of life to develop a malignancy, as well as a larger proportion of actively dividing cells in the radiosensitive phase of the cell cycle.

Hall EJ, Giaccia AJ. Radiation carcinogenesis. In: Hall EJ, Giaccia AJ, eds. *Radiobiology for the Radiologist*. 7th ed. Philadelphia, PA: Lippincott Williams & Wilkins; 2012:135–153.
Thompson DE, Mabuchi K, Ron E, et al. Cancer incidence in atomic bomb survivors. Part II: Solid tumors, 1958–1987. *Radiat Res*. 1994;137:17–67.

Question 9 *What is the Childhood Cancer Survivor study? In this study, an increased incidence of which types of cancers were observed in children who received radiation therapy (RT)?*

Answer 9

The Childhood Cancer Survivor Study is a retrospective cohort study of 14,000 5-year survivors of childhood cancer who were diagnosed between 1970 and 1986, with the goal of identifying the long-term adverse health and quality of life outcomes from surgery, RT, and chemotherapy. An increased incidence of skin cancer, sarcoma, meningioma, breast cancer, and thyroid cancer were all observed in children who received RT as part of management.

Armstrong GT, Stovall M, Robinson LL. Long-term effects of radiation exposure among adult survivors of childhood cancer: results from the Childhood Cancer Survivor Study. *Radiat Res*. 2010;174:840–850.

Question 10 *What organ has the highest sensitivity for radiation carcinogenesis in children?*

Answer 10

The thyroid gland is the most sensitive organ to radiation carcinogenesis in children. These malignancies tend to be well-differentiated, indolent tumors, often managed by surgery alone. Historic examples of high incidences of radiation-induced thyroid cancer include child survivors of the atomic bomb attacks on Hiroshima and Nagasaki, children who ingested radioactive iodine after the Chernobyl accident, and children treated with x-rays for various conditions including enlarged thymus and tinea capitis.

Cardis E, Kesminiene A, Ivanov V, et al. Risk of thyroid cancer after exposure to 131I in childhood. *J Natl Cancer Inst*. 2005;10:724–732.

Question 11 *What is the most common type of cancer found in children who were exposed to radiation after the Chernobyl nuclear power plant accident in 1986?*

Answer 11

Thyroid cancer is the most common type of cancer found in children who lived near the Chernobyl nuclear power plant in 1986. High concentrations of radioactive iodine were released into the environment, which was preferentially taken up by the thyroid.

Sadetzki S, Mandelzweig L. Childhood exposure to external ionizing radiation and solid cancer risk. *Br J Cancer*. 2009;100:1021–1025.

Question 12

Radiation of the scalp was a common therapy for children with tinea capitis until the 1950s. An increased incidence of what types of malignancies has been observed from this practice?

Question 13

What percentage of lung cancer deaths in the United States are attributed to radon exposure?

Question 14

Which diseases were historically treated with radium-224? What is the most common type of malignancy observed in these patients?

Question 15

What is the half-life of radium-224 and where is the majority of its dose to bone typically deposited?

Question 12 *Radiation of the scalp was a common therapy for children with tinea capitis until the 1950s. An increased incidence of what types of malignancies has been observed from this practice?*

Answer 12

An increased incidence of thyroid cancer, brain tumors, salivary gland tumors, skin cancer, and leukemia was observed in a population of patients treated in Israel. However, a similar population of children who were treated in New York was found to have an increased incidence of only thyroid tumors (benign and malignant) and skin cancer.

Hall EJ, Giaccia AJ. Radiation carcinogenesis. In: Hall EJ, Giaccia AJ, eds. *Radiobiology for the Radiologist*. 7th ed. Philadelphia, PA: Lippincott Williams & Wilkins; 2012:135–153.

Question 13 *What percentage of lung cancer deaths in the United States are attributed to radon exposure?*

Answer 13

Of the 150,000 lung cancer deaths annually in the United States, an estimated 10% are attributed to radon exposure. Radon is the first identified environmental cause for lung cancer, an association first identified through studies of underground miners in the 1920s. Radon is an inert, colorless, and odorless gas, which is found in rocks and soil. It is naturally produced from radium in the decay series of uranium. A meta-analysis of 13 case-control studies in Europe demonstrated an 8.4% increase in the risk of lung cancer per 100 Becquerels/m^3 increase in radon.

Darby S, Hill D, Auvinen A, et al. Radon in homes and risk of lung cancer: collaborative analysis of individual data from 13 European case-control studies. *BMJ*. 2005;330:223–228.
Schwartz AG, Cote ML. Epidemiology of lung cancer. *Adv Exp Med Biol*. 2016;893:21–41.

Question 14 *Which diseases were historically treated with radium-224? What is the most common type of malignancy observed in these patients?*

Answer 14

Patients with tuberculosis and ankylosing spondylitis were historically treated with injections of radium-224. The "Speiss Study" followed 899 patients who received injections of radium-224 between the years of 1945 and 1955. An increased incidence of malignant bone tumors was observed in this population, with a peak around 8 years after exposure. Osteosarcoma was the most common histological type observed.

Nekolla EA, Walsh L, Spiess H. Incidence of malignant diseases in humans injected with radium-224. *Radiat Res*. 2010;174:377–386.

Question 15 *What is the half-life of radium-224 and where is the majority of its dose to bone typically deposited?*

Answer 15

The half-life of radium-224 is relatively short, 3.6 days. Radium emits α-particles that follow the metabolic pathways of calcium, which is eventually deposited in bone. Given the short half-life, the majority of the dose is delivered to the surface endosteal cells of bones. Osteosarcomas typically arise from these surface endosteal cells. In fact, the dose delivered to the endosteal cells is 9 times higher with radium-224 than the average dose delivered to the remaining bone. On the other hand, the half-life of radium-226 and radium-228 are longer; therefore, more dose is distributed throughout the bone over the course of radioactive decay.

Kellerer AM, Spiess H, Chmelevsky D. Dose and dose-rate dependence for bone sarcomas in radium-224 patients. *Int J Radiat Biol*. 1990;58:864–866.

Question 16

What is the half-life of radium-226 and radium-228 and which population was historically exposed to high levels of these isotopes?

Question 17

According to the Committee on the Biological Effects of Ionizing Radiation (BEIR), what is the lifetime excess cancer risk due to exposure to ionizing radiation?

Question 18

According to data analysis of survivors of the atomic bomb attacks on Hiroshima and Nagasaki, what is the lowest dose of radiation exposure at which a significant excess cancer risk was identified?

Question 19

Of patients who develop fatal cancers after undergoing total body irradiation, what percentage of these fatal cancers are leukemia?

Question 20

What is the dose and dose-rate effectiveness factor (DDREF)?

Question 16 *What is the half-life of radium-226 and radium-228 and which population was historically exposed to high levels of these isotopes?*

Answer 16

The half-life of radium-226 is 1,600 years and the half-life of radium-228 is 6 years. Female factory workers who would paint the dials of watches and clocks would ingest paint containing radium-226 and radium-228 when licking their brushes to form a sharp point for painting. A high incidence of bone sarcomas, paranasal sinus, carcinomas, and nasopharyngeal carcinomas has been observed in this population.

Hall EJ, Giaccia AJ. Radiation carcinogenesis. In: Hall EJ, Giaccia AJ, eds. *Radiobiology for the Radiologist.* 7th ed. Philadelphia, PA: Lippincott Williams & Wilkins; 2012:135–153.

Question 17 *According to the Committee on the Biological Effects of Ionizing Radiation (BEIR), what is the lifetime excess cancer risk due to exposure to ionizing radiation?*

Answer 17

There is an estimated 1% lifetime excess cancer risk per 100 mSv of exposure to ionizing radiation. Epidemiological evidence exists that suggests a linear relationship between radiation exposure and solid malignancy development between doses of 0.15 and 1.5 Gy, approximately.

Preston DL, Cullings H, Suyama A, et al. Solid cancer incidence in atomic bomb survivors exposed in utero or as young children. *J Natl Cancer Inst.* 2008;100:428–436.

Question 18 *According to data analysis of survivors of the atomic bomb attacks on Hiroshima and Nagasaki, what is the lowest dose of radiation exposure at which a significant excess cancer risk was identified?*

Answer 18

Individuals who were exposed to an average dose of 34 mSv or higher demonstrated a statistically significant excess incidence of cancer. Average dose exposures below this level did not demonstrate a statistically significant difference in excess cancer risk when compared to a control population.

Hall EJ, Giaccia AJ. Radiation carcinogenesis. In: Hall EJ, Giaccia AJ, eds. *Radiobiology for the Radiologist.* 7th ed. Philadelphia, PA: Lippincott Williams & Wilkins; 2012:135–153.

Question 19 *Of patients who develop fatal cancers after undergoing total body irradiation, what percentage of these fatal cancers are leukemia?*

Answer 19

For patients who have undergone total body irradiation and developed a fatal cancer, 15% are leukemias.

Miller RW. Delayed effects of external radiation exposure: a brief history. *Radiat Res.* 1995;144:160–169.

Question 20 *What is the dose and dose-rate effectiveness factor (DDREF)?*

Answer 20

The United Nations Scientific Committee on the Effects of Atomic Radiation (UNSCEAR) and Biological Effects of Ionizing Radiation (BEIR) identify that the risk of malignancy is lower if there is a lower dose rate over a longer period of time compared to a high-dose rate, acute exposure. The DDREF is the factor by which radiation-induced cancer risk should be reduced when the radiation is delivered at a low-dose rate or in a lower dose per fraction compared to if it is delivered in a higher dose rate or large, acute doses.

Hall EJ, Giaccia AJ. Radiation carcinogenesis. In: Hall EJ, Giaccia AJ, eds. *Radiobiology for the Radiologist.* 7th ed. Philadelphia, PA: Lippincott Williams & Wilkins; 2012:135–153.

Question 21
What is the quantitative value of the dose and dose-rate effectiveness factor (DDREF)?

Question 22
What is the estimated lifetime risk of fatality from cancer by radiation exposure in the working population of both sexes and how does it differ between low-dose-rate and high-dose-rate exposure?

Question 23
How does the estimated lifetime risk of fatality from cancer by radiation exposure differ for the entire population compared to the working population?

Question 24
In a Surveillance, Epidemiology and End Results (SEER) analysis by Brenner et al. of patients who underwent surgery or radiation therapy (RT) for prostate cancer, what was the difference in risk of development of a second solid tumor between patients who underwent surgery and patients who underwent RT?

Question 21 *What is the quantitative value of the dose and dose-rate effectiveness factor (DDREF)?*

Answer 21

The magnitude of the dose-rate effect is described as a range from 2 to 10 based on animal data. The Internal Commission on Radiological Protection (ICRP) recommends a DDREF of two for doses below 0.2 Gy at any dose rate. Using a lower DDREF allows for conservative estimations.

Hall EJ, Giaccia AJ. Radiation carcinogenesis. In: Hall EJ, Giaccia AJ, eds. *Radiobiology for the Radiologist*. 7th ed. Philadelphia, PA: Lippincott Williams & Wilkins; 2012:135–153.

Question 22 *What is the estimated lifetime risk of fatality from cancer by radiation exposure in the working population of both sexes and how does it differ between low-dose-rate and high-dose-rate exposure?*

Answer 22

The lifetime risk of fatality from radiation-induced cancer is 8×10^{-2}/Sv for high dose and high-dose-rate radiation. The lifetime risk of fatality from radiation-induced cancer is 4×10^{-2}/Sv for low dose and low-dose-rate radiation.

Hall EJ, Giaccia AJ. Radiation carcinogenesis. In: Hall EJ, Giaccia AJ, eds. *Radiobiology for the Radiologist*. 7th ed. Philadelphia, PA: Lippincott Williams & Wilkins; 2012:135–153.

Question 23 *How does the estimated lifetime risk of fatality from cancer by radiation exposure differ for the entire population compared to the working population?*

Answer 23

The estimated lifetime risk of fatality from cancer by radiation exposure increases for the entire population compared to the working population. The lifetime risk of fatality from radiation-induced cancer is 10×10^{-2}/Sv for high dose and high-dose-rate radiation. The lifetime risk of fatality from radiation-induced cancer is 5×10^{-2} for low dose and low-dose-rate radiation. This effect is due to increased radiation sensitivity in children.

Hall EJ, Giaccia AJ. Radiation carcinogenesis. In: Hall EJ, Giaccia AJ, eds. *Radiobiology for the Radiologist*. 7th ed. Philadelphia, PA: Lippincott Williams & Wilkins; 2012:135–153.

Question 24 *In a Surveillance, Epidemiology and End Results (SEER) analysis by Brenner et al. of patients who underwent surgery or radiation therapy (RT) for prostate cancer, what was the difference in risk of development of a second solid tumor between patients who underwent surgery and patients who underwent RT?*

Answer 24

Brenner et al. conducted a SEER analysis comparing 51,584 men who received RT for prostate cancer and 70,539 men who received surgery for prostate cancer. There was a statistically significant increase in the risk of solid tumors (6%; $P = .02$) in the patients who received RT.

Brenner DJ, Curtis RE, Hall EJ, Ron E. Second malignancies in prostate patients after radiotherapy compared with surgery. *Cancer*. 2000;88:398–406.

Question 25

In the Surveillance, Epidemiology and End Results (SEER) analysis of men receiving radiation therapy (RT) or surgery for prostate cancer by Brenner et al., what were the most common second solid tumors observed after RT? Were all malignancies within the treated radiation field?

Question 26

What is the dose–response relationship curve for radiation-induced malignancies proposed by Gray in the 1960s? Is this model still accepted today?

Question 27

What is the estimated annual dose of radiation that early radiologists (1897–1979) were exposed to in the United States and Britain?

Question 25 *In the Surveillance, Epidemiology and End Results (SEER) analysis of men receiving radiation therapy (RT) or surgery for prostate cancer by Brenner et al., what were the most common second solid tumors observed after RT? Were all malignancies within the treated radiation field?*

Answer 25

There was an increased relative risk of bladder and rectal carcinomas, as well as sarcomas within the treatment field. Interestingly, there was also an increased relative risk of lung carcinoma. The lung was typically exposed to a low dose of 0.5 Gy compared to the bladder and rectum, which was subject to much higher doses. On the other hand, sarcomas only developed within the radiation treatment field. This finding suggests that carcinomas, which arise from actively dividing cells, can be induced from relatively low doses of radiation. On the other hand, sarcomas, which arise from dormant mesenchymal cells, are induced from higher doses, generally close to the treatment volume.

Brenner DJ, Curtis RE, Hall EJ, Ron E. Second malignancies in prostate patients after radiotherapy compared with surgery. *Cancer*. 2000;88:398–406.

Question 26 *What is the dose–response relationship curve for radiation-induced malignancies proposed by Gray in the 1960s? Is this model still accepted today?*

Answer 26

Gray proposed a bell-shaped model, in which the probability of radiation-induced malignancies would increase at low doses and decrease at higher doses. He proposed that high doses of radiation prevent sublethal repair of DNA damage and increase the probability of cell kill, preventing carcinogenesis. This model is controversial today, in that several large studies have demonstrated a significant increase in the risk of malignancy with increasing radiation dose. For example, a pooled analysis of atomic bomb survivors, exposed to low-dose radiation, and children who underwent prophylactic intracranial radiation therapy (RT) for acute lymphoblastic leukemia, demonstrated no evidence of decrease in cancer incidence at high doses. There was evidence of a plateau or increase in the incidence of cancer at high doses.

Hall EJ, Giaccia AJ. Radiation carcinogenesis. In: Hall EJ, Giaccia AJ, eds. *Radiobiology for the Radiologist*. 7th ed. Philadelphia, PA: Lippincott Williams & Wilkins; 2012:135–153.

Question 27 *What is the estimated annual dose of radiation that early radiologists (1897–1979) were exposed to in the United States and Britain?*

Answer 27

It is estimated that early radiologists were exposed to 1 Gy per year. In the current era, with shielding, annual doses are more than a thousand-fold lower.

Brenner DJ, Hall EJ. Mortality patterns in British and US radiologists: what can we really conclude? *Br J Radiol*. 2003;76:1–2.

Question 28

An obstetric x-ray has been shown to increase the risk of childhood cancer in a fetus in utero by what percentage?

Question 29

In which trimester is low-dose irradiation of a fetus in utero associated with the greatest risk of childhood malignancy?

Question 28 *An obstetric x-ray has been shown to increase the risk of childhood cancer in a fetus in utero by what percentage?*

Answer 28

Several British studies in the 1950s and 1960s established the increased risk of leukemia and childhood cancer in pregnant women who underwent pelvic x-rays. Radiation dose was only about 10 mGy; however, an estimated 40% increased risk of childhood cancer has been reported.

Stewart A, Kneale GW. Changes in the cancer risk associated with obstetric radiography. *Lancet.* 1968;1:104–107.

Question 29 *In which trimester is low-dose irradiation of a fetus in utero associated with the greatest risk of childhood malignancy?*

Answer 29

Low-dose irradiation in the third trimester is associated with the greatest risk of childhood malignancy. Animal studies suggest that the early stages of blastogenesis and organogenesis are less sensitive to radiation. Below 0.05 Gy of radiation exposure in utero, the estimated childhood cancer incidence is 0.3% to 1%.

Hall EJ, Giaccia AJ. Radiation carcinogenesis. In: Hall EJ, Giaccia AJ, eds. *Radiobiology for the Radiologist.* 7th ed. Philadelphia, PA: Lippincott Williams & Wilkins; 2012:135–153.

18

EFFECTS OF RADIATION ON HEREDITARY DAMAGE, MUTATIONS, AND CHROMOSOME ABERRATIONS

CAMILLE BERRIOCHOA, C. MARC LEYRER, AND ANTHONY MASTROIANNI

Question 1

Why might a male who has received 0.20 Gy (20 rad) to the testicles remain fertile for 6 weeks before noting a diminished sperm count?

Question 2

How does fractionation affect testicular gonadal function?

Question 3

What data exist to prove that male patients are at greater risk of sterility with fractionated radiation therapy (RT) than with single-dose treatment of an equal or greater dose?

Turn page to see the answers.

Question 1 *Why might a male who has received 0.20 Gy (20 rad) to the testicles remain fertile for 6 weeks before noting a diminished sperm count?*

Answer 1

Doses as low as 0.15 Gy (15 rad) cause oligospermia (diminished sperm count). Cells that have already undergone spermatogenesis are relatively radioresistant, in contrast to stem cells, which are more sensitive. Therefore, a male may have functional sperm for up to 6 weeks, with fertility waning once mature sperm have died or been expelled.

Hall EJ, Giaccia AJ. Heritable effects of radiation. In: Hall EJ, Giaccia AJ, eds. *Radiobiology for the Radiologist*. 7th ed. Philadelphia, PA: Lippincott Williams & Wilkins; 2012:159–173.

Question 2 *How does fractionation affect testicular gonadal function?*

Answer 2

For most tissues/organs of the body, dividing a particular dose into an increasing number of fractions results in a number of beneficial radiobiological effects (reassortment, reoxygenation, and repair). The repair of nontumor tissue/organs in the radiation treatment field is one of the fundamental underlying rationales for fractionation and tends to reduce some of the acute and late radiation toxicities. However, this is not true with testicular tissue, which is more sensitive to increased fractionation secondary to the long cell cycle of testicular stem cells (~16 days); the interval between fractions is too short to allow for sublethal repair.

Hall EJ, Giaccia AJ. Heritable effects of radiation. In: Hall EJ, Giaccia AJ, eds. *Radiobiology for the Radiologist*. 7th ed. Philadelphia, PA: Lippincott Williams & Wilkins; 2012:159–173.

Question 3 *What data exist to prove that male patients are at greater risk of sterility with fractionated radiation therapy (RT) than with single-dose treatment of an equal or greater dose?*

Answer 3

Studies on human male prisoner populations performed in the 1970s demonstrated that a single fraction of 6 Gy to the testes caused azoospermia (absence of living spermatozoa). Multiple studies have demonstrated that doses as low as 2.5 to 3 Gy delivered over a 2- to 4-week fractionated regimen can cause permanent azoospermia.

Centola GM, Keller JW, Henzler M, Rubin P. Effect of low-dose testicular irradiation on sperm count and fertility in patients with testicular seminoma. *J Androl*. 1994;15:608–613.

Hall EJ, Giaccia AJ. Heritable effects of radiation. In: Hall EJ, Giaccia AJ, eds. *Radiobiology for the Radiologist*. 7th ed. Philadelphia, PA: Lippincott Williams & Wilkins; 2012:159–173.

Sinno-Tellier S, Bouyer J, Ducot B, Geoffroy-Perez B, Spira A, Slama R. Male gonadal dose of ionizing radiation delivered during x-ray examinations and monthly probability of pregnancy: a population-based retrospective study. *BMC Public Health*. 2006;6:1–12.

Speiser B, Rubin P, Casarett G. Aspermia following lower truncal irradiation in Hodgkin's disease. *Cancer*. 1973;32:692–698.

Question 4
What radiation dose delivered to female gonadal structures is necessary to cause permanent sterility?

Question 5
What are several ways in which radiation therapy (RT) to the gonads differs between men and women?

Question 6
Why are male patients recommended to wait 6 months following chemotherapy or radiation therapy (RT) prior to attempting conception?

Question 4 *What radiation dose delivered to female gonadal structures is necessary to cause permanent sterility?*

Answer 4

The effect of dose on female sterility depends on the woman's inherent fertility at that point in her life. The absolute dose necessary to induce permanent sterility in women varies among various sources. Per Hall's seventh edition, in a prepubertal female, 12 Gy is required to induce sterility, whereas 2 Gy is sufficient in premenopausal patients. Other studies have demonstrated that 4 to 7 Gy in 1 to 4 fractions increased rates of sterility in premenopausal women greater than 40 years of age, whereas fractionated doses of 20 to 30 Gy in prepubertal females were necessary to cause permanent sterility. In summary, while the absolute threshold may vary among various studies, the underlying finding is that lower doses of radiation induce sterility in premenopausal than in prepubertal females. This decrement in dose necessary to cause sterility is directly related to the decline of functional oocytes as a female ages. Females have approximately 2 million oocytes at birth; this number decreases to 300,000 at puberty and declines further with each passing year, thus making female gonadal structures increasingly susceptible to radiation damage due to decreased ovarian reserve.

Hall EJ, Giaccia AJ. Heritable effects of radiation. In: Hall EJ, Giaccia AJ, eds. *Radiobiology for the Radiologist.* 7th ed. Philadelphia, PA: Lippincott Williams & Wilkins; 2012:159–173.
Ogilvy-Stuart AL, Shalet SM. Effect of radiation on the human reproductive system. *Environ Health Perspect.* 1993;101(suppl 2):109–116.

Question 5 *What are several ways in which radiation therapy (RT) to the gonads differs between men and women?*

Answer 5

Male testicular function is more susceptible to fractionated RT compared to a single fraction, whereas female ovarian function is less sensitive to fractionated RT. There is a latent period between males' exposure to radiation and manifestation of sterility, whereas female sterility is typically immediate. Males do not experience significant hormonal or libido-related toxicity following radiation-induced sterility, whereas females will often manifest the typical menopausal symptoms when sterility is induced. Ovaries are unable to generate additional new oocytes after birth, whereas sperm reserves are continually replenished. The radiation-induced sterility threshold is very age dependent in women, whereas it is relatively age independent in men.

Hall EJ, Giaccia AJ. Heritable effects of radiation. In: Hall EJ, Giaccia AJ, eds. *Radiobiology for the Radiologist.* 7th ed. Philadelphia, PA: Lippincott Williams & Wilkins; 2012:159–173.
Ogilvy-Stuart AL, Shalet SM. Effect of radiation on the human reproductive system. *Environ Health Perspect.* 1993;101(suppl 2):109–116.

Question 6 *Why are male patients recommended to wait 6 months following chemotherapy or radiation therapy (RT) prior to attempting conception?*

Answer 6

Several studies have demonstrated increased rates of spermatid aneuploidy in the period immediately following treatment for testicular cancer. Animal studies have been designed to quantify structural chromosomal aberrations and aneuploidy in mouse embryos after spermatozoa were exposed to radiation. While the exact duration of continued radiation-induced aneuploidy in the human is debated, the accepted recommendation is that male patients wait approximately 6 months after radiation exposure before attempting conception to allow for two complete cycles of a 3-month process of spermatogenesis and renewal of nonexposed sperm.

De Mas P, Daudin M, Vincent MC, et al. Increased aneuploidy in spermatozoa from testicular tumour patients after chemotherapy with cisplatin, etoposide and bleomycin. *Hum Reprod.* 2001;16:1204–1208.
Hall EJ, Giaccia AJ. Heritable effects of radiation. In: Hall EJ, Giaccia AJ, eds. *Radiobiology for the Radiologist.* 7th ed. Philadelphia, PA: Lippincott Williams & Wilkins; 2012:159–173.
Martin RH, Ernst S, Rademaker A, Barclay L, Ko E, Summers N. Chromosomal abnormalities in sperm from testicular cancer patients before and after chemotherapy. *Hum Genet.* 1997;99:214–218.
Tateno H, Kusakabe H, Kamiguchi Y. Structural chromosomal aberrations, aneuploidy, and mosaicism in early cleavage mouse embryos derived from spermatozoa exposed to gamma-rays. *Int J Radiat Biol.* 2001;87:320–329.

Question 7

What was the "megamouse project" and how did it help elucidate radiation-induced hereditary effects in mice?

Question 8

What is the estimated doubling dose of radiation proposed to markedly increase radiation-induced hereditary effects?

Question 9

What does the International Commission on Radiological Protection (ICRP) propose are the estimated risks of hereditary effects from radiation for the general population versus the population of radiation workers? Why are these numbers different?

Question 7 *What was the "megamouse project" and how did it help elucidate radiation-induced hereditary effects in mice?*

Answer 7

This project, led by the husband and wife team of William and Liane Russell at Oak Ridge National Laboratory in Tennessee, evaluated the hereditary effects of radiation on approximately 7 million mice. Investigators found that fractionating a total dose resulted in fewer mutations than if the total dose were given in a single fraction. This finding was in contrast to the dose-rate effect observed in drosophila. Investigators also found that increasing the time interval between radiation exposure and conception decreased the mutation rates found within offspring. Investigators proposed that immediate attempts at conception relied on mature spermatids that were unable to undergo post-radiation therapy (RT) repair, thus leading to higher mutation rates, whereas waiting several weeks from exposure to attempted conception likely allowed those spermatids that had been exposed in a primitive state to undergo repair.

Hall EJ, Giaccia AJ. Heritable effects of radiation. In: Hall EJ, Giaccia AJ, eds. *Radiobiology for the Radiologist*. 7th ed. Philadelphia, PA: Lippincott Williams & Wilkins; 2012:159–173.

Question 8 *What is the estimated doubling dose of radiation proposed to markedly increase radiation-induced hereditary effects?*

Answer 8

The dose is 1 Gy per Biological Effects of Ionizing Radiation (BEIR) V and UN Scientific Committee on the Effects of Atomic Radiation (UNSCEAR) based on low–dose-rate exposure, meaning that for every 1 Gy of fractionated radiation therapy (RT), the rate of hereditary effects doubles (i.e., it is twice the spontaneous mutation incidence rate). This calculation was also extrapolated from the Russells' megamouse project.

Hall EJ, Giaccia AJ. Heritable effects of radiation. In: Hall EJ, Giaccia AJ, eds. *Radiobiology for the Radiologist*. 7th ed. Philadelphia, PA: Lippincott Williams & Wilkins; 2012:159–173.

Question 9 *What does the International Commission on Radiological Protection (ICRP) propose are the estimated risks of hereditary effects from radiation for the general population versus the population of radiation workers? Why are these numbers different?*

Answer 9

This number is based on UN Scientific Committee on the Effects of Atomic Radiation (UNSCEAR) calculations, all of which refer to a reproductive population. These values are described in units of Sievert rather than units of gray. The unit *Sievert* is an SI unit representing the energy absorbed by 1 kg of biological tissue; like Gy, its units are J/kg, but it represents the biological impact of dose. For reference, 1 Gy = 1 Sv. The hereditary risk for the general population is 0.2%/Sv, whereas the risk for the population working in radiation facilities is 0.1%/Sv. These risk rates may initially seem counterintuitive as one might think that the overall risk should be higher for those working in radiation facilities than for those in the general population. To explain this, consider that the total Sieverts to which a radiation worker will be exposed over his or her lifetime is greater than the total for someone in the general population, thereby increasing the absolute risk for those working in radiation facilities. Additionally, radiation workers are not allowed to work in this environment until the age of 18, whereas the general population has no control of their "general risk" and may be exposed for a longer period of time (from age 0 to age 35, an arbitrary age selected to represent the age at which most individuals stop procreating). Therefore, radiation workers' risk spans about 17 years (from age 18 to 35), whereas the general population's risk spans about 35 years. Since the time interval is about 50% less for radiation workers, their percent per Sievert is commensurately lower. Of note, the probability of a hereditary disorder in the first generation born to parents exposed to radiation is estimated to be 0.002%/Sv.

Boice JD, Jr., Tawn EJ, Winther JF, et al. Genetic effects of radiotherapy for childhood cancer. *Health Phys*. 2003;85:65–80.
Hall EJ, Giaccia AJ. Heritable effects of radiation. In: Hall EJ, Giaccia AJ, eds. *Radiobiology for the Radiologist*. 7th ed. Philadelphia, PA: Lippincott Williams & Wilkins; 2012:159–173.

Question 10

What is the average dose to the gonads received by individuals of child-bearing potential due to diagnostic radiology in the United States?

Question 11

What is the number of genetic disorders secondary to exposure to diagnostic radiology procedures given the following numbers for the average population of the United States (in which the number of live births per year is ~3×10^6)?

Question 12

How should one describe the shape of the dose–response curve for heritable effects: linear quadratic, linear and no threshold, or convex upward?

Question 13

Which type of DNA break, single stranded versus double stranded, has a significant biological consequence and why?

Question 10 *What is the average dose to the gonads received by individuals of child-bearing potential due to diagnostic radiology in the United States?*

Answer 10

0.3 mSv. This dose is called the "genetically significant dose" (GSD) and is believed to be the average radiation *exposure* to which the general population is subjected.

Hall EJ, Giaccia AJ. Radiation carcinogenesis. In: Hall EJ, Giaccia AJ, eds. *Radiobiology for the Radiologist*. 7th ed. Philadelphia, PA: Lippincott Williams & Wilkins; 2006:135–153.

Question 11 *What is the number of genetic disorders secondary to exposure to diagnostic radiology procedures given the following numbers for the average population of the United States (in which the number of live births per year is ~3 × 10⁶)?*

Answer 11

Consider the following equation: number of genetic disorders = average exposure to diagnostic radiation × risk of heritable effects per Sv × number of live births per year. Recall that the average exposure is about 0.3 mSv and the risk of heritable effects is 0.2%/Sv (see question 9) for the general population. Convert 0.2% into an absolute number (0.002), include the approximate number of years in a generation (about 30 years), and make sure that all units cross out. The risk of genetic disorders = (0.002 risk/Sv in 1 generation) × (3.0 × 10⁶ births/year) × (0.3 mSv/year) × (1 Sv/1,000 mSv) × 30 year generation = 54.

Hall EJ, Giaccia AJ. Heritable effects of radiation. In: Hall EJ, Giaccia AJ, eds. *Radiobiology for the Radiologist*. 7th ed. Philadelphia, PA: Lippincott Williams & Wilkins; 2012:159–173.

Question 12 *How should one describe the shape of the dose–response curve for heritable effects: linear quadratic, linear and no threshold, or convex upward?*

Answer 12

It is linear and has no threshold. The rate of double-stranded DNA breaks is a linear-quadratic phenomenon; the specific effect of radiation on cell viability is described in this way. However, the *heritable effects* of radiation fall into a stochastic model in which the consequences are all or none. The likelihood of heritable effects is directly related to the dose of radiation.

Hall EJ, Giaccia AJ. Heritable effects of radiation. In: Hall EJ, Giaccia AJ, eds. *Radiobiology for the Radiologist*. 7th ed. Philadelphia, PA: Lippincott Williams & Wilkins; 2012:159–173.

Question 13 *Which type of DNA break, single stranded versus double stranded, has a significant biological consequence and why?*

Answer 13

Double-stranded DNA breaks occur when chromatin snaps into two pieces and are of greater biological consequence than those that are single stranded. When a single-stranded break occurs, it can be easily repaired using the opposite strand as a template preserving the integrity of the helix. If both strands are broken, but these breaks are far apart, DNA integrity can again be preserved because these two breaks can be managed separately. However, if the double-stranded breaks occur opposite or within a few bases from one another, the repair process is more difficult and error prone, thereby predisposing the cell to cell death, mutations, or carcinogenesis.

Hall EJ, Giaccia AJ. Molecular mechanisms of DNA and chromosome damage and repair. In: Hall EJ, Giaccia AJ, eds. *Radiobiology for the Radiologist*. 7th ed. Philadelphia, PA: Lippincott Williams & Wilkins; 2012:12–34.

Question 14

What is the ratio of single-stranded to double-stranded breaks for a given dose? How does increased dose impact the number of strand breaks?

Question 15

What is a fundamental difference between the gel preparations used to evaluate single-stranded versus double-stranded DNA breaks?

Question 16

What are the three most commonly used modalities by which DNA strand breaks are measured? Describe the way in which these three methods work.

Question 14 *What is the ratio of single-stranded to double-stranded breaks for a given dose? How does increased dose impact the number of strand breaks?*

Answer 14

The yield of double-stranded breaks is approximately 1/25th the amount of single-stranded breaks for a given dose. Both increase *linearly* with dose, which suggests that they are formed by single tracks of radiation.

Hall EJ, Giaccia AJ. Molecular mechanisms of DNA and chromosome damage and repair. In: Hall EJ, Giaccia AJ, eds. *Radiobiology for the Radiologist*. 7th ed. Philadelphia, PA: Lippincott Williams & Wilkins; 2012:12–34.

Question 15 *What is a fundamental difference between the gel preparations used to evaluate single-stranded versus double-stranded DNA breaks?*

Answer 15

Evaluating single-stranded breaks requires that the DNA double helix be denatured. Using a strong alkaline preparation disrupts the bonds between strands. Double-stranded breaks are measured by using a neutral preparation, since DNA can remain annealed. Both gels utilize a porous substrate. Since smaller strands are able to move further in the porous gel, the further the DNA travels in the gel, the more breaks which must have occurred. This is compared against a standard representative gel.

Hall EJ, Giaccia AJ. Molecular mechanisms of DNA and chromosome damage and repair. In: Hall EJ, Giaccia AJ, eds. *Radiobiology for the Radiologist*. 7th ed. Philadelphia, PA: Lippincott Williams & Wilkins; 2012:12–34.

Question 16 *What are the three most commonly used modalities by which DNA strand breaks are measured? Describe the way in which these three methods work.*

Answer 16

The three methods are pulsed field gel electrophoresis (PFGE), single cell electrophoresis, and DNA damage-induced nuclear foci. In the first two assays, cells are exposed to ionizing radiation, then embedded in agarose and lysed under specific buffer conditions (either neutral or alkaline; see question 13). PFGE is a technique that built upon standard gel electrophoresis; the latter technique was able to separate DNA strands of various sizes up to a point but could not separate very large molecules of DNA effectively. Schwartz and Cantor at Columbia University found that an alternating voltage gradient could improve the resolution of larger molecules. Instead of utilizing a constant voltage, voltage is periodically switched and allows for separation of DNA fragments according to size, up to the megabase pair size range.

Single cell electrophoresis, also called the *comet assay*, can detect differences in DNA damage at the single cell level that is advantageous when a biopsy sample containing only a small amount of tissue is available. The comet assay can measure both single-stranded and double-stranded breaks depending on whether an alkaline or neutral buffer solution has been used. If the cell is undamaged, then the DNA will not migrate significantly since it is a fairly large size. However, if the cell's DNA has been broken by radiation, it will migrate through the gel, with increased migration directly correlated to increased cell breakage. This migration takes on the appearance of a comet's tail, which lends to the "comet" name for this technique.

Lastly, the DNA damage-induced nuclear foci assay relies on the use of antibodies specific to certain repair proteins that localize to sites of DNA strand breaks in the nucleus of a cell.

Hall EJ, Giaccia AJ. Molecular mechanisms of DNA and chromosome damage and repair. In: Hall EJ, Giaccia AJ, eds. *Radiobiology for the Radiologist*. 7th ed. Philadelphia, PA: Lippincott Williams & Wilkins; 2012:12–34.
Schwartz DC, Cantor CR. Separation of yeast chromosome-sized DNAs by pulsed field gradient gel electrophoresis. *Cell*. 1984;37:67–75.

Question 17

How would you describe the DNA damage-induced nuclear foci assay, its typical antibody targets, and its advantages over the pulsed field gel electrophoresis (PFGE) and comet assays?

Question 18

What is a Western blot and how does this relate to the DNA damage-induced nuclear foci assay?

Question 19

What is the difference between a chromosome aberration and a chromatid aberration?

Question 17 *How would you describe the DNA damage-induced nuclear foci assay, its typical antibody targets, and its advantages over the pulsed field gel electrophoresis (PFGE) and comet assays?*

Answer 17

The DNA damage-induced nuclear foci assay capitalizes on the presence of characteristic repair proteins that are deployed when ionizing radiation damage occurs. Cells/tissues are incubated with antibodies against characteristic repair proteins. A second fluorescently labeled antibody then localizes to the first antibody and thus illustrates the presence or absence of repair proteins. The most commonly used repair proteins targeted are gamma-H2AX and 53BP1. These two proteins are similar in that both are phosphorylated in response to damage. Antibodies to both forms (H2AX and gamma-H2AX; 53BP and phosphorylated 53BP1) can be utilized. Other proteins that may be used in the DNA damage nuclear foci assay are ataxia telangiectasia mutated (ATM), replication protein A (RPA), RAD51, and BRCA1. Additionally, flow cytometry can be performed to quantify the amount of DNA repair proteins that have been deployed. Advantages of this assay include ease of use and the fact that it can be applied for both tissue sections and individual cell preparations.

Hall EJ, Giaccia AJ. Molecular mechanisms of DNA and chromosome damage and repair. In: Hall EJ, Giaccia AJ, eds. *Radiobiology for the Radiologist*. 7th ed. Philadelphia, PA: Lippincott Williams & Wilkins; 2012:12–34.

Question 18 *What is a Western blot and how does this relate to the DNA damage-induced nuclear foci assay?*

Answer 18

Southern, Northern and Western blots each assess a different type of biological material. To remember the ways in which these blots differ, use the mnemonic SNoW DRoP—Southern analyzes **D**NA, Northern analyzes **R**NA, and **W**estern analyzes **p**roteins (S for Southern, N for Northern, W for Western; D for DNA, R for RNA, P for protein). A Western blot is a gel electrophoresis used to detect specific proteins, either based on 3D structure (if proteins are intact) or based on size (if proteins have been denatured). Once they have run through the gel, proteins are then transferred to a membrane, where they are stained with antibodies specific to the target protein. Western blots are relevant to the DNA damage-induced nuclear foci assay as this is one way by which these seminal repair proteins (gamma-H2AX, 53BP1) are detected. Of note, if the antibody is directed toward the H2AX histone protein (rather than the phosphorylated gamma-H2AX protein), an unchanged band is seen on the Western blot, whereas staining for the gamma-H2AX protein produces a discrete band representative of activation of DNA damage proteins.

Hall EJ, Giaccia AJ. Molecular mechanisms of DNA and chromosome damage and repair. In: Hall EJ, Giaccia AJ, eds. *Radiobiology for the Radiologist*. 7th ed. Philadelphia, PA: Lippincott Williams & Wilkins; 2012:12–34.
Le T, Bushan V. *First Aid for the USMLE step 1 2011*. New York, NY: McGraw Hill Education; 2011.

Question 19 *What is the difference between a chromosome aberration and a chromatid aberration?*

Answer 19

To answer this question, one must recall the difference between a chromosome and a chromatid. A chromosome refers to the collection of genetic material found in the nucleus during nonreplicative stages. Chromatid refers to one of the sister arms of the stereotypically x-shaped chromatid pair that is formed during mitosis, with each arm attached to the other at the midpoint via a centromere. A chromosome aberration occurs if a cell is subject to radiation in early interphase, prior to cell division, whereas a chromatid aberration occurs during mitosis. This is important to note because chromosome aberrations will ultimately be duplicated to make two identically mutated sister chromatids and will thus affect both daughter cells, whereas a chromatid aberration affects only one of the daughter cells. Whether the aberration affects the chromosome or the chromatid also impacts what specific kind of radiation-induced aberration develops (dicentric chromosome, ring chromosome, and anaphase bridge).

Hall EJ, Giaccia AJ. Molecular mechanisms of DNA and chromosome damage and repair. In: Hall EJ, Giaccia AJ, eds. *Radiobiology for the Radiologist*. 7th ed. Philadelphia, PA: Lippincott Williams & Wilkins; 2012:12–34.

Question 20

What is the telomerase enzyme and how does it relate to cancer cells?

Question 21

What are the three types of genetic aberrations that are lethal to the cell? Name and describe them.

Question 22

What are the two types of genetic rearrangements that permit cell viability but may be associated with carcinogenesis?

Question 20 *What is the telomerase enzyme and how does it relate to cancer cells?*

Answer 20

Telomerase is a reverse transcriptase found in stem cells in self-renewing tissues. It transcribes a DNA sequence that is complementary to the long array of TTAGGG repeats found in mammalian telomeres. Recall that telomeres are located at the terminal ends of chromosomes and are there to protect these ends during chromosomal replication. If not present, the essential genetic material on the lagging strand would be shortened with each replication because DNA polymerase cannot synthesize new DNA in the absence of an RNA primer. However, even when present, telomeres ultimately degrade (typically after ~50 cell divisions) given the repetitive truncation that occurs with each chromosomal replication. Telomerase helps make telomeres essentially immortal since the protective DNA "cap" is continually restored following each replication. Investigators have found that telomerase is activated in many cancer cells and contributes to their longevity.

Hall EJ, Giaccia AJ. Molecular mechanisms of DNA and chromosome damage and repair. In: Hall EJ, Giaccia AJ, eds. *Radiobiology for the Radiologist*. 7th ed. Philadelphia, PA: Lippincott Williams & Wilkins; 2012:12–34.

Question 21 *What are the three types of genetic aberrations that are lethal to the cell? Name and describe them.*

Answer 21

The three types are the dicentric, the ring, and the anaphase bridge. Dicentrics and rings both result from aberrations in prereplication chromosomes, whereas the anaphase bridge occurs after replication of the chromosome into two sister chromatids. All three types are due to "two hit aberrations." Dicentric chromosomes develop from breaks in two separate chromosomes in which one dicentric and one acentric chromosome result. The acentric chromosome will be lost at the subsequent mitosis because its lack of a centromere means that it cannot migrate to either pole at mitosis. Ring chromosomes develop when there is a break in each arm of the *same* chromosome. The two sticky ends of the original chromosome then join to form a ring. The other originally separate truncated portions join to create a linear chromosome with significantly less genetic material. At replication, two overlapping rings and two acentric fragments are created. An anaphase bridge occurs *following* replication (typically in late G2) and is thus a defect in the two *chromatids* of one chromosome. The ends of two sister chromatids get severed and then reconnect to form an acentric ring chromosome. The sticky ends of the residual chromatid pair will combine such that one end of the attached sister chromatids is separate but the other end is now attached so as to appear like a horseshoe on that side.

Hall EJ, Giaccia AJ. Molecular mechanisms of DNA and chromosome damage and repair. In: Hall EJ, Giaccia AJ, eds. *Radiobiology for the Radiologist*. 7th ed. Philadelphia, PA: Lippincott Williams & Wilkins; 2012:12–34.

Question 22 *What are the two types of genetic rearrangements that permit cell viability but may be associated with carcinogenesis?*

Answer 22

The two types are symmetric translocations and small interstitial deletions. Symmetric translocations arise due to breaks in the ends of separate chromosomes, which then recombine with one another to produce a new, now-mutated chromosome. Examples of these translocations include Burkitt lymphoma [t(8:14)], follicular lymphoma [t(14:18)], and mantle cell lymphoma [t(11:14)], as well as translocations involved in a number of leukemias. Small interstitial deletions are also compatible with cell viability. These occur when two breaks develop in a segment of double-stranded DNA. Now the small segment has two sticky ends that often rejoin into a ring, whereas the larger DNA segment will also reconnect. As aforementioned, since the ring (created by the two sticky ends) does not have a centromere, it will be lost at subsequent mitosis.

Hall EJ, Giaccia AJ. Molecular mechanisms of DNA and chromosome damage and repair. In: Hall EJ, Giaccia AJ, eds. *Radiobiology for the Radiologist*. 7th ed. Philadelphia, PA: Lippincott Williams & Wilkins; 2012:12–34.

Question 23

How can these stereotypical chromosome abnormalities be used clinically by a radiation safety officer?

Question 24

How would you describe base excision repair (BER)? What clinical syndrome is secondary to a defect in a BER protein?

Question 25

How would you describe nucleotide excision repair (NER) and its two main pathways? Additionally, describe what clinical syndrome is secondary to a defect in an NER protein.

Question 23 *How can these stereotypical chromosome abnormalities be used clinically by a radiation safety officer?*

Answer 23

Dicentric and ring chromosomes become particularly useful in this regard as ionizing radiation produces these abnormalities in peripheral lymphocytes and can serve as a surrogate for radiation exposure to those not wearing radiation dosimeters. Since these chromosome aberrations are only lethal at the time of mitosis, and since mature T lymphocytes do not undergo further mitoses, these peripheral blood abnormalities may persist for weeks to months after exposure. Peripheral blood can be collected and metaphases scored to determine the number of aberrations. The minimum dose of whole body radiation therapy (RT) detected through measurement of dicentric chromosomes in lymphocytes is 0.25 Gy.

Hall EJ, Giaccia AJ. Molecular mechanisms of DNA and chromosome damage and repair. In: Hall EJ, Giaccia AJ, eds. *Radiobiology for the Radiologist.* 7th ed. Philadelphia, PA: Lippincott Williams & Wilkins; 2012:12–34.

Question 24 *How would you describe base excision repair (BER)? What clinical syndrome is secondary to a defect in a BER protein?*

Answer 24

BER is deployed when a single base has been paired incorrectly (e.g., C with T). There are a number of steps and proteins required to undergo BER. Cockayne syndrome is a disorder characterized by mutations in two genes important in the BER pathway: CSA and CSB. When normal, CSA and CSB interact closely with apurinic endonuclease 1 (APE1), an enzyme that is essential to base removal. Recall that Cockayne syndrome is due to a defect in BER and manifests as impaired CNS development, photosensitivity, ocular disorders, and premature aging. Of note, CSA and CSB are also important in nucleotide excision repair (NER) (see Question 25).

Hall EJ, Giaccia AJ. Molecular mechanisms of DNA and chromosome damage and repair. In: Hall EJ, Giaccia AJ, eds. *Radiobiology for the Radiologist.* 7th ed. Philadelphia, PA: Lippincott Williams & Wilkins; 2012:12–34.

Question 25 *How would you describe nucleotide excision repair (NER) and its two main pathways? Additionally, describe what clinical syndrome is secondary to a defect in an NER protein.*

Answer 25

NER removes bulky adducts in DNA, classically thymidine dimers, and adducts secondary to alkylating chemotherapy agents. Xeroderma pigmentosum (XP) is a genetic disorder that results from damage to the *XPC* and *XPE* genes, both of which are important in NER repair. Ultraviolet (UV) radiation often induces pyrimidine dimers; thus, XP patients are hypersensitive to UV light. In these patients, multiple skin malignancies occur by a young age with metastatic melanoma and squamous cell carcinoma being the two most common causes of death in XP patients. NER is divided into two pathways: global genome repair (GGR), which surveys the entire genome, both active and inactive, and transcription coupled repair (TCR), which only removes lesions in DNA whose strands are actively transcribing. GGR relies on the XPC–XPE protein complexes, whereas TCR is activated by the stalled RNA polymerase (which has been obstructed by the bulky adduct) in concert with CSA and CSB.

Hall EJ, Giaccia AJ. Molecular mechanisms of DNA and chromosome damage and repair. In: Hall EJ, Giaccia AJ, eds. *Radiobiology for the Radiologist.* 7th ed. Philadelphia, PA: Lippincott Williams & Wilkins; 2012:12–34.
Halpern J, Hopping B, Brostoff JM. Photosensitivity, corneal scarring and developmental delay: xeroderma pigmentosum in a tropical country. *Cases J.* 2008;1:1–3.

Question 26
What are the two processes by which DNA double-stranded breaks can be repaired?

Question 27
Describe the six essential steps involved in nonhomologous end joining (NHEJ).

Question 28
In what normal body system is nonhomologous end joining (NHEJ) an advantageous DNA repair method?

Question 26 *What are the two processes by which DNA double-stranded breaks can be repaired?*

Answer 26

The two processes are homologous recombination repair (HRR) and nonhomologous end joining (NHEJ). The use of HRR versus NHEJ is largely dependent upon the cell's stage in the cell cycle. Homologous recombination occurs in late S/G2 when the chromosome has multiplied into two sister chromatids. Since an undamaged sister chromatid is available to serve as a template, HRR is essentially error free. Note that RPA is an important protein involved in HRR, serving to coat single-stranded DNA regions generated during homologous recombination to prevent degradation. Rad51 and BRCA are also important HRR repair proteins to remember. In contrast to HRR, NHEJ is an error prone process and likely results in the premutagenic lesions induced in human cells after ionizing radiation. The repair protein 53BP1 (see question 17), in addition to the cell's phase in the cell cycle, helps regulate whether HRR or NHEJ will take place.

Hall EJ, Giaccia AJ. Molecular mechanisms of DNA and chromosome damage and repair. In: Hall EJ, Giaccia AJ, eds. *Radiobiology for the Radiologist*. 7th ed. Philadelphia, PA: Lippincott Williams & Wilkins; 2012:12–34.
Li X, Heyer WD. Homologous recombination in DNA repair and DNA damage tolerance. *Cell Res*. 2008;18:99–113.

Question 27 *Describe the six essential steps involved in nonhomologous end joining (NHEJ).*

Answer 27

(a) ATM, MRE (meiotic recombination), Rad50, and Nbs1 alert the cell about the presence of DNA damage. (b) The Ku70/Ku80 heterodimer (named as such because one is a 70 kDa unit and the other is an ~80 kDa unit) has a high affinity for DNA ends and forms a close fitting asymmetrical ring that attaches to the broken (and now free) end of radiation-damaged DNA. (c) The Ku heterodimer helps recruit DNA-PK, which is in the phosphatidyl inositol 3' kinase-related kinases (PIKK) family. When associated with the Ku heterodimer, DNA-PK becomes the DNA-PK holoenzyme and is activated to DNA-PKcs (catalytic subunit). This Ku heterodimer also attracts Artemis (an endonuclease) to form a physical complex. The DNA-PK holoenzyme can then phosphorylate Artemis and activate its endonuclease activity. (d) End processing then occurs via Artemis's activity in cleaving residual DNA loops or hairpins that develop during NHEJ. (e) Fill-in synthesis takes place via DNA polymerase. (f) The DNA-PK holoenzyme then recruits the ligase complex (XRCC4/XLF/LIGIV/PNK) to engage in the final ligation step.

Hall EJ, Giaccia AJ. Molecular mechanisms of DNA and chromosome damage and repair. In: Hall EJ, Giaccia AJ, eds. *Radiobiology for the Radiologist*. 7th ed. Philadelphia, PA: Lippincott Williams & Wilkins; 2012:12–34.

Question 28 *In what normal body system is nonhomologous end joining (NHEJ) an advantageous DNA repair method?*

Answer 28

NHEJ is an ideal repair method in the body's physiological generation of diverse antibodies. NHEJ is very important in the V(D)J recombination of human antibodies, whose variety is enhanced precisely by the error-prone nature of NHEJ.

Hall EJ, Giaccia AJ. Molecular mechanisms of DNA and chromosome damage and repair. In: Hall EJ, Giaccia AJ, eds. *Radiobiology for the Radiologist*. 7th ed. Philadelphia, PA: Lippincott Williams & Wilkins; 2012:12–34.

19

EFFECTS OF RADIATION ON THE EMBRYO AND FETUS

YVONNE PHAM AND STEVEN OH

Question 1
What are some effects that radiation can have on a developing embryo and fetus?

Question 2
Are the effects of irradiation during gestation considered deterministic or stochastic in nature?

Question 3
What is the baseline incidence of congenital abnormalities for infants in the general human population?

Question 4
What are the three developmental stages in utero that are typically considered in the context of radiation exposure?

Turn page to see the answers.

Question 1 *What are some effects that radiation can have on a developing embryo and fetus?*

Answer 1

Radiation can cause lethal effects (prenatal or neonatal death), hereditary defects, carcinogenesis, congenital malformations, growth disturbances, and mental retardation to occur in a developing embryo and fetus.

Hall EJ, Giaccia AJ. Effects of radiation on the embryo and fetus. In: Hall EJ, Giaccia AJ, eds. *Radiobiology for the Radiologist.* 7th ed. Philadelphia, PA: Lippincott Williams & Wilkins; 2012:174–187.

Question 2 *Are the effects of irradiation during gestation considered deterministic or stochastic in nature?*

Answer 2

The effects of irradiation during gestation, such as prenatal death and congenital malformations, are considered deterministic in nature since certain dose thresholds are necessary to cause these effects and the degree of severity is dependent on dose. In contrast, carcinogenesis from in utero irradiation is considered a stochastic effect in that there is no threshold dose and the severity is independent of dose.

Hall EJ, Giaccia AJ. Effects of radiation on the embryo and fetus. In: Hall EJ, Giaccia AJ, eds. *Radiobiology for the Radiologist.* 7th ed. Philadelphia, PA: Lippincott Williams & Wilkins; 2012:174–187.

Question 3 *What is the baseline incidence of congenital abnormalities for infants in the general human population?*

Answer 3

The baseline risk of congenital abnormalities is 5% to 10%. Thus, it is difficult to determine if exposure to a small dose of radiation in utero is solely responsible for an existing congenital abnormality.

Hall EJ, Giaccia AJ. Effects of radiation on the embryo and fetus. In: Hall EJ, Giaccia AJ, eds. *Radiobiology for the Radiologist.* 7th ed. Philadelphia, PA: Lippincott Williams & Wilkins; 2012:174–187.

Question 4 *What are the three developmental stages in utero that are typically considered in the context of radiation exposure?*

Answer 4

1. Preimplantation is the period of time from fertilization to implantation of the embryo into the uterine wall and occurs during days 0 to 9 postconception.
2. Organogenesis is the period of development of major organs and takes place from day 10 to week 6 postconception.
3. The fetal period encompasses the growth of organs that have been formed and occurs from week 6 postconception until term.

Hall EJ, Giaccia AJ. Effects of radiation on the embryo and fetus. In: Hall EJ, Giaccia AJ, eds. *Radiobiology for the Radiologist.* 7th ed. Philadelphia, PA: Lippincott Williams & Wilkins; 2012:174–187.

Question 5
What stage of development in rats and mice is most sensitive to the lethal effects of radiation?

Question 6
Which stages of radiation exposure generally result in prenatal and neonatal death, respectively?

Question 7
What is considered the threshold radiation dose for animals in utero thought to produce growth retardation?

Question 8
What is considered the threshold dose for central nervous system (CNS) damage for a mouse in utero?

Question 9
Radiation exposure during which stages of gestation for a mouse would result in temporary and permanent growth inhibition, respectively?

Question 5 *What stage of development in rats and mice is most sensitive to the lethal effects of radiation?*

Answer 5

The preimplantation stage is most susceptible to the lethal effects of radiation in mice and rats. There is thought to be an "all or nothing" effect of radiation during this stage in which an irradiated preimplanted embryo will grow normally if it survives but will otherwise result in death of the embryo if too many cells are killed by irradiation.

Hall EJ, Giaccia AJ. Effects of radiation on the embryo and fetus. In: Hall EJ, Giaccia AJ, eds. *Radiobiology for the Radiologist.* 7th ed. Philadelphia, PA: Lippincott Williams & Wilkins; 2012:174–187.

Question 6 *Which stages of radiation exposure generally result in prenatal and neonatal death, respectively?*

Answer 6

Prenatal death, which occurs before birth, generally results from irradiation during the preimplantation period. Neonatal death, which occurs around the time of birth, generally results from irradiation during organogenesis.

Hall EJ, Giaccia AJ. Effects of radiation on the embryo and fetus. In: Hall EJ, Giaccia AJ, eds. *Radiobiology for the Radiologist.* 7th ed. Philadelphia, PA: Lippincott Williams & Wilkins; 2012:174–187.

Question 7 *What is considered the threshold radiation dose for animals in utero thought to produce growth retardation?*

Answer 7

1 Gy of x-rays is thought to produce growth retardation during organogenesis and the fetal period. Studies have shown that a dose of 0.25 Gy is not high enough to cause an observable effect on growth.

Hall EJ, Giaccia AJ. Effects of radiation on the embryo and fetus. In: Hall EJ, Giaccia AJ, eds. *Radiobiology for the Radiologist.* 7th ed. Philadelphia, PA: Lippincott Williams & Wilkins; 2012:174–187.

Question 8 *What is considered the threshold dose for central nervous system (CNS) damage for a mouse in utero?*

Answer 8

0.1 Gy is thought to produce CNS damage according to mouse data.

Hall EJ, Giaccia AJ. Effects of radiation on the embryo and fetus. In: Hall EJ, Giaccia AJ, eds. *Radiobiology for the Radiologist.* 7th ed. Philadelphia, PA: Lippincott Williams & Wilkins; 2012:174–187.

Question 9 *Radiation exposure during which stages of gestation for a mouse would result in temporary and permanent growth inhibition, respectively?*

Answer 9

Exposure to radiation during organogenesis will most likely result in temporary growth inhibition at birth, whereas irradiation during the fetal period will result in permanent growth retardation.

Hall EJ, Giaccia AJ. Effects of radiation on the embryo and fetus. In: Hall EJ, Giaccia AJ, eds. *Radiobiology for the Radiologist.* 7th ed. Philadelphia, PA: Lippincott Williams & Wilkins; 2012:174–187.

Question 10

What is suggested as the threshold dose at which a pregnant patient exposed to radiation should be counseled by a physician to discuss the risk of radiation-induced birth defects?

Question 11

Irradiation during which gestational stage carries the highest risk of congenital malformations?

Question 12

What weeks during human pregnancy have the highest incidence of congenital malformations when exposed to 1 Gy of x-ray?

Question 13

According to rodent data, what weeks have the highest incidence of congenital malformation when exposed to irradiation?

Question 14

What were the principal effects seen in atomic bomb survivors of Hiroshima and Nagasaki?

Question 10 *What is suggested as the threshold dose at which a pregnant patient exposed to radiation should be counseled by a physician to discuss the risk of radiation-induced birth defects?*

Answer 10

0.1 Gy to the developing embryo or fetus from day 10 to 25 weeks of gestation is generally considered the threshold dose at which a physician needs to discuss with a pregnant patient the risks of radiation-induced birth defects and possible actions to take, including a therapeutic abortion.

Stovall M, Blackwell CR, Cundiff J, et al. Fetal dose from radiotherapy with photon beams: report of AAPM Radiation Therapy Committee Task Group No. 36. *Med Phys.* 1995;22(1):63–82.

Question 11 *Irradiation during which gestational stage carries the highest risk of congenital malformations?*

Answer 11

Organogenesis is the period of development of major organs and carries the highest risk of congenital malformations when exposed to radiation. In this stage of development, the embryonic cells are differentiating and are particularly susceptible to the effects of radiation.

Hall EJ, Giaccia AJ. Effects of radiation on the embryo and fetus. In: Hall EJ, Giaccia AJ, eds. *Radiobiology for the Radiologist.* 7th ed. Philadelphia, PA: Lippincott Williams & Wilkins; 2012:174–187.

Question 12 *What weeks during human pregnancy have the highest incidence of congenital malformations when exposed to 1 Gy of x-ray?*

Answer 12

Weeks 2 to 4 correspond to early organogenesis in human gestation and have the highest incidence of congenital malformations when exposed to x-ray irradiation.

Hall EJ, Giaccia AJ. Effects of radiation on the embryo and fetus. In: Hall EJ, Giaccia AJ, eds. *Radiobiology for the Radiologist.* 7th ed. Philadelphia, PA: Lippincott Williams & Wilkins; 2012:174–187.

Question 13 *According to rodent data, what weeks have the highest incidence of congenital malformation when exposed to irradiation?*

Answer 13

Weeks 1 to 6 correspond to organogenesis in small rodents and have the highest incidence of congenital malformations when exposed to x-ray irradiation.

Hall EJ, Giaccia AJ. Effects of radiation on the embryo and fetus. In: Hall EJ, Giaccia AJ, eds. *Radiobiology for the Radiologist.* 7th ed. Philadelphia, PA: Lippincott Williams & Wilkins; 2012:174–187.

Question 14 *What were the principal effects seen in atomic bomb survivors of Hiroshima and Nagasaki?*

Answer 14

Microcephaly and mental retardation were the two most frequent consequences of in utero exposure to radiation; both most often occurred from exposure during 8 to 15 weeks of gestation.

Hall EJ, Giaccia AJ. Effects of radiation on the embryo and fetus. In: Hall EJ, Giaccia AJ, eds. *Radiobiology for the Radiologist.* 7th ed. Philadelphia, PA: Lippincott Williams & Wilkins; 2012:174–187.

Question 15
Irradiation during which gestational stage carries the highest risk of mental retardation?

Question 16
What threshold dose is thought to cause mental retardation?

Question 17
What is the intelligence quotient (IQ) decrement per Gy from atomic bomb survivor data?

Question 18
What is the National Council on Radiological Protection and Measurements (NCRP) monthly dose limit to the embryo once a pregnancy is declared for occupationally exposed women?

Question 15 *Irradiation during which gestational stage carries the highest risk of mental retardation?*

Answer 15

The early fetal period, which occurs during weeks 8 to 15 of gestation in humans, carries the highest risk for mental retardation when exposed to radiation.

Hall EJ, Giaccia AJ. Effects of radiation on the embryo and fetus. In: Hall EJ, Giaccia AJ, eds. *Radiobiology for the Radiologist.* 7th ed. Philadelphia, PA: Lippincott Williams & Wilkins; 2012:174–187.

Question 16 *What threshold dose is thought to cause mental retardation?*

Answer 16

Mental retardation is considered deterministic in nature and a threshold dose of 0.3 Gy is necessary to kill enough cells for mental retardation to manifest. Deterministic effects are those that have dose thresholds to cause the effect and where the degree of severity increases with dose.

Hall EJ, Giaccia AJ. Effects of radiation on the embryo and fetus. In: Hall EJ, Giaccia AJ, eds. *Radiobiology for the Radiologist.* 7th ed. Philadelphia, PA: Lippincott Williams & Wilkins; 2012:174–187.

Question 17 *What is the intelligence quotient (IQ) decrement per Gy from atomic bomb survivor data?*

Answer 17

IQ loss is approximately 21 points per Gy during gestational weeks 8 to 15 and approximately 13 points per Gy during gestational weeks 16 to 25. In contrast, there was no evidence of radiation-related IQ decrement for individuals exposed to radiation within 0 to 7 weeks of fertilization or from the 26th week of gestation and beyond.

Schull WJ, Otake M. *Effects on Intelligence of Prenatal Exposure to Ionizing Radiation.* Hiroshima, Japan: Radiation Effects Research Foundation; 1986.
Schull WJ, Otake M, Yoshimaru H. *Effect on Intelligence Test Score of Prenatal Exposure to Ionizing Radiation in Hiroshima and Nagasaki.* Hiroshima, Japan: Radiation Effects Research Foundation; 1988.

Question 18 *What is the National Council on Radiological Protection and Measurements (NCRP) monthly dose limit to the embryo once a pregnancy is declared for occupationally exposed women?*

Answer 18

0.5 mSv per month is the recommendation and is designed to minimize the risk of mental retardation, congenital malformations, and carcinogenesis.

Hall EJ, Giaccia AJ. Effects of radiation on the embryo and fetus. In: Hall EJ, Giaccia AJ, eds. *Radiobiology for the Radiologist.* 7th ed. Philadelphia, PA: Lippincott Williams & Wilkins; 2012:174–187.

Question 19
What generalizations can be made regarding pelvic irradiation during pregnancy?

Question 20
When does the thyroid of a developing fetus incorporate radioactive iodine?

Question 21
What should a physician document when a pregnant patient is to receive radiation therapy (RT)?

Question 22
What is the approximate radiation dose to a fetus from a CT scan of the pelvis and abdomen?

Question 23
In a pregnant patient receiving breast irradiation for breast cancer (without shielding), what is the approximate dose exposed to the fetus from internal scatter?

Question 19 *What generalizations can be made regarding pelvic irradiation during pregnancy?*

Answer 19

Large doses of radiation delivered during preimplantation and early implantation may result in the abortion of embryos and are unlikely to produce severe abnormalities in children who survive. Irradiation between 4 and 11 weeks of gestation may result in severe abnormalities of many organs sensitive to radiation including the brain, eyes, genitals, and skeletal systems. Between 12 and 16 weeks, stunted growth, microcephaly, and mental retardation are frequently present, whereas irradiation between 16 and 19 weeks may lead to a milder degree of these abnormalities. Irradiation beyond 20 weeks of gestation is unlikely to produce gross organ or system abnormalities.

Dekaban AS. Abnormalities in children exposed to x-radiation during various stages of gestation: tentative timetable of radiation injury to the human fetus. Part I. *National Inst of Health*, 1968;9(9):471–477.

Question 20 *When does the thyroid of a developing fetus incorporate radioactive iodine?*

Answer 20

The thyroid of a developing fetus will incorporate radioactive iodine from about the 10th week of gestation onward.

Hyer S, Pratt B, Newbold K, Hamer C. Outcome of pregnancy after exposure to radioiodine in utero. *Endocr Pract.* 2011;1–10.
Shanklin DR. Pathologic studies of fetal thyroid development. *Adv Perinat Thyroidol.* 1991;299:27–46 (Springer US).

Question 21 *What should a physician document when a pregnant patient is to receive radiation therapy (RT)?*

Answer 21

The physician should document the following: time of gestation, estimated dose to fetus, geometry of shielding, basis of recommendations to patient with full references, and informed consent.

Stovall M, Blackwell CR, Cundiff J, et al. Fetal dose from radiotherapy with photon beams: report of AAPM Radiation Therapy Committee Task Group No. 36. *Medical Physics.* 1995;22(1):63–82.

Question 22 *What is the approximate radiation dose to a fetus from a CT scan of the pelvis and abdomen?*

Answer 22

The dose to the fetus from a CT of the abdomen and pelvis is typically about 0.01 to 0.04 Gy.

International Commission on Radiological Protection. Pregnancy and medical radiation. *Ann ICRP.* 2000;30:1–43.

Question 23 *In a pregnant patient receiving breast irradiation for breast cancer (without shielding), what is the approximate dose exposed to the fetus from internal scatter?*

Answer 23

A fetus that is in the true pelvis will be exposed to 0.1% to 0.3% of the total dose, or 0.05 to 0.15 Gy, for a typical regimen of 50 Gy. Later in pregnancy, a larger fetus may receive more than 2 Gy due to closer proximity to the radiation field.

Fenig E, Mishaeli M, Kalish Y, et al. Pregnancy and radiation. *Cancer Treat Rev.* 2001;27(1):1–7.

Question 24

What is the risk of childhood cancers and leukemia after in utero exposure to radiation?

Question 25

What types of growth retardation are seen after exposure to in utero irradiation?

Question 24 *What is the risk of childhood cancers and leukemia after in utero exposure to radiation?*

Answer 24

At a fetal dose of 0.01 Gy, the risk of developing a childhood cancer or leukemia is 3 to 4 per 1,000 persons compared to a baseline incidence in the general population of 2 to 3 per 1,000 persons.

Kal HB, Struikmans H. Radiotherapy during pregnancy: fact and fiction. *Lancet Oncol.* 2005;6(5):328–333.

Question 25 *What types of growth retardation are seen after exposure to in utero irradiation?*

Answer 25

Based on data from children exposed in utero in Hiroshima and Nagasaki, growth retardation can be seen in height, weight, and head diameter. By comparing children exposed within 1,500 m of the hypocenter versus more than 3,000 m, those closer to the hypocenter were 2.25 cm shorter in height, 3 kg lighter in weight, and 1.1 cm smaller in head diameter. These differences persisted into adulthood.

Hall EJ, Giaccia AJ. Effects of radiation on the embryo and fetus. In: Hall EJ, Giaccia AJ, eds. *Radiobiology for the Radiologist.* 7th ed. Philadelphia, PA: Lippincott Williams & Wilkins; 2012:174–187.

20

DOSES AND RISKS IN NONRADIATION ONCOLOGY SUBSPECIALTIES

FRANK DONG, KEVIN WUNDERLE, AND SALIM BALIK

Question 1

What is the standardized computed tomography (CT) dose metric?

Question 2

How are computed tomography dose index (CTDI) and $CTDI_w$ measured?

Turn page to see the answers.

Question 1 *What is the standardized computed tomography (CT) dose metric?*

Answer 1

The CT dose index (CTDI) is the standardized CT dose metric that is recognized internationally by the International Electrotechnical Commission (IEC). CTDI is measured in 1 of 2 cylindrical phantoms made of polymethyl methacrylate (PMMA), also called acrylic; the attenuation properties of this material closely resemble those of soft tissue. One phantom (the body CTDI phantom) has a diameter of 32 cm, which represents an average human torso. The other phantom (the head CTDI phantom) has a diameter of 16 cm and represents an average adult head. The IEC 60601-2-44 standard recommends that the CTDI for an adult human torso be determined using the 32-cm body phantom and that the CTDI for a head (adult or pediatric) be determined using the 16-cm head phantom. Currently, the CTDI used for a pediatric torso varies, with some vendors using the 16-cm head phantom and others using the 32-cm body phantom. The recently revised IEC 60601-2-44 standard recommends using the 32-cm body phantom for both adult and pediatric bodies to avoid confusion.

IEC 60601-2-44:2009 Medical electrical equipment—Part 2-44: Particular requirements for the basic safety and essential performance of x-ray equipment for CT. February 2009.

McCollough C, Cody D, Edyvean S, et al. *The Measurement, Reporting, and Management of Radiation Dose in CT.* AAPM Report No. 96; January, 2008.

Question 2 *How are computed tomography dose index (CTDI) and CTDI$_w$ measured?*

Answer 2

CTDI is defined as the integrated absorbed dose along the z-axis of the CTDI phantom, normalized by the total beam collimation. The integrated radiation exposure is measured by a 100-mm pencil ion chamber and then converted to the absorbed dose to the phantom. The measured CTDI value is labeled as CTDI$_{100}$, where "100" represents the length of the ion chamber in mm. CTDI$_{100}$ is measured at both center and peripheral positions in the phantom; the ion chamber can be inserted into holes at those locations (the holes are usually plugged with pins made of the same acrylic material). The weighted average of the peripheral and central dose values (CTDI$_w$) is calculated as:

$$CTDI_w = \frac{2}{3} \times CTDI_{100}(\text{peripheral}) + \frac{1}{3} \times CTDI_{100}(\text{center})$$

Bauhs JA, Vrieze TJ, Primak AN, Bruesewitz MR, McCollough CH. CT dosimetry: comparison of measurement techniques and devices. *Radiographics.* 2008;28:245–253.

McCollough C, Cody D, Edyvean S, et al. *The Measurement, Reporting, and Management of Radiation Dose in CT.* AAPM Report No. 96; January, 2008.

McNitt-Gray M. AAPM/RSNA physics tutorial for residents: radiation dose in CT. *Radiographics.* 2002;22: 1541–1553.

Question 3

How is computed tomography dose index volume ($CTDI_{vol}$) defined?

Question 4

Is computed tomography dose index volume ($CTDI_{vol}$) the same as patient dose?

Question 3 *How is computed tomography dose index volume (CTDI$_{vol}$) defined?*

Answer 3

CTDI$_w$ is the weighted average of the dose absorbed by the phantom during an axial scan without table movement. However, most clinical CT scans use helical mode, in which x-ray exposure is turned on as the patient table moves. To account for the table movement, a helical pitch factor (table movement per revolution/total beam collimation) is used to scale the CTDI$_w$ so that a volume-averaged CTDI (CTDI$_{vol}$) can be calculated:

$$CTDI_{vol} = \frac{CTDI_w}{Pitch\ factor}$$

All commercial CT vendors are required to display CTDI$_{vol}$ as one of the radiation dose metrics for each scan (the other metric is dose-length product [DLP], discussed in Question 5) and must also save this information in a radiation dose structured report.

Bauhs J, Vrieze T, Primak A, et al. CT dosimetry: comparison of measurement techniques and devices. *Radiographics.* 2008;28:245–253.

McCollough C, Cody D, Edyvean S, et al. *The Measurement, Reporting, and Management of Radiation Dose in CT.* AAPM Report No. 96; January, 2008.

McNitt-Gray M. AAPM/RSNA physics tutorial for residents: radiation dose in CT. *Radiographics.* 2002;22: 1541–1553.

Question 4 *Is computed tomography dose index volume (CTDI$_{vol}$) the same as patient dose?*

Answer 4

Because CTDI$_{vol}$ is defined as the volume-averaged radiation dose to a standard-sized cylindrical phantom, it is not equivalent to the radiation dose received by a patient. CTDI$_{vol}$ is used for three main applications: (a) to quantify a CT scanner's radiation exposure output, (b) to perform scanner quality control, and (c) to compare exposure between makes or models for similar protocol settings or between different protocols on the same scanner.

Patient-specific dose can be estimated based on CTDI$_{vol}$ and other acquisition parameters such as tube potential, tube current, and scan coverage and patient-specific information such as patient weight, age, sex, and location relative to the x-ray tube. Monte Carlo simulation is often used to estimate patient-specific dose based on CT images or realistic patient models.

McNitt-Gray M. AAPM/RSNA physics tutorial for residents: radiation dose in CT. *Radiographics.* 2002;22: 1541–1553.

Question 5

What is dose-length product (DLP) and how can it be used to estimate effective dose?

Question 6

What are the radiation risks associated with computed tomography (CT) examinations?

Question 5 *What is dose-length product (DLP) and how can it be used to estimate effective dose?*

Answer 5

DLP is defined as the product of computed tomography dose index volume ($CTDI_{vol}$) and scan length. DLP is proportional to the total energy deposited in a patient from a CT scan. In general, DLP values for multiple scans of the same body region can be added.

DLP from a CT examination can be used to estimate effective dose for the purpose of radiation risk assessment. To convert DLP to effective dose in mSv, a conversion factor (k-factor) can be used (see the following table). k-Factors are determined from Monte Carlo simulations and depend on the body region (organs irradiated) and patient age. For example, the k-factor for an adult head CT scan is 0.0021 mSv/(mGy*cm), whereas the k-factor for a newborn is 0.011 mSv/(mGy*cm), indicating that the newborn is more sensitive to radiation than is the adult patient.

Table of age-dependent conversion factor *k* for the effective dose from DLP

Region of Body	k (mSv mGy^{-1} cm^{-1})				
	0-Year-Old	1-Year-Old	5-Year-Old	10-Year-Old	Adult
Head and neck	0.013	0.0085	0.0057	0.0042	0.0031
Head	0.011	0.0067	0.0040	0.0032	0.0021
Neck	0.017	0.012	0.011	0.0079	0.0059
Chest	0.039	0.026	0.018	0.013	0.014
Abdomen/pelvis	0.049	0.030	0.020	0.015	0.015
Trunk	0.044	0.028	0.019	0.014	0.015

Source: Reprinted with permission from AAPM. *The Measurement, Reporting, and Management of Radiation Dose in CT.* AAPM Report No. 96. College Park, MD: American Association of Physicists in Medicine; January 2008.

McCollough C, Cody D, Edyvean S, et al. *The Measurement, Reporting, and Management of Radiation Dose in CT.* AAPM Report No. 96; January, 2008.

McNitt-Gray M. AAPM/RSNA physics tutorial for residents: radiation dose in CT. *Radiographics.* 2002;22:1541–1553.

Question 6 *What are the radiation risks associated with computed tomography (CT) examinations?*

Answer 6

Radiation-related risks can be deterministic (e.g., skin burn, hair loss), stochastic (e.g., cancer, genetic mutation), or both. Deterministic effects are very rare with diagnostic imaging procedures using ionizing radiation and are usually due to a malfunction or operator error. In a properly performed CT study, the skin entrance dose is generally much less than 2 Gy, which is near the dose threshold to induce transient erythema.

Effective dose is often used to assess the risk of stochastic effects, including carcinogenesis. The typical effective dose from a CT study is well under 50 mSv. According to a position statement on the radiation risks for medical imaging procedures from the American Association of Physicists in Medicine (AAPM), "Risks of medical imaging at effective doses below 50 mSv for single procedures or 100 mSv for multiple procedures over short periods are too low to be detectable and may be nonexistent. Predictions of hypothetical cancer incidence and deaths in patient populations exposed to such low doses are highly speculative and should be discouraged."

Even though the risk from a single CT examination is minimal or may be unknown, it is still prudent to follow the "as low as reasonably achievable" (ALARA) rule, especially for pediatric patients.

Bushberg JT, Seibert JA, Leidholdt EM, Boone JM. *Chapter 20 Radiation Biology, in the Essential Physics of Medical Imaging.* 3rd ed. Philadelphia, PA: Lippincott Williams & Wilkins; 2012:751–836.

Hall EJ, Giaccia AJ. Radiation carcinogenesis. In: Hall EJ, Giaccia AJ, eds. *Radiobiology for the Radiologist.* 7th ed. Philadelphia, PA: Lippincott Williams & Wilkins; 2006:135–153.

Sadetzki S, Mandelzweig L. Childhood exposure to external ionizing radiation and solid cancer risk. *Br J Cancer.* 2009;100:1021–1025.

Question 7
Would the radiation risk from multiple computed tomography (CT) examinations be cumulative?

Question 8
How much does computed tomography (CT) contribute to the population dose among diagnostic medical imaging procedures?

Question 7 *Would the radiation risk from multiple computed tomography (CT) examinations be cumulative?*

Answer 7

In general, the radiation risk from a CT examination follows a stochastic risk model if the examination is performed properly. In a stochastic model, the probability that an adverse event will occur (not the size of the event) is proportional to the insult (the amount of radiation dose) that the target receives.

All four major radiation protection agencies (International Commission on Radiological Protection [ICRP], National Council on Radiation Protection and Measurements [NCRP], Biological Effects of Ionizing Radiation [BEIR], and United Nations Scientific Committee on the Effects of Atomic Radiation [UNSCEAR]) support the linear no-threshold (LNT) risk model as a reasonable risk predictor for radiation protection purposes. The LNT risk model indicates that there is no threshold to radiation-induced risk: all radiation exposure is assumed to carry some risk for cancer, and thus there is no safe level of radiation in terms of carcinogenesis. The other assumption of the LNT model is that excessive cancer risk (above the natural occurrence rate of cancer, which is ~ 42% in the United States) is linearly proportional to the amount of radiation dose. When cancer risk prediction is based on the LNT stochastic model, each radiation event is independent, and only the probability of cancer occurrence is proportional to the radiation dose. With this model, the risk of cancer occurrence from the next CT examination is not increased or decreased based on the number of CT examinations performed previously. The decision to order another CT scan should therefore not be based on the number of previous CT examinations performed if CT is the best diagnostic tool for the patient.

Durand D, Dixon R, Morin R. Utilization strategies for cumulative dose estimates: a review and rational assessment. *J Am Coll Radiol.* 2012;9:480–485.

Question 8 *How much does computed tomography (CT) contribute to the population dose among diagnostic medical imaging procedures?*

Answer 8

Because of its superior image quality, fast scan time, and relative ease of operation, CT use has increased more quickly than the use of any other diagnostic imaging modality. According to one statistic, more than 80 million CT examinations were performed in the United States in 2008. From 1990 to 2006, CT use increased more than 10% each year. This rapid increase in CT use has also contributed to an overall increase in population dose (the annual collective effective dose divided by the size of the U.S. population) from the medical use of radiation. In 2009, CT contributed approximately 50% of the medical-related population dose from diagnostic imaging procedures.

Brenner DJ, Hall EJ. Computed tomography: an increasing source of radiation exposure. *N Engl J Med.* 2007;357(22):2277–2284.

Brenner DJ, Shuryak I, Einstein AJ. Impact of reduced patient life expectancy on potential cancer risks from radiologic imaging. *Radiology.* 2011;261(1):193–198.

Question 9

What are the typical effective doses from a routine abdomen/pelvis scan and head scan?

Question 10

What are the common techniques used to reduce the computed tomography (CT) radiation dose?

Question 9 *What are the typical effective doses from a routine abdomen/pelvis scan and head scan?*

Answer 9

The effective dose from a routine abdomen/pelvis scan ranges from 7 mSv (abdomen) to 12 mSv (abdomen + pelvis). The effective dose from a routine head scan ranges from 1 mSv to 3 mSv. The following table reports effective doses from typical x-ray radiographic and computed tomography (CT) examinations:

Typical effective dose for several common imaging procedures

Non-CT Typical Effective Dose Values (mSv)		CT Typical Effective Dose Values (mSv)	
Hand radiograph	< 0.1	Head CT	1–2
Dental bitewing	< 0.1	Chest CT	5–7
Chest radiograph	0.1–0.2	Abdomen CT	5–7
Mammogram	0.3–0.6	Pelvis CT	3–4
Lumbar spine radiograph	0.5–1.5	Abdomen and pelvis CT	8–14
Barium enema exam	3–6	Coronary artery calcium CT	1–3
Coronary angiogram (diagnostic)	5–10	Coronary CT angiography	5–15
Sestamibi myocardial perfusion	13–16		
Thallium myocardial perfusion	35–40		
Average U.S. background		3.0	

Source: Reprinted with permission from AAPM. *The Measurement, Reporting, and Management of Radiation Dose in CT.* AAPM Report No. 96. College Park, MD: American Association of Physicists in Medicine; January 2008.

Mettler F, Huda W, Yoshizumi T, et al. Effective doses in radiology and diagnostic nuclear medicine. *Radiology.* 2008;248:254–263.

Question 10 *What are the common techniques used to reduce the computed tomography (CT) radiation dose?*

Answer 10

Common techniques available from most CT vendors to reduce or optimize the CT radiation dose include (a) automatic tube current modulation (also called automatic exposure control [AEC]) and (b) patient size specific protocols.

Patient attenuation to x-ray photons varies along the longitudinal direction and within the imaging plane (e.g., different anteroposterior [AP] vs lateral patient thickness). CT scanners should be able to modulate the tube current (and hence the dose) automatically based on attenuation changes. Attenuation changes depend on the anatomy being imaged and total attenuation through that anatomy (e.g., larger lateral attenuation requires greater output than AP).

Patient size specific protocols are commonly used to reduce the dose for small patients, especially for the pediatric patient population. Pediatric patients are more vulnerable to radiation damage because some of their organs may still be under development; they also have a longer life span ahead of them during which any damage from radiation can be expressed. It is imperative, therefore, to reduce the radiation dose to this patient population, as proposed by the Image Gently campaign. The radiation dose delivered by CT examination to the pediatric patient should be based on either the age or the weight of the child. Some vendors even provide organ-based tube current modulation to reduce the dose to the gonads and/or breasts.

McCollough C, Cody D, Edyvean S, et al. *The Measurement, Reporting, and Management of Radiation Dose in CT.* AAPM Report No. 96; January, 2008.
McNitt-Gray M. AAPM/RSNA physics tutorial for residents: radiation dose in CT. *Radiographics.* 2002;22: 1541–1553.

Question 11

How do new technologies help reduce the computed tomography (CT) radiation dose?

Question 12

How does the dose distribution inside a patient differ between a computed tomography (CT) scan and a general x-ray radiograph?

Question 11 *How do new technologies help reduce the computed tomography (CT) radiation dose?*

Answer 11

In the past, cardiac CT examinations were among the diagnostic studies with the highest radiation exposure because of the challenge posed by heart motion. With the advent of new technologies such as wider detector coverage, fast gantry rotation, and ECG-gated tube modulation, radiation dose from a typical coronary CT angiogram has been reduced to a few mSv as compared to previous doses of 20 to 30 mSv.

CT iterative reconstruction is a feature that uses the information acquired during the scan and repeated reconstruction steps to produce an image with less noise or better image quality (e.g., higher spatial resolution or decreased artifacts) than is achievable using filtered back projection, the standard image reconstruction technique. Iterative reconstruction can therefore help to maintain a clinically acceptable image quality at a reduced CT radiation dose to the patient. The degree of dose reduction is dependent on the diagnostic task. For example, the radiation dose required to image kidney stones is less than that required to detect a low-contrast liver lesion; therefore, aggressive dose reduction in conjunction with iterative reconstruction has been used for kidney stones, whereas only minimal dose reduction can be achieved for liver lesion detection even with a very aggressive iterative reconstruction algorithm.

McCollough C, Cody D, Edyvean S, et al. *The Measurement, Reporting, and Management of Radiation Dose in CT.* AAPM Report No. 96; January, 2008.
McNitt-Gray M. AAPM/RSNA physics tutorial for residents: radiation dose in CT. *Radiographics.* 2002;22: 1541–1553.

Question 12 *How does the dose distribution inside a patient differ between a computed tomography (CT) scan and a general x-ray radiograph?*

Answer 12

A typical CT scan consists of multiple gantry rotations around the target region of the body with ~1,000 x-ray projections every 360°, whereas a general x-ray radiograph is a single-projection acquisition (i.e., the tube does not rotate around the target region). Because the body region is irradiated 360° during a CT scan, the dose distribution is more uniform around the target region inside the patient; the dose distribution is not uniform from a general x-ray radiograph, with the highest dose occurring at the body surface closest to the x-ray tube.

McNitt-Gray M. AAPM/RSNA physics tutorial for residents: radiation dose in CT. *Radiographics.* 2002;22: 1541–1553.

Question 13

During a head computed tomography (CT) scan, it is critical to reduce or minimize the dose to the eye lens. How well does the computed tomography dose index volume (CTDI$_{vol}$) measured on a head CTDI phantom approximate the dose to the eye lens?

Question 14

What is the typical conceptus dose from a single computed tomography (CT) acquisition for an abdomen/pelvis examination?

Question 13 *During a head computed tomography (CT) scan, it is critical to reduce or minimize the dose to the eye lens. How well does the computed tomography dose index (CTDI$_{vol}$) measured on a head CTDI phantom approximate the dose to the eye lens?*

Answer 13

CT neuroimaging perfusion scans are capable of delivering a high radiation dose to the skin and eye lenses. If precautions are not taken, the radiation dose can reach levels capable of causing deterministic injuries to the eye lens, such as cataracts. Compared with Monte Carlo simulation using computerized patient models, CTDI$_{vol}$ overestimates the dose to the eye lens by 33% to 106% depending on the tube potential, scanner make/model, and patient size. Therefore, using CTDI$_{vol}$ as an approximation of the eye lens dose is overly conservative.

Zhang D, Cagnon CH, Villablanca JP, et al. Estimating peak skin and eye lens dose from neuroperfusion examinations: use of Monte Carlo based simulations and comparisons to CTDI$_{vol}$, AAPM Report No. 111, and ImPACT dosimetry tool values. *Medical Physics*. 2013;40(9):091901-1-9.

Question 14 *What is the typical conceptus dose from a single computed tomography (CT) acquisition for an abdomen/pelvis examination?*

Answer 14

CT is associated with higher radiation exposure than general x-ray radiography. It is important to estimate the fetal dose before an abdomen/pelvis CT examination is performed, as the scan may overlap the fetus. The conceptus dose from a CT examination is highly dependent on the location of the uterus relative to the axial scan planes, the gestational age of the conceptus, CT acquisition parameters, and patient habitus.

For CT abdomen/pelvis examinations, the conceptus is most likely within the scan coverage. In a study of 24 pregnant patients who underwent abdominal/pelvic examinations with conceptus gestational ages ranging from 5 to 36 weeks, the image data were used to generate 24 models of maternal and fetal anatomy and Monte Carlo simulation was used to estimate the fetal dose based on these patient models. The average fetal dose from the simulation (tube potential at 120 kVp) was 10.8 mGy/100 mAs. For a typical abdomen/pelvis examination, 200 mAs is often used, which would result in a fetal dose of 22 mGy.

According to American College of Radiology (ACR) guidelines for imaging pregnant patients, any diagnostic imaging procedure delivering less than 50 mGy of fetal dose has essentially no deterministic effect on a conceptus of any gestational age. Most diagnostic imaging procedures (including CT and nuclear medicine) fall into this category, except for some fluoroscopically guided interventional procedures.

Angel E, Wellnitz CV, Goodsitt MM, et al. Radiation dose to the fetus for pregnant patients undergoing multidetector CT imaging: Monte Carlo simulations estimating fetal dose for a range of gestational age and patient size. *Radiology*. 2008;249:220–227.

Pollack MS, Ali S, Bigongiari LR, et al. ACR-SPR practice guideline for imaging pregnant or potentially pregnant adolescents and women with ionizing radiation. *Resolution*. 48, revised 2013.

Question 15

During a chest computed tomography (CT) scan, would wrapping a lead apron around a pregnant patient's pelvis reduce the radiation dose to the fetus?

Question 16

For a mammography scan, what is the average glandular dose (AGD) limit set by the American College of Radiology (ACR)?

Question 17

What is the radiation dose from x-ray radiography compared to the doses from computed tomography (CT) or fluoroscopically guided interventional procedures?

Question 15 *During a chest computed tomography (CT) scan, would wrapping a lead apron around a pregnant patient's pelvis reduce the radiation dose to the fetus?*

Answer 15

It is true that wrapping a lead apron around a pregnant patient's pelvic area will reduce the overall radiation dose to the fetus. However, because most of the radiation dose to the fetus from a chest CT scan is due to internal scatter (i.e., the scatter from internal organs), using a lead apron may have a limited effect on reducing scatter radiation to the fetus. Lead apron shielding does provide the patient with a sense of protection and reassurance even though the dose reduction to the fetus with this technique is minimal.

McCollough CH, Schueler BA, Atwell TD, et al. Radiation exposure and pregnancy: when should we be concerned? *Radiographics*. 2007;27:909–918.

Question 16 *For a mammography scan, what is the average glandular dose (AGD) limit set by the American College of Radiology (ACR)?*

Answer 16

If a grid is used, the AGD limit (for a 4.2-cm thick breast) set by the ACR is less than 3 mGy per image. If no grid is used, the AGD is less than 1 mGy per image. In general, both screening and diagnostic mammography deliver low radiation doses to the patient. However, as healthy patients are the targeted population for screening mammography, it is imperative to follow the "as low as reasonably achievable (ALARA)" rule to minimize radiation risk.

Bushberg JT, Seibert JA, Leidholdt EM, Boone JM. *Mammography, in the Essential Physics of Medical Imaging.* 3rd ed. Philadelphia, PA: Lippincott Williams & Wilkins; 2012:238–281.

Question 17 *What is the radiation dose from x-ray radiography compared to the doses from computed tomography (CT) or fluoroscopically guided interventional procedures?*

Answer 17

In general, the effective dose from a general radiography examination is lower than doses from CT scans, fluoroscopically guided interventional procedures targeted at the same body region, and most nuclear medicine procedures. For example, chest x-ray radiography (two views) has a typical effective dose of 0.1 mSv, whereas a chest CT scan can deliver more than 7 mSv. Depending on the complexity of the fluoroscopically guided interventional procedure, the effective dose can be much higher, such as 40 or 50 mSv.

Mettler F, Huda W, Yoshizumi T, et al. Effective doses in radiology and diagnostic nuclear medicine. *Radiology*. 2008;248:254–263.

Question 18

What are typical measures used in general x-ray imaging to reduce radiation dose to the patient?

Question 19

What are typical measures used in diagnostic imaging procedures to protect radiation workers?

Question 20

Exposure index (EI) and deviation index (DI) are often used in x-ray radiography to indicate whether the digital detector is overexposed or underexposed. Can EI and DI be used as radiation dose metrics? What are the other radiation dose metrics used in conventional x-ray radiography?

Question 18 *What are typical measures used in general x-ray imaging to reduce radiation dose to the patient?*

Answer 18

In general x-ray imaging, automatic exposure control (AEC) is used to maintain image quality while reducing unnecessary radiation to the patient. AEC systems use radiation detectors to measure the dose incident on the image receptor. For a large patient, AEC will require increased radiation output to provide a sufficient radiation dose to the detector, whereas for a smaller patient, AEC will require less radiation output.

Matching the size of collimation with the anatomical region of interest also helps to reduce overall radiation exposure to the patient. In pediatric imaging, some technologists may open up the collimator to full size so that the entire torso is covered (resulting in a so-called "baby gram"). This type of practice unnecessarily increases the radiation exposure to the pediatric patient.

When young adult and pregnant patients are imaged, lead aprons are often provided to shield the sensitive organs from radiation.

Chaparian A, Kanani A, Baghbanian M. Reduction of radiation risks in patients undergoing some x-ray examinations by using optimal projections: a Monte Carlo program-based mathematical calculation. *J Med Phys*. 2014;39(1):32–39.

Question 19 *What are typical measures used in diagnostic imaging procedures to protect radiation workers?*

Answer 19

Three basic factors are involved in minimizing radiation exposure for workers: time, distance, and shielding.

- Time: Workers should try to minimize the amount of time they stay inside the scanning room. The total radiation dose is proportional to the duration of exposure.
- Distance: The radiation flux is inversely proportional to the square of the distance between the radiation source and the worker. Therefore, workers should stay as far away as possible from the x-ray source or radioactive materials.
- Shielding: Shielding includes structural shielding such as lead-lined doors/walls and concrete floors. Shielding also includes mobile shields and hanging drapes.

Numerous protection tools are also available for radiation workers. Most frequently used is the lead apron. For some interventional procedures, operators should use equipment such as lead glasses and thyroid shields to protect sensitive organs.

Bushberg JT, Seibert JA, Leidholdt EM, Boone JM. Radiation protection. In: Bushberg JT, Seibert JA, Leidholdt EM, Boone JM, eds. *The Essential Physics of Medical Imaging*. 3rd ed. Philadelphia, PA: Lippincott Williams & Wilkins; 2012:837–909; chap 21.

Question 20 *Exposure index (EI) and deviation index (DI) are often used in x-ray radiography to indicate whether the digital detector is overexposed or underexposed. Can EI and DI be used as radiation dose metrics? What are the other radiation dose metrics used in conventional x-ray radiography?*

Answer 20

For screen film radiography, overexposure or underexposure can be easily detected by visual observation of developed films. However, in the era of digital radiography, image brightness and contrast are no longer directly related to exposure, as both can be easily altered by postprocessing. EI and DI are intended as indicators for radiographers and radiologists to determine whether the technique used to acquire a radiograph was appropriate. If the DI is 0, the exposure matched perfectly with the target exposure, whereas a negative DI indicates a lower exposure than the target and a positive value indicates a higher exposure than the target.

Entrance skin dose, cumulative air kerma ($K_{a,r}$), and dose-area product (DAP) are often used as radiation dose metrics for conventional radiography systems.

Shepard S, Wang J, Flynn M, et al. An exposure indicator for digital radiography. American Association of Physicists in Medicine Task Group Report No. 116, July 2009:14–20.

Question 21

What is the $K_{a,r}$ and how does it relate to the patient skin entrance dose? Fluoroscopes manufactured after 2012 are required to provide either the $K_{a,r}$ or the air kerma-area-product (AKAP).

Question 22

What is the air kerma-area-product (AKAP) and how does it relate to the patient skin entrance dose? Fluoroscopes manufactured after 2012 are required to provide either the $K_{a,r}$ or AKAP.

Question 23

Are radiation-induced tissue reactions from diagnostic energy x-ray beams possible?

Question 21 *What is the $K_{a,r}$ and how does it relate to the patient skin entrance dose? Fluoroscopes manufactured after 2012 are required to provide either the $K_{a,r}$ or the air kerma-area-product (AKAP).*

Answer 21

The $K_{a,r}$ is the cumulative air kerma at the interventional reference plane or point (IRP) for a given procedure. The IRP is defined in relation to the isocenter of the c-Arm (for c-Arm type fluoroscopes) and may or may not represent the location of the skin entrance. Additionally, $K_{a,r}$ is the sum of air kerma contributions from all projections, irrespective of gantry angulation (cranial/caudal) or rotation (right anterior oblique [RAO]/left anterior oblique [LAO]). As the name implies, the $K_{a,r}$ is a quantity expressed in air and also differs from the skin entrance dose by the ratio of the mass attenuation coefficients $(((\mu/\rho)_{tissue})/((\mu/\rho)_{air}))$. For these and other reasons, $K_{a,r}$ does not directly represent the patient skin entrance dose.

Jones AK, Pasciak AS. Calculating the peak skin dose resulting from fluoroscopically guided interventions. Part I: Methods. *JACMP*. 2011;12(4):231–244.

National Council on Radiation Protection and Measurement. *Radiation Dose Management for Fluoroscopically-Guided Interventional Medical Procedures*. NCRP Report No. 168; 2010.

Wunderle KA, Gill AS. Radiation-related injuries and their management: an update. *Semin Intervent Radiol.* 2015;32:156–162.

Question 22 *What is the air kerma-area-product (AKAP) and how does it relate to the patient skin entrance dose? Fluoroscopes manufactured after 2012 are required to provide either the $K_{a,r}$ or the AKAP.*

Answer 22

The AKAP is a step further removed from the skin entrance dose than $K_{a,r}$. AKAP is the product of the air kerma at a location in the beam path and the x-ray beam field size in the same plane. This quantity is proportional to the total amount of radiation imparted to the patient. The AKAP is independent of the distance from the focal spot. Although the radiation dose rate decreases by $1/r^2$, the diverging x-ray beam increases in area as r^2; therefore, the two factors offset each other. The AKAP is poorly correlated with the skin entrance dose; however, it is better correlated with effective dose than $K_{a,r}$ given the anatomy irradiated.

National Council on Radiation Protection and Measurement. *Radiation Dose Management for Fluoroscopically-Guided Interventional Medical Procedures*. NCRP Report No. 168; 2010.

Question 23 *Are radiation-induced tissue reactions from diagnostic energy x-ray beams possible?*

Answer 23

Yes, although such reactions are rare. Skin doses in fluoroscopically guided interventions (interventional radiology, vascular surgery, cardiac catheterization, and cardiac electrophysiology) can exceed the threshold for causing erythema, epilation, dry or moist desquamation, and even necrosis.

National Council on Radiation Protection and Measurement. *Radiation Dose Management for Fluoroscopically-Guided Interventional Medical Procedures*; NCRP Report No. 168; 2010.

Wunderle KA, Gill AS. Radiation-related injuries and their management: an update. *Semin Intervent Radiol.* 2015;32:156–162.

Question 24
What are the two primary modes of operation of a fluoroscope?

Question 25
Are there dose-rate limitations for fluoroscopes?

Question 26
What is the goal of the automatic dose-rate control (ADRC) of a fluoroscope?

Question 27
What is spectral filtration and what is it used for?

Question 24 *What are the two primary modes of operation of a fluoroscope?*

Answer 24

Fluoroscopes have two primary modes of operation: fluoroscopy mode and acquisition mode. The fluoroscopic mode is the most commonly used mode; with this mode, images do not need to be recorded and are instead viewed live. Acquisition mode operates at much higher dose rates, and images must be recorded with this mode.

National Council on Radiation Protection and Measurement. *Radiation Dose Management for Fluoroscopically-Guided Interventional Medical Procedures*. NCRP Report No. 168; 2010.

Wunderle KA, Rakowski JT, Dong FF. Approaches to interventional fluoroscopic dose curves. *JACMP*. 2016;17(1): 342–352.

Question 25 *Are there dose-rate limitations for fluoroscopes?*

Answer 25

Yes, but the limitations apply only to the fluoroscopic mode of imaging. The limitations are 88 mGy/min for normal fluoroscopic imaging and 176 mGy/min for high-dose fluoroscopic imaging under a predefined geometry. In the acquisition mode, there are no dose-rate limitations set by regulations; the only limitations are those imposed by the chosen protocol or hardware limitations.

National Council on Radiation Protection and Measurement. *Radiation Dose Management for Fluoroscopically-Guided Interventional Medical Procedures*. NCRP Report No. 168; 2010.

Question 26 *What is the goal of the automatic dose-rate control (ADRC) of a fluoroscope?*

Answer 26

The goal of the ADRC is to maintain a constant dose to a region of the x-ray detector for the purpose of consistent image quality. The ADRC is responsible for automatically changing the x-ray technique factors (e.g., kVp, mA, pulse width, and copper filtration) to maximize image quality at the lowest skin entrance dose rate possible while maintaining a constant dose rate to the image receptor.

Lin PJ. The operation logic of automatic dose control of fluoroscopy system in conjunction with spectral shaping filters. *Med Phys*. 2007;34(8):3169–3172.

Wunderle KA, Rakowski JT, Dong FF. Approaches to interventional fluoroscopic dose curves. *JACMP*. 2016;17(1): 342–352.

Question 27 *What is spectral filtration and what is it used for?*

Answer 27

All modern fluoroscopes used for interventional procedures utilize spectral filters (copper filters located in the collimator) to preferentially remove low-energy x-ray photons from the beam. The result of using spectral filters is harder x-ray beams; this reduces the skin entrance dose per unit dose to the detector. Typically, larger amounts of spectral filtration are used at lower kVps; higher kVp beams are naturally harder.

Lin PJ. The operation logic of automatic dose control of fluoroscopy system in conjunction with spectral shaping filters. *Med Phys*. 2007;34(8):3169–3172.

Wunderle KA, Rakowski JT, Dong FF. Approaches to interventional fluoroscopic dose curves. *JACMP*. 2016;17(1): 342–352.

Question 28
Is the skin entrance dose well localized or is it distributed over large anatomical regions?

Question 29
How does magnification affect the radiation dose rate to the patient?

Question 30
What are the source and magnitude of the radiation dose to a physician or operator required to be in the procedure room during fluoroscopic imaging?

Question 31
What are the three primary methods for acquiring radionuclides used in nuclear medicine?

Question 28 *Is the skin entrance dose well localized or is it distributed over large anatomical regions?*

Answer 28

This is highly dependent on the type of clinical procedure being performed and, to a lesser extent, on the operator. The following is an example of the two-dimensional (2D) radiation dose distribution for a vascular surgery procedure. The darker the area, the higher the dose (the scale at the top is for reference and ranges from 0 to 20 Gy).

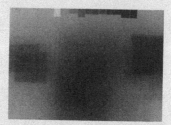

2D radiation dose distribution on a GafChromic film

Wunderle KA, Gill AS. Radiation-related injuries and their management: an update. *Semin Intervent Radiol.* 2015;32:156–162.

Question 29 *How does magnification affect the radiation dose rate to the patient?*

Answer 29

As greater magnification (smaller field of view [FOV]) is selected, the dose rate to the patient generally increases. The magnitude of the increase depends on the type of image receptor. Older image-intensifier–based systems demonstrate a well-defined relationship between the FOV and the dose. For these systems, the dose rate is proportional to the area of the image receptor being irradiated. For example, transitioning from a 9-inch FOV to a 6-inch FOV results in a $(9/6)^2 = 2.25$ increase in the dose rate. For digital detectors, the relationship is not necessarily as straightforward, but in general, greater magnification equals greater dose rate.

National Council on Radiation Protection and Measurement. *Radiation Dose Management for Fluoroscopically-Guided Interventional Medical Procedures.* NCRP Report No. 168; 2010.

Question 30 *What are the source and magnitude of the radiation dose to a physician or operator required to be in the procedure room during fluoroscopic imaging?*

Answer 30

The primary source of radiation to a person in the fluoroscopy suite during irradiation is the patient. The patient's skin entrance is the source of the highest scatter flux and, for all intents and purposes, represents the source of radiation to the operator. The rule of thumb is that the air kerma rate at 1 m laterally from the patient's skin entrance is 1/1,000 of the skin entrance air kerma.

National Council on Radiation Protection and Measurement. *Radiation Dose Management for Fluoroscopically-Guided Interventional Medical Procedures.* NCRP Report No. 168; 2010.

Question 31 *What are the three primary methods for acquiring radionuclides used in nuclear medicine?*

Answer 31

The three primary methods are cyclotron bombardment, nuclear reactor (fission products and neutron activation), and generators.

Bushberg JT, Seibert JA, Leidholdt EM, Boone JM. The *Essential Physics of Medical Imaging.* 2nd ed. Philadelphia, PA: Lippincott Williams & Wilkins; 2012:603–626.

Question 32
How are the radionuclides produced in cyclotron?

Question 33
How are the nuclear reactors utilized in radionuclide production?

Question 34
How is the ^{99m}Tc produced in a generator?

Question 32 *How are the radionuclides produced in cyclotron?*

Answer 32

With the cyclotron bombardment method, heavy charged particles such as protons are reaccelerated in circular paths to high kinetic energies to overcome the repulsive Coulomb barrier of the target nuclei. The collision of the accelerated particles with the target nuclei causes nuclear reactions and in general produces short-lived unstable nuclei of interest. Most cyclotron-produced radionuclides are neutron poor and decay by electron capture or positron emission, making this the method of choice for producing PET radionuclides. These radionuclides include ^{18}F, ^{67}Ga, ^{201}Tl, ^{123}I, ^{11}C, ^{15}O, ^{13}N, ^{111}In, and ^{57}Co.

Bushberg JT, Seibert JA, Leidholdt EM, Boone JM. *The Essential Physics of Medical Imaging*. 2nd ed. Philadelphia, PA: Lippincott Williams & Wilkins; 2012:603–626.

Hall EJ, Giaccia AJ. Dose and risks in diagnostic radiology, interventional radiology and cardiology, and nuclear medicine. In: Hall EJ, Giaccia AJ, eds. *Radiobiology for the Radiologist*. 7th ed. Philadelphia, PA: Lippincott Williams & Wilkins; 2012:222–252.

Question 33 *How are the nuclear reactors utilized in radionuclide production?*

Answer 33

Fission products: Because neutrons are uncharged particles, they can easily penetrate the target nucleus without being accelerated. Absorption of neutrons by heavy nuclei induces splitting of the nuclei (fission). The fission of uranium creates more than 200 radionuclides. The three fission products most often used in nuclear medicine are ^{99}Mo, ^{131}I, and ^{133}Xe.

Neutron activation: Neutrons produced by the fission of uranium are captured by stable nuclei. This results in the production of various radionuclides used in nuclear medicine such as ^{32}P, ^{51}Cr, ^{125}I, ^{89}Sr, ^{58}Co, ^{59}Fe, and ^{153}Sm.

Bushberg JT, Seibert JA, Leidholdt EM, Boone JM. *The Essential Physics of Medical Imaging*. 2nd ed. Philadelphia, PA: Lippincott Williams & Wilkins; 2012:603–626.

Hall EJ, Giaccia AJ. Dose and risks in diagnostic radiology, interventional radiology and cardiology, and nuclear medicine. In: Hall EJ, Giaccia AJ, eds. *Radiobiology for the Radiologist*. 7th ed. Philadelphia, PA: Lippincott Williams & Wilkins; 2012:222–252.

Question 34 *How is the ^{99m}Tc produced in a generator?*

Answer 34

Generators are devices in which a parent radionuclide is kept and the daughter is extracted for clinical use. For example, ^{99m}Tc is one of the most important radionuclides used in nuclear medicine, but because of its short half-life (6 hours), it is difficult to store for clinical use. This problem is overcome by keeping the parent radionuclide, ^{99}Mo, in a generator; this radionuclide decays to produce ^{99m}Tc. Another example is ^{82}Rb, which is obtained from the decay of ^{82}Sr.

Bushberg JT, Seibert JA, Leidholdt EM, Boone JM. *The Essential Physics of Medical Imaging*. 2nd ed. Philadelphia, PA: Lippincott Williams & Wilkins; 2012:603–626.

Hall EJ, Giaccia AJ. Dose and risks in diagnostic radiology, interventional radiology and cardiology, and nuclear medicine. In: Hall EJ, Giaccia AJ, eds. *Radiobiology for the Radiologist*. 7th ed. Philadelphia, PA: Lippincott Williams & Wilkins; 2012:222–252.

Question 35

How does the ratio of neutrons and protons change for stable nuclei?

Question 36

What are the two main diagnostic imaging modalities that use radionuclides? What are their basic principles of operation?

Question 35 *How does the ratio of neutrons and protons change for stable nuclei?*

Answer 35

Stable nuclides with a low mass number have an approximately equal number of neutrons and protons. As the mass number increases, there will be more neutrons than protons in stable nuclides. For example, the tungsten nucleus (^{184}W) has 74 protons and 110 neutrons.

Huda W, Slone RM. *Review of Radiologic Physics*. 3rd ed. Philadelphia, PA: Lippincott Williams & Wilkins; 2003:139–158.

Question 36 *What are the two main diagnostic imaging modalities that use radionuclides? What are their basic principles of operation?*

Answer 36

Depending on the purpose of the scan, the radionuclide is injected, swallowed, or inhaled and allowed to accumulate in the target organ or whole body. The distribution of radioactive emissions from the radionuclide is identified by detectors or cameras surrounding the patient. Nuclear medicine images lack sufficient anatomical detail and are therefore often coregistered to CT or MRI data sets.

Single-photon emission computed tomography (SPECT): Radionuclides used in SPECT imaging emit either gamma rays after isomeric transition or characteristic x-rays after electron capture decay. SPECT uses a circular array of detectors or a rotating gamma camera system with up to four detector heads to detect the emitted radiation. The most commonly used radionuclide in SPECT is ^{99m}Tc. This agent has a half-life of 6 hours, which allows for same-day scanning procedures while keeping patient radiation exposure low. The typical spatial resolution of clinical SPECT images ranges from ~8 to 12 mm.

PET: PET imaging is based on the simultaneous detection of a pair of 511-keV photons arising from the annihilation of a positron and electron. The most common radionuclide used in PET imaging is ^{18}F in the form of fluorodeoxyglucose (FDG). PET imaging systems contain rings of scintillators surrounding the patient that are coupled to photomultiplier tubes. The typical spatial resolution of PET images ranges from 4 to 6 mm.

Bushberg JT, Seibert JA, Leidholdt EM, Boone JM. *The Essential Physics of Medical Imaging*. 2nd ed. Philadelphia, PA: Lippincott Williams & Wilkins; 2012:703–736.

Hall EJ, Giaccia AJ. Dose and risks in diagnostic radiology, interventional radiology and cardiology, and nuclear medicine. In: Hall EJ, Giaccia AJ, eds. *Radiobiology for the Radiologist*. 7th ed. Philadelphia, PA: Lippincott Williams & Wilkins; 2012:222–252.

Khalil MM, Tremoleda JL, Bayomy TB, Gsell W. Molecular SPECT imaging: an overview. *Int J Mol Imaging*. 2011;15.

Question 37
What are the associated risks of administering radionuclides for diagnostic scans?

Question 38
Which organs receive the highest dose from a typical [^{18}F]FDG PET procedure?

Question 39
What is the typical activity administered during the [^{18}F]FDG PET procedure, its effective dose, and the associated radiation-induced cancer risk?

Question 40
Which nuclear medicine diagnostic procedure requires more shielding for occupational exposure precautions, positron emission tomography (PET) or single-photon emission computed tomography (SPECT)? Why?

Question 37 *What are the associated risks of administering radionuclides for diagnostic scans?*

Answer 37

The primary risk from radiation delivered during nuclear medicine imaging is a stochastic risk of radiation-induced leukemia and/or cancer. The risk is related to the effective dose. Because different organs have different sensitivities to radiation, doses to critical organs are particularly important and are dependent on the biodistribution and resident time of the radiopharmaceutical.

Hall EJ, Giaccia AJ. Dose and risks in diagnostic radiology, interventional radiology and cardiology, and nuclear medicine. In: Hall EJ, Giaccia AJ, eds. *Radiobiology for the Radiologist*. 7th ed. Philadelphia, PA: Lippincott Williams & Wilkins; 2012:222–252.

Question 38 *Which organs receive the highest dose from a typical [¹⁸F]FDG PET procedure?*

Answer 38

The bladder wall typically receives the highest dose (~70 mGy per 10 mCi) because of the accumulation of the radionuclide in the bladder for biological clearance. Other organs that receive relatively higher doses are the heart, spleen, brain, and kidneys, organs that use large amounts of glucose or are involved in waste clearance.

Hall EJ, Giaccia AJ. Dose and risks in diagnostic radiology, interventional radiology and cardiology, and nuclear medicine. In: Hall EJ, Giaccia AJ, eds. *Radiobiology for the Radiologist*. 7th ed. Philadelphia, PA: Lippincott Williams & Wilkins; 2012:222–252.

Question 39 *What is the typical activity administered during the [¹⁸F]FDG PET procedure, its effective dose, and the associated radiation-induced cancer risk?*

Answer 39

Typically, 370 MBq (10 mCi) is administered. According to the International Commission on Radiological Protection (ICRP) publication 53, the effective dose is approximately 11 mSv. The associated radiation-induced risk of cancer is 8%/Sv × 0.011 mSv ~0.09%.

Hall EJ, Giaccia AJ. Dose and risks in diagnostic radiology, interventional radiology and cardiology, and nuclear medicine. In: Hall EJ, Giaccia AJ, eds. *Radiobiology for the Radiologist*. 7th ed. Philadelphia, PA: Lippincott Williams & Wilkins; 2012:222–252.
ICRP Publication 53. Radiation dose to patients from radiopharmaceuticals. *Ann. ICRP*. 1988;18:1–4.

Question 40 *Which nuclear medicine diagnostic procedure requires more shielding for occupational exposure precautions, positron emission tomography (PET) or single-photon emission computed tomography (SPECT)? Why?*

Answer 40

Because of the relatively high-energy photons (511 keV) that are emitted after electron–positron annihilation, shielding requirements are an important consideration in the design of a PET facility. Also, large initial activities must be prepared because of the short half-life of the radionuclides used in PET imaging. This causes the occupational radiation exposure to be higher for PET technologists. The energy of emitted radiation for radionuclides used in SPECT imaging is much lower and is mainly attenuated by the patient's body.

Hall EJ, Giaccia AJ. Dose and risks in diagnostic radiology, interventional radiology and cardiology, and nuclear medicine. In: Hall EJ, Giaccia AJ, eds. *Radiobiology for the Radiologist*. 7th ed. Philadelphia, PA: Lippincott Williams & Wilkins; 2012:222–252.

Question 41

How is the absorbed dose to internal organs from nuclear medicine procedures calculated?

Question 42

What is the main concern following radioactive iodine 131 (I-131) therapy for the treatment of thyroid cancer?

Question 43

What is the risk of developing leukemia and thyroid cancer after I-131 therapy for the treatment of hyperthyroidism in adults?

Question 41 *How is the absorbed dose to internal organs from nuclear medicine procedures calculated?*

Answer 41

The internal dosimetry calculation for nuclear medicine procedures consists of three major steps:
(a) estimation of the amount of activity and time spent by the radioactivity in various source organs,
(b) estimation of the total amount of energy emitted by the radioactivity in the source organs, and
(c) estimation of the fraction of energy emitted by the source organs that is absorbed by the target organ.

Currently, there are two systems for internal dosimetry calculation: the Medical Internal Radiation Dose (MIRD) method and the International Commission on Radiological Protection (ICRP) method. The systems are similar in terms of their assumptions and defining equations but use different terminology and notation. The MIRD method is a computational technique in which doses to specific target organs from radioactive emissions originating from source organs are calculated and the associated risks are assessed. The ICRP method is based on the Biological Effects of Ionizing Radiation (BEIR), with calculated doses based on the biological data (BEIR Reports), organ/tissue models, and their weighting factors.

Bevelacqua JJ. *Appendix D: Internal Dosimetry in Health Physics in the 21st Century.* Weinheim, Germany: Wiley-VCH Verlag GmbH & Co. KGaA; 2008:483–496.

Question 42 *What is the main concern following radioactive iodine 131 (I-131) therapy for the treatment of thyroid cancer?*

Answer 42

In the treatment of thyroid cancer, the total-body dose received by patients is sufficient to cause severe depression of the bone marrow, which may limit the efficacy of the treatment. Because of the repeated administration of large doses of I-131, induction of myeloid leukemia is also a concern.

Hall EJ, Giaccia AJ. Dose and risks in diagnostic radiology, interventional radiology and cardiology, and nuclear medicine. In: Hall EJ, Giaccia AJ, eds. *Radiobiology for the Radiologist.* 7th ed. Philadelphia, PA: Lippincott Williams & Wilkins; 2012:222–252.

Question 43 *What is the risk of developing leukemia and thyroid cancer after I-131 therapy for the treatment of hyperthyroidism in adults?*

Answer 43

No excess of thyroid cancer has been observed in adults after I-131 treatments. According to the Cooperative Thyrotoxicosis Therapy Follow-Up Study, which was initiated in 1961, there is also no significant excess of leukemia after I-131 treatments.

Hall EJ, Giaccia AJ. Dose and risks in diagnostic radiology, interventional radiology and cardiology, and nuclear medicine. In: Hall EJ, Giaccia AJ, eds. *Radiobiology for the Radiologist.* 7th ed. Philadelphia, PA: Lippincott Williams & Wilkins; 2012:222–252.

Question 44

What are the advantages of radium-223 (Ra-223) therapy?

Question 44 *What are the advantages of radium-223 (Ra-223) therapy?*

Answer 44

Ra-223 selectively binds to areas of increased bone turnover in bone metastases. Ra-223 emits 95% of its radiation in the form of alpha decay. Alpha particles have a very short range (<100 μm), which minimizes the dose to normal tissue. Alpha particles also have high linear energy transfer (LET) and induce a greater number of double-strand DNA breaks compared to low LET particles such as electrons, thus increasing the efficacy of this agent.

Parker C, Nilsson S, Heinrich D, et al. Alpha emitter radium-223 and survival in metastatic prostate cancer. *N Engl J Med.* 2013;369:213–223.

21

RADIATION PROTECTION

TAORAN CUI AND PENG QI

Question 1

In the United States, which agency provides guidelines for radiation protection?

Question 2

According to the National Council for Radiation Protection and Measurements (NCRP), what are the two main objectives of radiation protection?

Question 3

What is the major difference between the deterministic effects and stochastic effects?

Question 4

Which quantities are used in the latest National Council for Radiation Protection and Measurements (NCRP) reports on radiation protection?

Turn page to see the answers.

Question 1 *In the United States, which agency provides guidelines for radiation protection?*

Answer 1

The National Council for Radiation Protection and Measurements (NCRP) provides recommendations for radiation protection. The NCRP recommendations are directly related to the Biological Effects of Ionizing Radiation (BEIR) reports, of which the latest is BEIR VII report of 2006.

National Council on Radiation Protection and Measurements. *Risk Estimates for Radiation Protection*. NCRP Report No. 115; Bethesda: MD; 1993.

Question 2 *According to the National Council for Radiation Protection and Measurements (NCRP), what are the two main objectives of radiation protection?*

Answer 2

1. To prevent clinically significant radiation-induced deterministic effects by adhering to dose limits that are below the apparent or practical threshold.
2. To reduce the probability of stochastic effects as a result of occupational exposure to ionizing radiation.

National Council on Radiation Protection and Measurements. *Risk Estimates for Radiation Protection*. NCRP Report No. 115, Bethesda, MD; 1993.

Question 3 *What is the major difference between the deterministic effects and stochastic effects?*

Answer 3

Deterministic effect has a threshold of dose and the severity is dose dependent, whereas stochastic effect does not have a dose threshold and is not dose dependent. Examples of deterministic effects are skin erythema, hair loss, and cataracts. Stochastic effects include radiation carcinogenesis and hereditary effects.

Cember H, Johnson TE. Radiation safety guides. In: Cember H, Johnson TE, eds. *Introduction to Health Physics*. 4th ed. New York, NY: McGraw-Hill; 2009:344–347.

Question 4 *Which quantities are used in the latest National Council for Radiation Protection and Measurements (NCRP) reports on radiation protection?*

Answer 4

Equivalent dose and effective dose have been recommended by the internal organization: International Commission of Radiological Protection (ICRP). Other quantities have been used or are still used including exposure (unit: R), radiation absorbed dose (unit: rad or Gy), occupational exposure (unit: rem), and dose equivalent.

National Council on Radiation Protection and Measurements. *SI Units in Radiation Protection and Measurements*. NCRP Report No. 82, Bethesda, MD; 1985.

Question 5
What is equivalent dose?

Question 6
What are the latest recommended values for radiation weighting factor w_R by the International Commission on Radiological Protection (ICRP)?

Question 7
What is effective dose?

Question 5 *What is equivalent dose?*

Answer 5

Equivalent dose (H_T) is defined as the radiation-weighted sum of the absorbed dose in a tissue or organ ($D_{T,R}$), given by the expression:

$$H_T = \sum w_R \times D_{T,R}$$

where w_R is the radiation weighting factor. The unit of equivalent dose is given the special name Sievert (Sv), and 1 Sv is equal to 1 J/kg.

Hall EJ, Giaccia AJ. Radiation protection. In: Hall EJ, Giaccia AJ, eds. *Radiobiology for the Radiologist*. 7th ed. Philadelphia, PA: Lippincott Williams & Wilkins; 2006:224–239.

Question 6 *What are the latest recommended values for radiation weighting factor w_R by the International Commission on Radiological Protection (ICRP)?*

Answer 6

Type and Energy Range	Radiation Weighting Factor W_R
Photons	1
Electrons	1
Protons	2
α-particles, fission fragments, heavy nuclei	20
Neutrons	A continuous function of neutron on energy

Valentin J. The 2007 recommendations of the International Commission on Radiological Protection: Publication 103. *Ann. ICRP* 2010;37(2–4):1–332

Question 7 *What is effective dose?*

Answer 7

Effective dose (E) is the sum of all the weighted (w_T) equivalent doses in all the organs or tissues irradiated, given by:

$$E = \sum w_T H_T \text{ or } E = \sum w_T \sum w_R D_{T,R}$$

The calculation of this quantity takes into account the sensitivity to radiation of different organs or tissues. The standard international (SI) unit of effective dose is the same as equivalent dose (unit: Sv). Both equivalent dose and effective dose are used to indicate the stochastic effects of ionizing radiation on the human body.

Hall EJ, Giaccia AJ. Radiation protection. In: Hall EJ, Giaccia AJ, eds. *Radiobiology for the Radiologist*. 7th ed. Philadelphia, PA: Lippincott Williams & Wilkins. 2006:224–239.

Question 8

What are the latest tissue weighting factors (w_T) recommended by the International Commission of Radiological Protection (ICRP)?

Question 9

Which quantity, equivalent dose or effective dose, should be used as the primary radiological protection quantity?

Question 10

What are the assumptions, simplifications, and approximations included in the definition of effective dose?

Question 8 *What are the latest tissue weighting factors (w$_T$) recommended by the International Commission of Radiological Protection (ICRP)?*

Answer 8

Tissue	w$_T$	Σw$_T$
Bone-marrow (red), colon, lung, stomach, breast	0.12	0.72
Gonads	0.08	0.08
Bladder, esophagus, liver, thyroid	0.04	0.16
Bone surface, brain, salivary glands, skin	0.01	0.04
		1

Valentin J. The 2007 recommendations of the International Commission on Radiological Protection: Publication 103. *Ann. ICRP* 2010;37(2–4):1–332

Question 9 *Which quantity, equivalent dose or effective dose, should be used as the primary radiological protection quantity?*

Answer 9

Effective dose has been introduced by the International Commission on Radiological Protection (ICRP) as the primary protection quantity. It is used for planning and optimizing radiation protection for workers and the public.

Harrison JD, Ortiz-Lopez PO. Use of effective dose in medicine. *Ann. ICRP* 2015; 44(1S):221–228.

Question 10 *What are the assumptions, simplifications, and approximations included in the definition of effective dose?*

Answer 10

1. The radiation sensitivities of tissues (w$_T$) assume only four different, nominal values ranging from 0.01 to 0.12.
2. The radiation weighting factors (w$_R$) assume only three different values—1, 2, 20—for all radiations and all energies except for neutrons.
3. A linear no threshold (LNT) model is used for stochastic effects in the low-dose range.
4. Committed dose calculation needs validation in the low-dose range.
5. Gender average is used to evaluate for dose conversion coefficients.

Menzel HG, Harrison JD. Effective dose: a radiation protection quantity. *Ann. ICRP* 2012;41(3/4):117–123.

Question 11
Should effective dose be used for the assessment of risks of individuals?

Question 12
Which phantoms are recommended by the International Commission of Radiological Protection (ICRP) to calculate organ or tissue absorbed doses?

Question 13
What is the monthly dose limit for a pregnant occupational worker?

Question 14
What is the risk estimate of the deleterious effects of radiation in terms of hereditary effects, carcinogenesis, and effects on the developing embryo and fetus?

Question 11 *Should effective dose be used for the assessment of risks of individuals?*

Answer 11

No. Because of the uncertainties in calculating effective dose (see question 9), effective dose is not suitable for the assessment of risks of individuals.

Menzel HG, Harrison JD. Effective dose: a radiation protection quantity. *Ann. ICRP* 2012;41(3/4):117–123.

Question 12 *Which phantoms are recommended by the International Commission of Radiological Protection (ICRP) to calculate organ or tissue absorbed doses?*

Answer 12

Instead of using a variety of mathematical models, reference computational phantoms of the human body based on tomographic images ("voxel phantom") are used.

Menzel HG, Clement C, DeLuca P. Realistic reference phantoms: an ICRP/ICRU joint effort: a report of adult reference computational phantoms. *Ann. ICRP* 2009;39(2):1–164. [Published correction appears in *Ann. ICRP* 2009;39(2):165.]

Question 13 *What is the monthly dose limits for a pregnant occupational worker?*

Answer 13

According to 10 CFR 20.1208(b), the monthly exposure rate limit to a declared pregnant worker is 5 mSv/month to the embryo/fetus. The National Council for Radiation Protection and Measurements (NCRP), however, recommends a lower limit which is 0.5 mSv to the embryo/fetus, although any monthly dose of greater than 0.5 mSv but less than 1 mSv may not be considered as a substantial violation.

National Council on Radiation Protection and Measurements. *Limitation of Exposure to Ionizing Radiation.* NCRP Report No. 116, Bethesda, MD; 1993.

Question 14 *What is the risk estimate of the deleterious effects of radiation in terms of hereditary effects, carcinogenesis, and effects on the developing embryo and fetus?*

Answer 14

End Point	Risk Estimate
Severe mental retardation: exposure of embryo/fetus (8–15 weeks)	40%/Sv
Carcinogenesis: general population (low dose, low dose rate)	5%/Sv
Hereditary effects: general population	0.2%/Sv

Source: Table adapted from:
Otake M. Threshold for radiation-related severe mental retardation in prenatally exposed A-bomb survivors: a re-analysis. *Int. J. Radiat. Biol.* 1996;70(6):755–763.
Valentin J. The 2007 Recommendations of the International Commission on Radiological Protection: Publication 103. *Ann. ICRP* 2010;37(2–4):50–57.

Hall EJ, Giaccia AJ. Radiation protection. In: Hall EJ, Giaccia AJ, eds. *Radiobiology for the Radiologist.* 7th ed. Philadelphia, PA: Lippincott Williams & Wilkins; 2006:224–239.

Question 15

What are the National Council for Radiation Protection and Measurements (NCRP) recommendations on the limits for the stochastic effects of occupational exposure?

Question 16

What is the "as low as reasonably achievable" (ALARA) principle?

Question 17

What are the three cardinal principles of radiation protection in practice?

Question 18

What materials are usually used for shielding the radiation?

Question 15 *What are the National Council for Radiation Protection and Measurements (NCRP) recommendations on the limits for the stochastic effects of occupational exposure?*

Answer 15

1. No occupational exposure should be permitted until the age of 18 years.
2. The effective dose in any year should not exceed 50 mSv.
3. The individual worker's lifetime effective dose should not exceed age in years times 10 mSv.

Hall EJ, Giaccia AJ. Radiation protection. In: Hall EJ, Giaccia AJ, eds. *Radiobiology for the Radiologist.* 7th ed. Philadelphia, PA: Lippincott Williams & Wilkins; 2006:224–239.

Question 16 *What is the "as low as reasonably achievable" (ALARA) principle?*

Answer 16

ALARA stands for "as low as reasonably achievable." This principle applies to all parties involved in the use of radiation. For example, quarterly investigation levels (Level I and II) are reviewed by radiation safety officers (RSO) to monitor occupational exposure to radiation workers.

Cember H, Johnson TE. Radiation safety guides. In: Cember H, Johnson TE, eds. *Introduction to Health Physics.* 4th ed. New York, NY: McGraw-Hill; 2009:346–348.

Question 17 *What are the three cardinal principles of radiation protection in practice?*

Answer 17

1. Minimize exposure time.
2. Maximize distance from the radiation source. The radiation dose of a point source is inversely proportional to the square of the distance from the source. This is often referred to as the inverse square law.
3. Maximize shielding.

Cember H, Johnson TE. External radiation safety. In: Cember H, Johnson TE, eds. *Introduction to Health Physics.* 4th ed. New York, NY: McGraw-Hill; 2009:513–514.

Question 18 *What materials are usually used for shielding the radiation?*

Answer 18

Materials with high atomic number (high-Z), such as lead, bismuth, and tin, are preferred to be used for shielding of high energy photons. Hydrogen-rich material, such as polyethylene and concrete, are ideal for neutron shielding.

Cember H, Johnson TE. External radiation safety. In: Cember H, Johnson TE, eds. *Introduction to Health Physics.* 4th ed. New York, NY: McGraw-Hill; 2009:522–545.

Question 19

What is the half-value layer (HVL) and tenth-value layer (TVL)?

Question 20

What is the National Council for Radiation Protection and Measurements (NCRP) recommendation on the limits for public exposure?

Question 21

What is the average exposure from background radiation per person per year in the United States?

Question 22

What are the approximate effective doses for diagnostic imaging procedures?

Question 19 *What is the half-value layer (HVL) and tenth-value layer (TVL)?*

Answer 19

HVL/TVL is defined as the thickness of a material required to reduce the radiation intensity to one half/tenth of its initial value. It is used to measure the attenuation of a material for a specific radiation. For example, TVL has been widely used for shielding design for medical linear accelerators.

Cember H, Johnson TE. Interaction of radiation with matter. In: Cember H, Johnson TE, eds. *Introduction to Health Physics.* 4th ed. New York, NY: McGraw-Hill; 2009:172–173.

Question 20 *What is the National Council for Radiation Protection and Measurements (NCRP) recommendation on the limits for public exposure?*

Answer 20

The annual public limit is 1 mSv for continuous or frequent exposure and 5 mSv for infrequent exposure.

National Council on Radiation Protection and Measurements. *Limitation of Exposure to Ionizing Radiation.* NCRP Report No. 116, Bethesda, MD; 1993.

Question 21 *What is the average exposure from background radiation per person per year in the United States?*

Answer 21

The average exposure from background radiation per person per year in the United States was about 3.1 mSv, out of a total annual exposure of 6.2 mSv.

National Council on Radiation Protection and Measurements. *Ionizing Radiation Exposure of the Population of the United States.* NCRP Report No. 160, Bethesda, MD; 2009.

Question 22 *What are the approximate effective doses for diagnostic imaging procedures?*

Answer 22

Procedure	Approximate Effective Dose (mSv)
Chest radiograph	0.1–0.2
Mammogram	0.3–0.6
CT	1–14
Coronary angiography	5–15
PET/CT	25

McCollough C, Cody D, Edyvean S, et al. The measurement, reporting, and management of radiation dose in CT. Report of AAPM Task Group 23, 2008.

Question 23
What are the possible biological effects of low doses of radiation less than 0.5 Gy?

Question 24
What are the most commonly used detectors in monitoring of radiation?

Question 25
What is the dose and dose-rate effectiveness factor (DDREF)?

Question 26
What is the annual limit on intake (ALI)?

Question 23 *What are the possible biological effects of low doses of radiation less than 0.5 Gy?*

Answer 23

1. Genetic effects: radiation-induced gene mutation, chromosome breaks, and anomalies
2. Neoplastic disease: leukemia, thyroid tumors, skin lesions
3. Effects on growth and development: fetus and young children
4. Effect on life span: diminishing life span or premature aging
5. Cataracts

National Research Council (US). Advisory Committee on the Biological Effects of Ionizing Radiations, and United States. Environmental Protection Agency. Radiation Office. The effects on populations of exposure to low levels of ionizing radiation: report. National Academies, 1972.

Question 24 *What are the most commonly used detectors in monitoring of radiation?*

Answer 24

The Geiger–Muller counter and ion-chamber survey meter are most commonly used.

Cember H, Johnson TE. Health physics instrumentation. In: Cember H, Johnson TE, eds. *Introduction to Health Physics*. 4th ed. New York, NY: McGraw-Hill; 2009:427–435.

Question 25 *What is the dose and dose-rate effectiveness factor (DDREF)?*

Answer 25

DDREF is defined as the ratio between the radiation detriment of risk (per unit effective dose) for high doses/high dose rates and that for low dose/low dose rates. It is used to estimate the risk for low dose/low dose rates from observations and epidemiological results at high doses/high dose rates. The International Commission on Radiological Protection (ICRP) 60 recommends using a value of 2 for the DDREF.

Valentin J. The 2007 Recommendations of the International Commission on Radiological Protection: Publication 103. *Ann. ICRP* 2010;37(2–4):1–332.

Question 26 *What is the annual limit on intake (ALI)?*

Answer 26

ALI is the activity of a radionuclide which, if taken in alone, would irradiate an individual to the annual occupational exposure limit of 0.05 Sv. ALI doesn't account for radiation time or dose rate.

Cember H, Johnson TE. Radiation safety guides. In: Cember H, Johnson TE, eds. *Introduction to Health Physics*. 4th ed. New York, NY: McGraw-Hill; 2009:351–356.

Question 27

What are the quantities used to evaluate the stochastic effects of an intake of radioactive materials on the human body?

Question 28

What is the collective effective dose (S)?

Question 27 *What are the quantities used to evaluate the stochastic effects of an intake of radioactive materials on the human body?*

Answer 27

The quantities used are committed equivalent dose ($E(\tau)$) and committed effective dose ($H_T(\tau)$).

Committed equivalent dose is the sum of the products of the committed organ or tissue equivalent doses and the appropriate tissue weighting factors (w_T). The commitment period is taken to be 50 years for adults and 70 years for children.

Committed effective dose is defined as the time integral of the equivalent dose rate in a particular tissue or organ that will be received by an individual following intake of radioactive material into the body by a reference person, where s is the integration time in years.

Valentin J. The 2007 Recommendations of the International Commission on Radiological Protection: Publication 103. *Ann. ICRP* 2010;37(2–4):1–332.

Question 28 *What is the collective effective dose (S)?*

Answer 28

The collective effective dose can be approximated as $S = \sum_i E_i(\tau)N_i$ where E_i is the average effective dose for a subgroup i, and N_i is the number of individuals in this subgroup. The time period (τ) and number of individuals over which the effective doses are summed should always be specified. The unit of the collective effective dose is Sievert (Sv) and 1 Sv is equal to 1 J/kg.

Valentin J. The 2007 Recommendations of the International Commission on Radiological Protection: Publication 103. *Ann. ICRP* 2010;37(2–4):1–332.

22

ALTERNATIVE RADIATION THERAPY MODALITIES

SUSAN KOST AND ANDREW GODLEY

Question 1
What types of alternative radiation therapies (RTs) use high linear energy transfer (LET) sources?

Question 2
Why do high linear energy transfer (LET) radiation sources have a greater relative biological effectiveness (RBE) compared to photons of low LET?

Question 3
How do neutrons impart dose to the tissue?

Question 4
How do the radiobiological properties of neutrons differ from x-rays?

Turn page to see the answers.

Question 1 *What types of alternative radiation therapies (RTs) use high linear energy transfer (LET) sources?*

Answer 1

RTs using high LET sources include fast neutron, boron neutron capture, proton, carbon, and heavy ion therapies. This is in comparison to megavoltage photons and electrons, which are considered low LET particles.

Hall EJ, Giaccia AJ. Linear energy transfer and relative biologic effectiveness. In: Hall EJ, Giaccia AJ, eds. *Radiobiology for the Radiologist*. 7th ed. Philadelphia, PA: Lippincott Williams & Wilkins; 2006:106–116.

Question 2 *Why do high linear energy transfer (LET) radiation sources have a greater relative biological effectiveness (RBE) compared to photons of low LET?*

Answer 2

High LET radiation is densely ionizing compared to the sparse ionization that occurs with low LET photons (megavoltage energies). The damage to DNA within a cell from the dense ionization of high LET radiation occurs more often, causing difficulty for the cell to repair itself. The diminution of cell repair correlates with increased efficiency in cell killing and decreased cell survival, leading to higher RBE.

Sørensen BS, Overgaard J, Bassler N. In vitro RBE-LET dependence for multiple particle types. *Acta Oncol.* 2011;50(6):757–762.

Question 3 *How do neutrons impart dose to the tissue?*

Answer 3

Neutrons are an indirectly ionizing form of radiation. Neutrons lose energy during interactions with the atomic nuclei in tissue to produce recoil protons, α-particles and other heavier nuclear fragments. The resultant charged particles are most likely to damage the DNA directly (direct action).

Hall EJ, Giaccia AJ. Physics and chemistry of radiation absorption. In: Hall EJ, Giaccia AJ, eds. *Radiobiology for the Radiologist*. 7th ed. Philadelphia, PA: Lippincott Williams & Wilkins; 2006:5–15.

Question 4 *How do the radiobiological properties of neutrons differ from x-rays?*

Answer 4

Studies irradiating cell cultures with fast neutron beams of various energies have shown that survival curves are more linear compared to x-rays (250 kVp). The smaller shoulder in the cell survival curve indicates little or no repair of neutron-induced sublethal damage. In addition, no change in the surviving fraction of cells irradiated by two doses separated by varying time intervals is observed. Neutrons have a reduced dependence on the presence of oxygen, with oxygen enhancement ratios of approximately 1.6 to 1.8, compared to a value of 3.4 for 250 kVp x-rays. Neutrons are also more insensitive to cell cycle. Studies have shown little variation in the survival curves of synchronized cells at different positions in the cell cycle for neutron irradiations compared to the variation observed with ^{60}Co gamma rays.

Gragg RL, Humphrey RM, Thames Jr HD, Meyn RE. The response of Chinese hamster ovary cells to fast neutron radiotherapy beams: III. variation in relative biological effectiveness with position in the cell cycle. *Radiat Res.* 1978;76(2):283–291.

Hall EJ, Rossi HH, Kellerer AM, Goodman L, Marino S. Radiobiological studies with monoenergetic neutrons. *Radiat Res.* 1973;54(3):431–443.

Ngo FQ, Han A, Utsumi H, Elkind MM. Comparative radiobiology of fast neutrons: relevance to radiotherapy and basic studies. *Int J Rad Oncol Biol Phys.* 1977;3:187–193.

Question 5

For what types of cancer have clinical trials proven an advantage for fast neutron therapy?

Question 6

What biological aspects of tumors can make them more susceptible to neutron therapy?

Question 7

What beam energies are used for fast neutron-based radiation therapy (RT)?

Question 8

What are the characteristics of the percent depth dose curve for neutron therapy?

Question 5 *For what types of cancer have clinical trials proven an advantage for fast neutron therapy?*

Answer 5

First generation Radiation Therapy Oncology Group (RTOG) neutron studies have resulted in statistically significant advantages for fast neutron radiation therapy (RT) over conventional (external photon and electron beam) therapy for salivary gland and prostate tumors. Other studies have shown a possible advantage to using neutron therapy for soft-tissue sarcomas.

Griffin TW. Fast neutron radiation therapy. *Crit Rev Oncol Hematol.* 1992;13(1):17–31.
Griffin TW, Pajak TF, Laramore GE, et al. Neutron vs photon irradiation of inoperable salivary gland tumors: results of an RTOG-MRC cooperative study. *Int J Rad Oncol Biol Phys.* 1988;15(5):1085–1090.
Laramore GE, Griffith JT, Boespflug M, et al. Fast neutron radiotherapy for sarcomas of soft tissue, bone, and cartilage. *Am J Clin Oncol.* 1989;12(4):320–326.
Russell KJ, Caplan RJ, Laramore GE, et al. Photon versus fast neutron external beam radiotherapy in the treatment of locally advanced prostate cancer: results of a randomized prospective trial. *Int J Rad Oncol Biol Phys.* 1994;28(1):47–54.

Question 6 *What biological aspects of tumors can make them more susceptible to neutron therapy?*

Answer 6

Tumors that respond to hypoxic sensitizers or slow growing tumors that have a slower rate of reoxygenation may respond favorably to neutron therapy. Slow growing tumors may be more responsive to neutron therapy because of the insensitivity of neutrons to the phase of the mitotic cycle as these tumors tend to have slow cycling and out-of-phase cell populations. Cells irradiated with neutrons exhibit less cell repair; therefore the fractionation schedule is of less importance. This may prove to be beneficial when treating fast proliferating tumors.

Wambersie A, Richard F, Breteau N. Development of fast neutron therapy worldwide: radiobiological, clinical and technical aspects. *Acta Oncol.* 1994;33(3):261–274.

Question 7 *What beam energies are used for fast neutron-based radiation therapy (RT)?*

Answer 7

Neutron beams from hospital-based generators have average particle energies between 18 and 70 MeV.

Griffin TW. Fast neutron radiation therapy. *Crit Rev Oncol Hematol.* 1992;13(1):17–31.

Question 8 *What are the characteristics of the percent depth dose curve for neutron therapy?*

Answer 8

The shape of the percent depth–dose curve for neutrons depends on many factors including the particle energy, field size, source-surface distance, and phantom material. The neutron percent depth–dose curve could also represent the total absorbed dose or only the neutron absorbed dose. Central axis dose measurements for clinical neutron beams, generated from deuterons on either a beryllium or tritium target, result in depth–dose curves similar to Co-60 with 50% dose values around 12 cm depth. The maximum dose occurs at depths of 7 to 15 mm. The entrance dose is around 60% of the maximum dose.

Mijnheer BJ, Zoetelief J, Broerse JJ. Build-up and depth–dose characteristics of different fast neutron beams relevant for radiotherapy. *Brit J Radiol.* 1978;51(602):122–126.

Question 9
What is the mechanism for delivering dose in boron neutron capture therapy (BNCT)?

Question 10
What neutron particle energies are used for boron neutron capture therapy (BNCT)?

Question 11
What are some disadvantages inherent with boron neutron capture therapy (BNCT)?

Question 12
How does the radiation biology of boron neutron capture therapy (BNCT) differ from conventional external beam radiation therapy (EBRT)?

Question 9 *What is the mechanism for delivering dose in boron neutron capture therapy (BNCT)?*

Answer 9

First, a boron-containing drug that is selectively taken up by malignant cells is administered to the patient. The patient is then exposed to a beam of thermal neutrons. The neutrons interact preferentially with the boron to produce alpha particles that intensely irradiate the tumor over a short range and spare normal tissue.

Hall EJ, Giaccia AJ. Alternative radiation modalities. In: Hall EJ, Giaccia AJ, eds. *Radiobiology for the Radiologist.* 7th ed. Philadelphia, PA: Lippincott Williams & Wilkins; 2006:407–418.

Question 10 *What neutron particle energies are used for boron neutron capture therapy (BNCT)?*

Answer 10

BNCT is based on the nuclear capture and fission reaction of boron-10 with low-energy thermal neutrons to yield high linear energy alpha particles. The neutron energy required for this interaction is around 0.025 eV. However, thermal neutrons do not deeply penetrate tissue, and instead epithermal neutrons of energies from 0.5 eV to 10 keV are used. These neutrons lose energy and fall into the thermal range as they travel deeper into the patient.

Barth RF, Coderre JA, Vicente MGH, Blue TE. Boron neutron capture therapy of cancer: current status and future prospects. *Clin Cancer Res.* 2005;11(11):3987.

Question 11 *What are some disadvantages inherent with boron neutron capture therapy (BNCT)?*

Answer 11

It is difficult to develop boron delivery agents that selectively bind to tumor cells. Furthermore, it is challenging to achieve boron concentrations sufficient to deliver therapeutic doses of radiation to the tumor without normal tissue toxicity. The low-energy neutrons required to interact with boron do not penetrate tissue effectively, which results in poor percent depth doses. Also, the dosimetry for BNCT is determined by the microdistribution of boron in the tumor. Currently, there is no adequate method for quantifying the concentration of boron in tissue, making it difficult to estimate delivered radiation doses to the tumor and correlate them to therapeutic response.

Barth RF, Coderre JA, Vicente MGH, Blue TE. Boron neutron capture therapy of cancer: current status and future prospects. *Clin Cancer Res.* 2005;11(11):3987.
Hall EJ, Giaccia AJ. Alternative radiation modalities. In: Hall EJ, Giaccia AJ, eds. *Radiobiology for the Radiologist.* 7th ed. Philadelphia, PA: Lippincott Williams & Wilkins; 2006:407–418.

Question 12 *How does the radiation biology of boron neutron capture therapy (BNCT) differ from conventional external beam radiation therapy (EBRT)?*

Answer 12

The radiation field in tissues during BNCT consists of a mixture of components with differing linear energy transfer (LET) characteristics. Three types of directly ionizing radiation are produced: low LET gamma rays, primarily from the capture of thermal neutrons by normal tissue hydrogen atoms, high LET protons from both scattering of fast neutrons and from the capture of thermal neutrons by nitrogen atoms, and high LET, heavier-charged α-particles generated by thermal neutron capture and fission reactions with ^{10}B. High LET particles generate a higher density of ionization events along their paths, leading to an increased biological effect compared with the same dose of low LET radiation as used in conventional external beam RT. The total delivered radiation dose can be expressed in photon-equivalent units as the sum of each of the dose components multiplied by their radiation weighting factors.

Coderre JA, Morris GM. The radiation biology of boron neutron capture therapy. *Radiat Res.* 1999;151(1):1–18.
Coderre JA, Turcotte JC, Riley KJ, Binns PJ, Harling OK, Kiger III WS. Boron neutron capture therapy: cellular targeting of high linear energy transfer radiation. *Technol Cancer Res Treat.* 2003;2(5):355–375.

Question 13

What are the different radiobiological properties of protons versus x-rays?

Question 14

What is the main advantage of radiation therapy (RT) using protons?

Question 15

What is a spread-out Bragg peak (SOBP) and why is it important in proton therapy?

Question 16

What relative biological effectiveness (RBE) value is used for determining the dose in proton therapy and what are some implications of using this generic value clinically?

Question 13 *What are the different radiobiological properties of protons versus x-rays?*

Answer 13

The radiobiological properties of protons are similar to those of x-rays. The relative biological effectiveness (RBE) for protons is the same as that of a 250 kV x-ray. Protons are only 10% to 15% more effective than Co-60 gamma rays or standard linear accelerator-generated megavoltage x-rays. The oxygen enhancement ratio of protons is also equivalent to x-rays (2.5–3.0). Thus, the biological effect of protons is similar to photons at the same absorbed dose.

Paganetti H, Niemierko A, Ancukiewicz M, et al. Relative biological effectiveness (RBE) values for proton beam therapy. *Int J Rad Oncol Biol Phys*. 2002;53(2):407–421.

Question 14 *What is the main advantage of radiation therapy (RT) using protons?*

Answer 14

Protons are an attractive modality for RT not because of their radiobiological characteristics but instead because of the behavior of the proton depth–dose curve. The dose deposited by a monoenergetic beam of protons increases slowly and then exhibits a sharp maximum (Bragg peak) at the end of the particle range with little dose deposition after the peak. The tumor can be treated by confining the volume within the Bragg peak, thus minimizing the dose to the normal tissue.

Miller DW. A review of proton beam radiation therapy. *Med Phys*. 1995;22:1943–1954.

Question 15 *What is a spread-out Bragg peak (SOBP) and why is it important in proton therapy?*

Answer 15

The shape of a monoenergetic proton depth-dose curve has a sharp and narrow maximum at the depth in tissue where the protons reach their end of range. When used for treatment, the narrow Bragg peak will concentrate the deposited dose in a very small, localized region within the tumor. In order to treat an extended tumor volume, the proton beam energy is modulated, causing the Bragg peak to spread out. This SOBP will deliver the same dose over a range of depths, allowing the tumor to be completely covered with a uniform dose distribution.

Chu WT. *Overview of Light Ion Beam Therapy, Dose Reporting in Ion Beam Therapy*. International Atomic Energy Agency, ed. 2006; vol. IAEA-TECDOC-1560.

Question 16 *What relative biological effectiveness (RBE) value is used for determining the dose in proton therapy and what are some implications of using this generic value clinically?*

Answer 16

There is a small but significant increase in the RBE of protons compared to x-rays. The International Commission on Radiation Units (ICRU) recommends reporting the prescribed dose of protons in RBE-weighted dose (denoted as Gy(RBE)). A Gy(RBE) prescribed dose represents the hypothetical photon dose distribution required to deliver the same biological effect. The assumed RBE value for proton therapy is 1.1 to 1.15 relative to ^{60}Co, based on the average of in vivo measurements at the middle of the SOBP. This value is applied to all tissues during treatment planning regardless of position along the depth–dose distribution. One concern is the potential for late responding tissues having a higher RBE, especially in distal regions of the treatment field. This may result in increased normal tissue toxicity due to underestimation of the dose.

Britten RA, Nazaryan V, Davis LK, et al. Variations in the RBE for cell killing along the depth–dose profile of a modulated proton therapy beam. *Radiat Res*. 2012;179(1):21–28.
ICRU Report 78. Prescribing, recording, and reporting proton-beam therapy. *J ICRU*. 2007;7(2):21–28.

Question 17
Why is the energy of carbon and other heavy-ion beams defined by the energy per nucleon?

Question 18
How does the relative biological effectiveness (RBE) of carbon and heavy ions depend on the distance from the Bragg peak (point of maximum dose deposition)?

Question 19
How does the local distribution of energy deposition for heavy ions differ from photons and why does this contribute to an enhanced biological effect?

Question 20
Why must relative biological effectiveness (RBE) be factored into treatment planning with heavy-ion therapy while it is not routinely used in proton therapy?

Question 17 *Why is the energy of carbon and other heavy-ion beams defined by the energy per nucleon?*

Answer 17

In order to treat deep-seated tumors, the heavy-ion beam energy must be greatly increased. For example, a 150 MeV proton beam can penetrate to a depth of 16 cm; the total beam energy for carbon ions to reach the same depth is 3,000 MeV. Thus, beam energies are typically reported per nucleon. The 3,000 MeV total energy carbon beam is reduced to 250 MeV/u (energy per nucleon, of which carbon has 12).

Jäkel O. Heavy ion radiotherapy. In: Schlegel W, Bortfeld T, Grosu AL, eds. *New Technologies in Radiation Oncology*. Heidelberg: Springer; 2006:365–378.

Question 18 *How does the relative biological effectiveness (RBE) of carbon and heavy ions depend on the distance from the Bragg peak (point of maximum dose deposition)?*

Answer 18

RBE is dependent on the linear energy transfer (LET) of the particle. For carbon and heavy ions, the LET increases as the particle energy decreases. At the Bragg peak, the charged particles are densely ionizing and energy loss is greater compared to entrance depths. The RBE is therefore greatest at the Bragg peak and decreases with distance from this maximum.

Kraji G. Tumor therapy with heavy charged particles. *Prog Part Nucl Phys*. 2000;45(2):S473–S544.

Question 19 *How does the local distribution of energy deposition for heavy ions differ from photons and why does this contribute to an enhanced biological effect?*

Answer 19

Heavy ions impart much of their energy in the center of the track. The energy is first transferred to electrons through interactions with atoms in the tissue. These electrons receive only a small amount of energy, which is absorbed locally, or they are scattered in the forward direction along the track. Thus, the radial dose distribution around a charged ion exhibits a steep gradient following an inverse square dependence on radial distance. This is in contrast to the much more homogeneous dose distribution from photons, which transfer energy sparsely by the photoelectric effect or Compton scattering. In the context of inflicting damage to a cell, heavy ions will deposit dose locally along their tracks, resulting in an increased probability of correlated and severe DNA damage. The distance between DNA damage is larger for photons with an evenly distributed local dose distribution and is potentially repairable. Therefore, the radiation damage is larger for heavy ions compared to photons and the biological response to radiation is increased for equivalent macroscopic doses.

Schardt D, Elsässer T, Schulz-Ertner D. Heavy-ion tumor therapy: physical and radiobiological benefits. *Rev Mod Phys*. 2010;82(1):383–425.

Question 20 *Why must relative biological effectiveness (RBE) be factored into treatment planning with heavy-ion therapy while it is not routinely used in proton therapy?*

Answer 20

Protons have similar radiobiological properties to x-rays and their RBE is estimated to be only 10% to 15% greater than megavoltage x-rays generated by clinical linear accelerators. Carbon and other heavy ions have much larger RBEs that are also dependent on the tissue type, dose level, atomic number, particle energy, and treatment depth. Furthermore, RBE values vary across the irradiated volume; different values must be assigned to different tissues in order to determine the biologically effective dose for both tumor and normal tissues in the treatment region.

Elsässer T, Weyrather WK, Friedrich T, et al. Quantification of the relative biological effectiveness for ion beam radiotherapy: direct experimental comparison of proton and carbon ion beams and a novel approach for treatment planning. *Int J Radiat Oncol Biol Phys*. 2010;78(4):1177–1183.

Weyrather WK, Kraft G. RBE of carbon ions: experimental data and the strategy of RBE calculation for treatment planning. *Radiother Oncol*. 2004;73:S161–S169.

Question 21

What are several treatment characteristics that may influence the biological effect of intraoperative radiation therapy (IORT)?

Question 22

What causes nonuniform dose distributions in intraoperative radiation therapy (IORT)?

Question 23

Why do low-energy x-rays (kV range) produce more lethal damage per unit dose than high-energy x-rays (MV range)?

Question 21 *What are several treatment characteristics that may influence the biological effect of intraoperative radiation therapy (IORT)?*

Answer 21

The beam energy, dose distribution, fraction size, dose delivery time, treatment depth, and time of application may influence the biological response of the tumor and normal tissue during IORT. IORT delivers a large dose of radiation directly to the tumor site during surgery. The goal is to eliminate potential malignant cells left behind by the surgery. The use of a single treatment fraction may decrease the therapeutic window between tumor control and adverse normal tissue effects that are typically mitigated through fractionation. Low-energy x-rays have a higher relative biological effectiveness (RBE) compared to conventional external beam RT due to their high linear energy transfer (LET). Also, the low-energy x-rays employed in IORT are delivered at a low dose rate with often nonuniform dose distributions that may affect the biological response to treatment.

Herskind C, Wenz F. Radiobiological aspects of intraoperative tumour-bed irradiation with low-energy x-rays (LEX-IORT). *Transl Cancer Res*. 2014;3(1):3–17.

Question 22 *What causes nonuniform dose distributions in intraoperative radiation therapy (IORT)?*

Answer 22

Low-energy (30–50 kV) x-rays used in IORT are absorbed more readily with lower penetration in tissue compared to the megavoltage x-rays produced by linear accelerators for conventional external beam RT. These low-energy x-rays deposit a larger proportion of dose closer to the beam source. The dose deposited at a given depth is dependent on both the inverse square law governing the spherical propagation of the isotropic field of x-rays generated by the source and the exponential attenuation of the beam in tissue. This steep radial dose gradient results in nonuniform dose distributions and possibly reduced tumor control depending on the depth of the treated tumor bed.

Herskind C, Wenz F. Radiobiological aspects of intraoperative tumour-bed irradiation with low-energy x-rays (LEX-IORT). *Transl Cancer Res*. 2014;3(1):3–17.

Question 23 *Why do low-energy x-rays (kV range) produce more lethal damage per unit dose than high-energy x-rays (MV range)?*

Answer 23

Dose in tissue is delivered primarily from free electrons created when a photon interacts with atoms in the tissue through ionization. Low-energy photons create more low-energy electrons compared to high-energy photons. These low-energy electrons deposit a larger proportion of their total energy at the end of their tracks. Cell damage is due to irreparable double-strand DNA breaks that occur more frequently at the end of the electron track in the region of dense ionizations. In contrast, high-energy x-rays induce more sparse ionizations along the majority of their track, until they lose enough energy to form the cluster of ionizations that will cause more double-strand DNA breaks and lethal cell damage. The types of damage caused by sparse ionization along most of the x-ray path are typically single-strand breaks and base damage that are completely repairable. Although both low-energy and high-energy x-rays produce the same types of cell damage, the number of lethal lesions per unit dose will be larger for low-energy than for high-energy x-rays.

Herskind C, Wenz F. Radiobiological aspects of intraoperative tumour-bed irradiation with low-energy x-rays (LEX-IORT). *Transl Cancer Res*. 2014;3(1):3–17.

Question 24

What role does hypoxia and tumor oxygenation play in intraoperative radiation therapy (IORT) and why?

Question 25

How do pions deposit their energy in tissue and how does this method affect the relative biological effectiveness (RBE) of pions?

Question 24 *What role does hypoxia and tumor oxygenation play in intraoperative radiation therapy (IORT) and why?*

Answer 24

IORT is a single-fraction therapy. Tumor response to a single fraction is predominately determined by the hypoxic cell fraction as well-oxygenated cells are typically more radiosensitive. Treatment failure can occur in tumors with even a small amount of hypoxic cells. Thus, several clinical approaches are aimed at reducing hypoxia prior to irradiation. Methods for tumor oxygenation include increasing the oxygen partial pressure by ventilating the patient with near pure oxygen and administering a dose of a radiosensitizing drug such as nitroimidazole.

Okunieff P, Sundararaman S, Metcalfe S, Chen Y. Biology of large dose per fraction irradiation. In: Gunderson LL, Willett CG, Calvo FA, Harrison LB, eds. *Intraoperative Irradiation*. New York: Humana Press; 2011:27–47.

Question 25 *How do pions deposit their energy in tissue and how does this method affect the relative biological effectiveness (RBE) of pions?*

Answer 25

Pions are particles that act to hold together the protons and neutrons in an atomic nucleus. The negative pion has the same charge as an electron but is over 200 times as massive. Because pions are charged particles, the range in tissue is directly related to their initial kinetic energy and the stopping power of the tissue. When negative pions come to rest in tissue, their negative charge attracts them to a nearby nucleus (typically an oxygen, nitrogen, or carbon atom). The pion is captured by this nucleus and its entire mass is converted to energy, causing the captured nucleus to explode and throw out nuclear fragments in a star formation. The nuclear fragments include protons, alpha particles, and heavier nuclei. These charged particles are densely ionizing and have a short range in tissue. Because these particles are densely ionizing, they deposit a large amount of energy close to the site where the pion was captured by the nucleus with increased cell killing ability. The RBE of the particles formed by pion capture is approximately three; thus, they are three times as effective at killing cells at the same dose compared to x-rays and gammas rays commonly used for RT.

Langham WH. The potential of negative pions in the therapy of cancer. *CA Cancer J Clin.* 1970;20(5):302–311.

23

BRACHYTHERAPY AND STEREOTACTIC RADIOSURGERY

SUDHA AMARNATH

Question 1
Why are blood vessels and vasculature important to tumors?

Question 2
How are tumor blood vessels formed?

Question 3
How would you describe the properties of tumor blood vessels?

Question 4
How are tumor blood vessels different from normal tissue blood vessels?

Turn page to see the answers. **379**

Question 1 *Why are blood vessels and vasculature important to tumors?*

Answer 1

Blood vessels provide nutrients and oxygen to cells in a growing tumor and directly control the intratumor microenvironment. Therefore, the survival and continued growth of a tumor are directly dependent on adequate blood flow via blood vessels to the tumor.

Song SW, Park H, Griffin R, Levitt SH. Radiobiology of stereotactic radiosurgery and stereotactic body radiation therapy. In: Levitt SH, Purdy JA, Perez CA, Poortmans P, eds. *Technical Basis of Radiation Therapy*. Berlin/Heidelberg: Springer-Verlag; 2012:51–61.

Question 2 *How are tumor blood vessels formed?*

Answer 2

Tumor blood vessels can be formed via three different mechanisms: angiogenesis, vasculogenesis, or co-opting nearby blood vessels from normal tissues. Blood vessels are formed through angiogenesis by sprouting or intussusceptive microvascular growth; in vasculogenesis, blood vessels are formed by progenitor and other stem-like cells found in the blood and bone marrow.

Song SW, Park H, Griffin R, Levitt SH. Radiobiology of stereotactic radiosurgery and stereotactic body radiation therapy. In: Levitt SH, Purdy JA, Perez CA, Poortmans P, eds. *Technical Basis of Radiation Therapy*. Berlin/Heidelberg: Springer-Verlag; 2012:51–61.

Question 3 *How would you describe the properties of tumor blood vessels?*

Answer 3

Blood vessels found in tumors are typically formed quite hastily compared to those found in normal tissues and tend to be more like immature capillaries. They are composed of a single layer of endothelial cells (often with gaps between the endothelial cells filled with tumor cells) with no basement membrane. These gaps cause tumor blood vessels to be quite leaky compared to normal tissue blood vessels.

Song SW, Park H, Griffin R, Levitt SH. Radiobiology of stereotactic radiosurgery and stereotactic body radiation therapy. In: Levitt SH, Purdy JA, Perez CA, Poortmans P, eds. *Technical Basis of Radiation Therapy*. Berlin/Heidelberg: Springer-Verlag; 2012:51–61.

Question 4 *How are tumor blood vessels different from normal tissue blood vessels?*

Answer 4

Tumor blood vessels, in addition to being highly leaky compared to normal tissue blood vessels, are often without innervations and therefore are unable to autoregulate in response to external stresses (i.e., ionizing radiation). Because tumor vasculature is formed so hastily, tumor blood vessels are often irregular in diameter, tortuous, sharply bent, and branched with dead ends. This leads to sluggish, and sometimes stationary, blood flow through a tumor and arterio-venous (A-V) shunting of tumor perfusion. Lastly, poor lymphatic drainage and increased leakiness of the tumor blood vessels lead to elevated intratumoral interstitial pressure that can cause temporary or permanent collapse of the tumor blood vessels. These properties of tumor blood vessels are more common in faster growing tumors than in slower growing tumors.

Song SW, Park H, Griffin R, Levitt SH. Radiobiology of stereotactic radiosurgery and stereotactic body radiation therapy. In: Levitt SH, Purdy JA, Perez CA, Poortmans P, eds. *Technical Basis of Radiation Therapy*. Berlin/Heidelberg: Springer-Verlag; 2012:51–61.

Question 5
How do the differences in tumor vasculature compared to normal tissue vasculature affect the response of each of these tissues to ionizing radiation?

Question 6
What are the implications to tumor vasculature after a single fraction of ionizing radiation greater than 10 Gy based on animal tumor and human xenograft models?

Question 7
By what mechanism/pathway does high-dose radiation (>10 Gy) lead to apoptosis of endothelial cells?

Question 5 *How do the differences in tumor vasculature compared to normal tissue vasculature affect the response of each of these tissues to ionizing radiation?*

Answer 5

The differences in vascular properties, primarily the abnormal structure and organization of tumor blood vessels compared to normal tissue blood vessels, likely account for the hypoxia, nutritional depletion, and acidic intratumor microenvironment that leads to a differential response between tumors and normal tissues to ionizing radiation.

Song SW, Park H, Griffin R, Levitt SH. Radiobiology of stereotactic radiosurgery and stereotactic body radiation therapy. In: Levitt SH, Purdy JA, Perez CA, Poortmans P, eds. *Technical Basis of Radiation Therapy.* Berlin/Heidelberg: Springer-Verlag; 2012:51–61.

Question 6 *What are the implications to tumor vasculature after a single fraction of ionizing radiation greater than 10 Gy based on animal tumor and human xenograft models?*

Answer 6

Most of the data on the effects of high-dose radiation on tumor vasculature comes from studies in animal tumor models and human xenograft models. These studies show the functional vascularity in tumors undergoes a rapid decline within several hours after irradiation of greater than 10 Gy. This is thought to be due, in part, to death of endothelial cells and also to collapse of the tumor vessels due to increased interstitial pressure caused by extravasation of plasma protein. With doses of 8 to 10 Gy, studies have also shown ceramide-mediated apoptosis of tumor endothelial cells, leading to indirect tumor kill. Lastly, tumor shrinkage by high-dose irradiation can cause disruption and disorganization of tumor vascular networks.

Song SW, Park H, Griffin R, Levitt SH. Radiobiology of stereotactic radiosurgery and stereotactic body radiation therapy. In: Levitt SH, Purdy JA, Perez CA, Poortmans P, eds. *Technical Basis of Radiation Therapy.* Berlin/Heidelberg: Springer-Verlag; 2012:51–61.

Question 7 *By what mechanism/pathway does high-dose radiation (>10 Gy) lead to apoptosis of endothelial cells?*

Answer 7

Endothelial cell apoptosis is mediated via the sphingomyelin pathway. In this pathway, exposure to high-dose radiation (>10 Gy) leads to translocation of acid sphingomyelinase (ASMase) to the plasma membrane of endothelial cells, where it helps generate ceramide from sphingomyelin. The release of ceramide leads to activation of the BCL-2 associated X protein (BAX) proapoptotic protein (part of the Bcl-2 family), which then causes release of mitochondrial cytochrome c and consequently commits the cell to apoptosis via the intrinsic pathway. Endothelial cell apoptosis peaks at about 6 hours postradiation exposure and leads to vascular dysfunction. This combination of vascular dysfunction and DNA damage after a high-dose radiation exposure leads to the increased tumor cell kill and high local control rates demonstrated with stereotactic radiosurgery (SRS)/stereotactic body radiation therapy (SBRT).

Balagamwala EH, Chao ST, Suh JH. Principles of radiobiology of stereotactic radiosurgery and clinical applications in the central nervous system. *Technol Cancer Res Treat.* 2012;11(1):3–13.

Question 8
How is ceramide produced with radiation exposures greater than 17 Gy?

Question 9
How do vascular endothelial growth factor (VEGF) inhibitors act as potential radiosensitizing agents in stereotactic radiosurgery (SRS)/stereotactic body radiation therapy (SBRT)?

Question 10
Does ionizing radiation damage blood vessels within the tumor in an equal distribution?

Question 8 *How is ceramide produced with radiation exposures greater than 17 Gy?*

Answer 8

At higher doses of ionizing radiation (>17 Gy), in addition to the ASMase pathway described in Question 7, ceramide is also produced by ceramide synthase. This second pathway is modulated by ataxia telangiectasia-mutated (ATM) kinase, which typically represses ceramide synthase under normal conditions. The ceramide synthase pathway can also be activated by unrepaired double-stranded DNA breaks at lower doses of radiation exposure, also leading to apoptosis.

Balagamwala EH, Chao ST, Suh JH. Principles of radiobiology of stereotactic radiosurgery and clinical applications in the central nervous system. *Technol Cancer Res Treat.* 2012;11(1):3–13.

Question 9 *How do vascular endothelial growth factor (VEGF) inhibitors act as potential radiosensitizing agents in stereotactic radiosurgery (SRS)/stereotactic body radiation therapy (SBRT)?*

Answer 9

In cultured endothelial cells, the presence of VEGF has been shown to prevent radiation-induced ASMase activation, leading to decreased apoptosis of the endothelial cells. VEGF inhibitors (such as bevacizumab) allow unhindered activation of ASMase and the subsequent ceramide → BAX → mitochondrial cytochrome c pathway that ultimately leads to endothelial cell apoptotic death via the intrinsic pathway and consequent vascular dysfunction. The inhibition of VEGF must occur within 60 minutes before the high-dose radiation exposure to be effective.

Balagamwala EH, Chao ST, Suh JH. Principles of radiobiology of stereotactic radiosurgery and clinical applications in the central nervous system. *Technol Cancer Res Treat.* 2012;11(1):3–13.

Question 10 *Does ionizing radiation damage blood vessels within the tumor in an equal distribution?*

Answer 10

Studies in animal tumor models and human xenograft models have shown that irradiation leads to preferential destruction of vasculature in the inner regions of tumors as compared to those in the tumor periphery. This is likely due to the fact that blood vessels in the periphery are more likely to be vessels co-opted from normal tissues and therefore more stable and resistant to radiation damage. It has also been shown that blood vessels in smaller tumors tend to be more radiosensitive than those in larger tumors.

Song SW, Park H, Griffin R, Levitt SH. Radiobiology of stereotactic radiosurgery and stereotactic body radiation therapy. In: Levitt SH, Purdy JA, Perez CA, Poortmans P, eds. *Technical Basis of Radiation Therapy.* Berlin/Heidelberg: Springer-Verlag; 2012:51–61.

Question 11

Why have several clinical studies of high-dose hypofractionated radiation therapy (stereotactic radiosurgery [SRS] or stereotactic body radiation therapy [SBRT]) shown higher local control rates and tumor cell kill than what would be predicted by the *linear-quadratic (LQ)* model?

Question 12

Why does the total clonogenic cell death survival curve (assuming a 10% hypoxic fraction) differ after exposure to different doses of ionizing radiation in a single fraction: less than 5 Gy, 5 to 10 Gy, and greater than 10 Gy?

Question 13

How are cancer stem cells potentially affected by high-dose hypofractionated irradiation?

Question 11 *Why have several clinical studies of high-dose hypofractionated radiation therapy (stereotactic radiosurgery [SRS] or stereotactic body radiation therapy [SBRT]) shown higher local control rates and tumor cell kill than what would be predicted by the linear-quadratic (LQ) model?*

Answer 11

Many clinical studies with SRS and SBRT have shown local control rates of 80% to 95+% with fraction sizes greater than 10 Gy, but mathematical calculations assuming a 10% to 20% hypoxic fraction and other normal assumptions with the LQ model (alpha/beta ratio = 10, oxygen enhancement ratio (OER) = 3, no reoxygenation/repopulation during treatment) predict far less cell kill (in one study looking at the commonly used 20 Gy × 3 regimen for non-small cell lung cancer (NSCLC), the calculation predicts only 7.7 log cell kill, which would be insufficient to kill even small tumors). This implies that high-dose hypofractionated irradiation kills tumor cells via mechanisms other than just direct DNA damage and can overcome hypoxic radioprotection via other mechanisms such as vascular damage and immune response.

Song SW, Park H, Griffin R, Levitt SH. Radiobiology of stereotactic radiosurgery and stereotactic body radiation therapy. In: Levitt SH, Purdy JA, Perez CA, Poortmans P, eds. *Technical Basis of Radiation Therapy.* Berlin/Heidelberg: Springer-Verlag; 2012:51–61.

Question 12 *Why does the total clonogenic cell death survival curve (assuming a 10% hypoxic fraction) differ after exposure to different doses of ionizing radiation in a single fraction: less than 5 Gy, 5 to 10 Gy, and greater than 10 Gy?*

Answer 12

With a single dose of less than 5 Gy, there is an initial steep decline in the cell survival curve caused by direct killing of oxygenated cells. With a single fraction of 5 to 10 Gy, this steep decline is followed by a shallower phase of the survival curve that corresponds to the direct killing of hypoxic cells. With a single fraction of greater than 10 Gy, there is a second sharp decline in the cell survival curve after the initial two phases that corresponds to indirect cell death due to vascular damage.

Song SW, Park H, Griffin R, Levitt SH. Radiobiology of stereotactic radiosurgery and stereotactic body radiation therapy. In: Levitt SH, Purdy JA, Perez CA, Poortmans P, eds. *Technical Basis of Radiation Therapy.* Berlin/Heidelberg: Springer-Verlag; 2012:51–61.

Question 13 *How are cancer stem cells potentially affected by high-dose hypofractionated irradiation?*

Answer 13

Cancer stem cells have been identified as a self-renewing population of cells that tend to be radioresistant and can cause tumor relapse after radiation therapy has otherwise depleted the nonstem cell tumor population. These cancer stem cells live in the perivascular space of tumors, and tumor endothelial cells provide factors that maintain the cells in their self-renewing and undifferentiated state. High-dose hypofractionated radiation therapy (>10 Gy) causes damage and death to tumor endothelial cells, which may lead to the depletion of cancer stem cells, and therefore greater tumor control.

Song SW, Park H, Griffin R, Levitt SH. Radiobiology of stereotactic radiosurgery and stereotactic body radiation therapy. In: Levitt SH, Purdy JA, Perez CA, Poortmans P, eds. *Technical Basis of Radiation Therapy.* Berlin/Heidelberg: Springer-Verlag; 2012:51–61.

Question 14
What are the 4 R's of radiation biology?

Question 15
How is the reoxygenation effect different between conventional fractionated radiotherapy and stereotactic radiosurgery (SRS)/stereotactic body radiation therapy (SBRT)?

Question 16
How is the repair of sublethal radiation damage effect different between conventional fractionated radiotherapy and stereotactic radiosurgery (SRS)/stereotactic body radiation therapy (SBRT)?

Question 14 *What are the 4 R's of radiation biology?*

Answer 14

The 4 R's of radiation biology are: reoxygenation of hypoxic tumor cells, repair of sublethal radiation damage, redistribution/reassortment of cells in cell cycle phases, and repopulation of cells.

Hall EJ, Giaccia AJ. Time, dose, and fractionation in radiotherapy. In: Hall EJ, Giaccia AJ, eds. *Radiobiology for the Radiologist.* 7th ed. Philadelphia, PA: Lippincott Williams & Wilkins; 2012:391–411.

Question 15 *How is the reoxygenation effect different between conventional fractionated radiotherapy and stereotactic radiosurgery (SRS)/stereotactic body radiation therapy (SBRT)?*

Answer 15

In conventional fractionated radiotherapy (1.8–2.0 Gy/fraction), a single fraction of ionizing radiation will kill the oxic cells, but not the hypoxic cells. Between fractions, the hypoxic cells become oxygenated due to decreased oxygen demand from the death of the oxic tumor cells and the ability for oxygen to now diffuse and reach the cells in previously hypoxic areas of the tumor. These newly oxic cells will now be sensitive to radiation damage and cell death. In SRS/SBRT with doses greater than 10 Gy, there can be significant vascular damage that decreases the reoxygenation effect. Hypoxic cells are still killed in SBRT/SRS, but more typically as a secondary or indirect effect of the vascular damage. If doses less than 10 Gy are used in SBRT/SRS, then reoxygenation can still occur.

Song SW, Park H, Griffin R, Levitt SH. Radiobiology of stereotactic radiosurgery and stereotactic body radiation therapy. In: Levitt SH, Purdy JA, Perez CA, Poortmans P, eds. *Technical Basis of Radiation Therapy.* Berlin/Heidelberg: Springer-Verlag; 2012:51–61.

Question 16 *How is the repair of sublethal radiation damage effect different between conventional fractionated radiotherapy and stereotactic radiosurgery (SRS)/stereotactic body radiation therapy (SBRT)?*

Answer 16

In conventional fractionated radiotherapy (1.8–2.0 Gy/fraction), the time of delivery of radiation dose is extremely short; therefore, a negligible amount of repair of sublethal damage occurs during radiation exposure. In SRS/SBRT, however, there may be a more pronounced component of sublethal damage repair, because it takes a longer period of time to deliver high doses of radiation. Since the kinetics of sublethal radiation damage repair are biphasic (median half-time for faster components = 0.3 hours, median half-time for slower components = 4 hours), it has been estimated that at least 10% of biological effectiveness is lost due to sublethal damage repair when radiation exposures last greater than 30 minutes. However, repair may be hindered due to the hypoxic, acidic, and nutritionally depleted microenvironment created by vascular damage with SRS/SBRT.

Song SW, Park H, Griffin R, Levitt SH. Radiobiology of stereotactic radiosurgery and stereotactic body radiation therapy. In: Levitt SH, Purdy JA, Perez CA, Poortmans P, eds. *Technical Basis of Radiation Therapy.* Berlin/Heidelberg: Springer-Verlag; 2012:51–61.

Question 17

How is the reassortment effect different between conventional fractionated radiotherapy and stereotactic radiosurgery (SRS)/stereotactic body radiation therapy (SBRT)?

Question 18

How is the repopulation effect different between conventional fractionated radiotherapy and stereotactic radiosurgery (SRS)/stereotactic body radiation therapy (SBRT)?

Question 19

Is the linear-quadratic (LQ) model applicable to the dose and fractionation schemes used in stereotactic radiosurgery (SRS)/stereotactic body radiation therapy (SBRT)? Why or why not?

Question 17 *How is the reassortment effect different between conventional fractionated radiotherapy and stereotactic radiosurgery (SRS)/stereotactic body radiation therapy (SBRT)?*

Answer 17

After a low-to-moderate dose of ionizing radiation, cells will arrest in different phases of the cell cycle (phase of arrest determined by the dose) to help with repair of radiation-induced repair before progressing through the cell cycle. This is typically the G2 phase with lower doses of radiation. Eventually, though, the cycle arrest will disappear and the cells will again be reassorted into different phases of the cell cycle. This is the reassortment effect. With conventional fractionated radiation therapy (1.8–2.0 Gy/fraction), most damaged cells will transiently arrest in the G2 phase, leading to mitotic cell death. However, with very high single fraction doses of ionizing radiation (>15–20 Gy), cells are permanently arrested and killed in the phase of the cell cycle at which they were irradiated with no reassortment effect seen.

Song SW, Park H, Griffin R, Levitt SH. Radiobiology of stereotactic radiosurgery and stereotactic body radiation therapy. In: Levitt SH, Purdy JA, Perez CA, Poortmans P, eds. *Technical Basis of Radiation Therapy*. Berlin/Heidelberg: Springer-Verlag; 2012:51–61.

Question 18 *How is the repopulation effect different between conventional fractionated radiotherapy and stereotactic radiosurgery (SRS)/stereotactic body radiation therapy (SBRT)?*

Answer 18

With a conventional fractionated (1.8–2.0 Gy/fraction) course of radiotherapy, tumor cells and normal tissue cells that survive radiation exposure during the course of treatment can continue to grow and proliferate. This implies that the number of tumor cells that must be sterilized increases during a course of fractionated radiotherapy. This repopulation effect is typically noted at 3 to 4 weeks after the initiation of radiotherapy. With SRS/SBRT, the overall duration of treatment is quite short (typically ≤2 weeks), so repopulation is considered less significant.

Song SW, Park H, Griffin R, Levitt SH. Radiobiology of stereotactic radiosurgery and stereotactic body radiation therapy. In: Levitt SH, Purdy JA, Perez CA, Poortmans P, eds. *Technical Basis of Radiation Therapy*. Berlin/Heidelberg: Springer-Verlag; 2012:51–61.

Question 19 *Is the linear-quadratic (LQ) model applicable to the dose and fractionation schemes used in stereotactic radiosurgery (SRS)/stereotactic body radiation therapy (SBRT)? Why or why not?*

Answer 19

The LQ model is based on the principles of irreparable (alpha) and reparable (beta) DNA damage caused by ionizing radiation that lead to cell death. This model does not take into account any secondary cell death that may be caused by vascular damage and is therefore not particularly applicable for fraction sizes greater than 10 Gy. However, the LQ model is considered applicable for fraction sizes less than 10 Gy. Although other modified LQ models have been proposed to better fit clinically observed data, none of these models incorporate cell death due to vascular damage, so they are not considered applicable either.

Song SW, Park H, Griffin R, Levitt SH. Radiobiology of stereotactic radiosurgery and stereotactic body radiation therapy. In: Levitt SH, Purdy JA, Perez CA, Poortmans P, eds. *Technical Basis of Radiation Therapy*. Berlin/Heidelberg: Springer-Verlag; 2012:51–61.

Question 20

What is the definition of low-dose rate (LDR), medium-dose rate (MDR), and high-dose rate (HDR) brachytherapy?

Question 21

What is pulsed dose rate (PDR) brachytherapy?

Question 22

What is the difference between the dose rates used in external beam radiation therapy (EBRT) and brachytherapy?

Question 23

What is the difference between the dose gradients found in conventional external beam radiation therapy (EBRT) and those found in brachytherapy plans?

Question 20 *What is the definition of low-dose rate (LDR), medium-dose rate (MDR), and high-dose rate (HDR) brachytherapy?*

Answer 20

Brachytherapy is defined as radiotherapy delivered using nuclides placed within or in contact of the area to be treated. LDR is defined as less than or equal to 2 Gy/hr, but most commonly delivered at dose rates between 0.3 and 1 Gy/hr. MDR is defined as dose rates of 2 to 12 Gy/hr. MDR is rarely used in clinical applications. HDR is defined as dose rates greater than 12 Gy/hr.

Chang DS, Lasley FD, Das IJ, Mendonca MS, Dynlacht JR. Biology of brachytherapy, particle therapy, and alternative radiation modalities. In: *Basic Radiotherapy Physics and Biology*. New York, NY: Springer; 2014:292–296.

Question 21 *What is pulsed dose rate (PDR) brachytherapy?*

Answer 21

PDR brachytherapy delivers the dose in a large number of small fractions with short intervals (typically using a lower activity high-dose rate (HDR) source and afterloader), which allows only for incomplete repair of DNA damage, mimicking the biological effect of low-dose rate (LDR) radiotherapy over the same treatment time (typically a few days).

Chang DS, Lasley FD, Das IJ, Mendonca MS, Dynlacht JR. Biology of brachytherapy, particle therapy, and alternative radiation modalities. In: *Basic Radiotherapy Physics and Biology*. New York, NY: Springer; 2014:292–296.

Question 22 *What is the difference between the dose rates used in external beam radiation therapy (EBRT) and brachytherapy?*

Answer 22

EBRT (with total body irradiation being an exception) is typically delivered at a high-dose rate (HDR). Brachytherapy can be delivered via low-dose rate (LDR), HDR, pulsed dose rate (PDR), or very LDRs (using permanent implants).

Chang DS, Lasley FD, Das IJ, Mendonca MS, Dynlacht JR. Biology of brachytherapy, particle therapy, and alternative radiation modalities. In: *Basic Radiotherapy Physics and Biology*. New York, NY: Springer; 2014:292–296.

Question 23 *What is the difference between the dose gradients found in conventional external beam radiation therapy (EBRT) and those found in brachytherapy plans?*

Answer 23

In general, EBRT plans attempt to achieve more homogeneous and uniform dose distributions within the target volume. In contrast, in brachytherapy planning, dose is prescribed to an isodose encircling a small target volume. The dose distribution is extremely heterogeneous because of the inverse square relationship—in the very near vicinity of the source, the dose and dose rate are extremely high; the dose falls off rapidly as a function of the distance from the source. Because the dose is typically prescribed at the periphery of the tumor volume, the average dose received by the tumor itself is actually higher in brachytherapy applications.

Mazeron JJ, Scalliet P, Van Limbergen E, Lartigau E. Radiobiology of brachytherapy and the dose rate effect. In: *GEC-ESTRO Handbook of Brachytherapy*. http://www.estro.org/binaries/content/assets/estro/about/gec-estro/handbook-of-brachytherapy/e-4-23072002-radiobiology-print_proc.pdf. Accessed February 19, 2016.

Question 24

Why are normal tissue dose tolerance levels higher in brachytherapy applications than those considered acceptable with external beam radiation therapy?

Question 25

How are the 4 R's of radiobiology different with high-dose rate (HDR) brachytherapy compared to external beam radiation therapy (EBRT)?

Question 26

How are the 4 R's of radiobiology different with low-dose rate (LDR) brachytherapy compared to external beam radiation therapy (EBRT)?

Question 24 *Why are normal tissue dose tolerance levels higher in brachytherapy applications than those considered acceptable with external beam radiation therapy?*

Answer 24

The dose tolerance levels in brachytherapy applications are often much higher than those that would be considered acceptable in external beam radiation treatment planning because of the volume effect relationship, which states that very small volumes of tissue can tolerate very high-dose levels.

Mazeron JJ, Scalliet P, Van Limbergen E, Lartigau E. Radiobiology of brachytherapy and the dose rate effect. In: *GEC-ESTRO Handbook of Brachytherapy*. http://www.estro.org/binaries/content/assets/estro/about/gec-estro/handbook-of-brachytherapy/e-4-23072002-radiobiology-print_proc.pdf. Accessed February 19, 2016.

Question 25 *How are the 4 R's of radiobiology different with high-dose rate (HDR) brachytherapy compared to external beam radiation therapy (EBRT)?*

Answer 25

The biological effects of radiation are very strongly dependent on the dose rate of treatment delivery, so in general, the radiobiological effects of HDR brachytherapy are the same as those seen with fractionated external beam therapy, except for the volume effect noted in Question 24. Since the duration of treatment is short with HDR brachytherapy, repair, repopulation, and reoxygenation occur only between consecutive treatments. Reassortment does not play an important role in HDR applications. HDR brachytherapy is reasonably modeled by the linear-quadratic (LQ) model.

Mazeron JJ, Scalliet P, Van Limbergen E, Lartigau E. Radiobiology of brachytherapy and the dose rate effect. In: *GEC-ESTRO Handbook of Brachytherapy*. http://www.estro.org/binaries/content/assets/estro/about/gec-estro/handbook-of-brachytherapy/e-4-23072002-radiobiology-print_proc.pdf. Accessed February 19, 2016.

Question 26 *How are the 4 R's of radiobiology different with low-dose rate (LDR) brachytherapy compared to external beam radiation therapy (EBRT)?*

Answer 26

As noted earlier, the biological effects of radiation are strongly dependent on the dose rate of treatment delivered; the biological effect of radiation decreases as the dose rate decreases. With LDR brachytherapy, the duration of treatment is quite long (typically dose rates are ~0.3 to 1 Gy/hr, therefore, treatment is delivered over several days), and repair of sublethal damage occurs during treatment. This modifies the linear-quadratic (LQ) model to add a time factor that depends upon the half-time for repair and the duration of exposure. If the exposure time is protracted enough, then the quadratic component of the LQ model disappears and the survival curve is linear ($S = alpha * D$). This modified LQ model is termed the "incomplete repair model." Theoretically, reassortment also plays an important role in LDR tumor kill because cells have time to synchronize in the G2/M stages (due to G2 block) during treatment and therefore are more radiosensitive, leading to increased cell kill. There is experimental evidence to this effect. Reoxygenation effects due to a temporary increase in blood flow via recirculation through closed vessels have been implicated in LDR brachytherapy and the oxygen enhancement ratio (OER) is estimated to be as low as 1.6 to 1.7 with LDR irradiation (compared to OER of 3 with fractionated EBRT). Typically, reoxygenation effects due to tumor shrinkage secondary to elimination of oxic cells are not seen in LDR as compared to fractionated EBRT. Repopulation does not play an important role in LDR given the time frame of delivery over a few days.

Mazeron JJ, Scalliet P, Van Limbergen E, Lartigau E. Radiobiology of brachytherapy and the dose rate effect. In: *GEC-ESTRO Handbook of Brachytherapy*. http://www.estro.org/binaries/content/assets/estro/about/gec-estro/handbook-of-brachytherapy/e-4-23072002-radiobiology-print_proc.pdf. Accessed February 19, 2016.

Question 27

What is the effect of dose rate on cell survival in experimental studies?

Question 28

What is the optimal interval between external beam radiation therapy and brachytherapy boost?

Question 29

Is there an effect of dose rate on local outcomes in low-dose rate (LDR) brachytherapy?

Question 27 *What is the effect of dose rate on cell survival in experimental studies?*

Answer 27

In vitro studies from the 1960s have shown that considerably more dose is required to achieve the same cell kill with low-dose rates (LDRs) compared to high-dose rates (HDRs) of radiation (e.g., the dose needed for 99% cell kill is 1.5 to 3 times higher at 1 Gy/hr compared to the dose needed if delivered at 1 Gy/min). This effect can differ based on the cell type as well. In vivo studies have shown that in tumors, dose must be increased by a factor of 1.1 to 2 to achieve the same biological effect at 1 Gy/hr compared to 1 Gy/min; early responding normal tissues require two times higher dose, whereas late-responding normal tissues require 2.5 times higher dose. This translates to a relative protective effect on late-responding normal tissues with LDR irradiation.

Mazeron JJ, Scalliet P, Van Limbergen E, Lartigau E. Radiobiology of brachytherapy and the dose rate effect. In: *GEC-ESTRO Handbook of Brachytherapy*. http://www.estro.org/binaries/content/assets/estro/about/gec-estro/handbook-of-brachytherapy/e-4-23072002-radiobiology-print_proc.pdf. Accessed February 19, 2016.

Question 28 *What is the optimal interval between external beam radiation therapy and brachytherapy boost?*

Answer 28

No specific optimal interval has been reported; however, tumor repopulation effects can be the most pronounced in the weeks following external beam radiation, so minimizing the interval between external beam and a brachytherapy boost may maximize local control.

Mazeron JJ, Scalliet P, Van Limbergen E, Lartigau E. Radiobiology of brachytherapy and the dose rate effect. In: *GEC-ESTRO Handbook of Brachytherapy*. http://www.estro.org/binaries/content/assets/estro/about/gec-estro/handbook-of-brachytherapy/e-4-23072002-radiobiology-print_proc.pdf. Accessed February 19, 2016.

Question 29 *Is there an effect of dose rate on local outcomes in low-dose rate (LDR) brachytherapy?*

Answer 29

Over the decades, this has been an area of controversy, but the most recent data from the 1990s imply that there is a clear effect of dose rate on local outcomes in the 0.3 to 1 Gy/hr range. The effect is most pronounced for late-responding normal tissues rather than on tumor local control. Decreasing the dose rate increases the therapeutic ratio. Most experts feel that with LDR brachytherapy, the total dose should be kept high to maximize local control and the dose rate should be kept low (0.3–0.6 Gy/hr) to minimize late effects on normal tissues.

Mazeron JJ, Scalliet P, Van Limbergen E, Lartigau E. Radiobiology of brachytherapy and the dose rate effect. In: *GEC-ESTRO Handbook of Brachytherapy*. http://www.estro.org/binaries/content/assets/estro/about/gec-estro/handbook-of-brachytherapy/e-4-23072002-radiobiology-print_proc.pdf. Accessed February 19, 2016.

Question 30
What are some of the potential advantages of high-dose rate (HDR) brachytherapy over low-dose rate (LDR) brachytherapy?

Question 31
How can various high-dose rate (HDR) brachytherapy fractionation schemes be compared?

Question 30 *What are some of the potential advantages of high-dose rate (HDR) brachytherapy over low-dose rate (LDR) brachytherapy?*

Answer 30

Some of the potential advantages of HDR remote afterloading include: (a) patient treatment times and immobilization times are much shorter, which leads to decreased potential for complications from prolonged immobility/bed rest, such as pulmonary emboli. (b) Applicator geometry can be better optimized due to the shorter duration of treatment. Also, image verification of applicator geometry can be performed prior to treatment delivery, ensuring more accurate delivery of dose to target volumes. (c) Treatment can be delivered on an outpatient basis, reducing overall health care costs by eliminating the need for operating room time and hospitalization.

Martinez AA. Brachytherapy. In: Gunderson LL, Tepper JE, eds. *Clinical Radiation Oncology*. 2nd ed. Philadelphia, PA: Elsevier Churchill Livingstone; 2007:255–282.

Question 31 *How can various high-dose rate (HDR) brachytherapy fractionation schemes be compared?*

Answer 31

The American Brachytherapy Society has developed a linear-quadratic (LQ) model spreadsheet that allows clinicians to calculate the 2 Gy equivalent doses and biological effective dose of various HDR dose and fractionation schemes. It also allows for computing total doses of radiation delivered with combinations of external beam radiation therapy and HDR brachytherapy. It is available for download at: https://www.americanbrachytherapy.org/guidelines/LQ_spreadsheet.xls.

24

GENE THERAPY

HYEONJOO CHEON

Question 1
What is gene therapy?

Question 2
What are commonly used viral vectors for gene therapy? What are the pros and cons for each viral vector system?

Question 3
How are viruses modified for gene therapy?

Question 4
What is suicide gene therapy?

Question 1 *What is gene therapy?*

Answer 1

Gene therapy is the delivery of genetic materials (RNA or DNA) into cells so that genetic properties of cells change. One or multiple aberrant genes can be replaced or their expression levels adjusted. Gene therapy encompasses treatments using monoclonal antibodies or small-molecule chemicals to correct pathological phenotypes caused by gene mutations.

Hall EJ, Giaccia AJ. Gene therapy. In: Hall EJ, Giaccia AJ, eds. *Radiobiology for the Radiologist*. 6th ed. Philadelphia, PA: Lippincott Williams & Wilkins; 2006:432–437.

Question 2 *What are commonly used viral vectors for gene therapy? What are the pros and cons for each viral vector system?*

Answer 2

1. Retroviral vector
   Pros: Retroviral vector can be incorporated into the host genome, and thus the incorporated genes are replicated during cell division.
   Cons: The infection rate is low, because only dividing cells can be infected with retroviruses. Integration is random and can activate proto-oncogenes.
2. Lentiviral vector
   Pros: (a) Therapeutic genes are incorporated into the host genome and replicated during cell division. Lentiviruses are a subclass of retroviruses. (b) The infected cell ratio is high since lentiviruses infect dividing and nondividing cells.
3. Adenoviruses
   Pros: Adenoviruses infect both dividing and quiescent cells. Infected cell ratio is high.
   Cons: (a) Adenoviral DNA is not integrated into host genome. Thus, it is not replicated during cell division, and the therapeutic effects are short lived. (b) Adenoviruses induce immune responses, which limit repeat treatments.

Hall EJ, Giaccia AJ. Gene therapy. In: Hall EJ, Giaccia AJ, eds. *Radiobiology for the Radiologist*. 6th ed. Philadelphia, PA: Lippincott Williams & Wilkins; 2006:432–437.
Thomas CE, Ehrhardt A, Kay MA. Progress and problems with the use of viral vectors for gene therapy. *Nat Rev Genet*. 2003;4(5):346–358.

Question 3 *How are viruses modified for gene therapy?*

Answer 3

Viral vectors are engineered so that they cannot produce pathogenic viruses. A part of the viral genome critical for viral replication is deleted from viral vectors, so that they do not replicate.

Hall EJ, Giaccia AJ. Gene therapy. In: Hall EJ, Giaccia AJ, eds. *Radiobiology for the Radiologist*. 6th ed. Philadelphia, PA: Lippincott Williams & Wilkins; 2006:432–437.

Question 4 *What is suicide gene therapy?*

Answer 4

Suicide gene therapy needs two components. The first component is a gene that converts an inert prodrug into a toxic agent. The gene, contained in a viral vector, is injected into the tumor. The encoded protein is not toxic by itself if there is no prodrug in the tumor. The second component is a prodrug, which is converted into a toxic agent by the injected gene product. The prodrug, which is nontoxic in itself, is administered systemically. The prodrug does not harm the nontumor region, but is converted into a toxic agent in the tumor that expresses the converter gene. The tumor cells will be killed by the toxic agent upon conversion from the prodrug.

Hall EJ, Giaccia AJ. Gene therapy. In: Hall EJ, Giaccia AJ, eds. *Radiobiology for the Radiologist*. 6th ed. Philadelphia, PA: Lippincott Williams & Wilkins; 2006:432–437.

Question 5

How would you describe two commonly used suicide gene therapy systems?

Question 6

What is the advantage of suicide gene therapy as an adjunct over chemotherapeutic agents?

Question 7

A "bystander effect" in which neighboring cells are killed can be seen with suicide gene therapy. What are the causes of the bystander effect?

Question 8

Adenovirus varieties are used not only as a viral vector for gene therapy but also can function as an oncolytic virus. How does adenoviral protein E1b contribute to virus propagation in infected human cells expressing wild-type p53?

Question 5 *How would you describe two commonly used suicide gene therapy systems?*

Answer 5

1. The most commonly used suicide gene system consists of herpes simplex virus thymidine kinase gene (*HSK-tk*, a gene injected into the tumor) plus ganciclovir (GCV, a prodrug administered systematically). In cells containing the thymidine kinase gene (*HSK-tk*), the prodrug (GCV) is activated to become a toxic agent. HSV-tk phosphorylates GCV, converting it to a nucleoside analogue that inhibits DNA synthesis. This system inhibits repair of DNA double-strand breaks.
2. An alternative suicide gene system involves *cytosine deaminase* (*CD*, a gene injected into the tumor), which converts 5-fluorocytosine (5-FC, a prodrug administered systemically) to 5-fluorouracil (5-FU, a toxic agent that kills tumor cells). The 5-FU induces DNA strand breaks.

Hall EJ, Giaccia AJ. Gene therapy. In: Hall EJ, Giaccia AJ, eds. *Radiobiology for the Radiologist.* 6th ed. Philadelphia, PA: Lippincott Williams & Wilkins; 2006:432–437.

Question 6 *What is the advantage of suicide gene therapy as an adjunct over chemotherapeutic agents?*

Answer 6

In suicide gene therapy, the cytotoxic molecules are produced locally within the tumor by the gene directly injected into the tumor. Thus, it can avoid systemic toxicity that is often observed with traditional chemoradiotherapy.

Hall EJ, Giaccia AJ. Gene therapy. In: Hall EJ, Giaccia AJ, eds. *Radiobiology for the Radiologist.* 6th ed. Philadelphia, PA: Lippincott Williams & Wilkins; 2006:432–437.

Question 7 *A "bystander effect" in which neighboring cells are killed can be seen with suicide gene therapy. What are the causes of the bystander effect?*

Answer 7

1. The toxic agent produced in the initially transduced cells is transported to neighboring cells through gap junctions.
2. When the initially transduced cells die and are lysed, the toxic agent is released and spread to surrounding cells.
3. When tumor cells die in response to toxic agents, additional antigens are released, inducing the activation of T cells and B cells that can attack tumor cells, including those in remote locations.

Hall EJ, Giaccia AJ. Gene therapy. In: Hall EJ, Giaccia AJ, eds. *Radiobiology for the Radiologist.* 6th ed. Philadelphia, PA: Lippincott Williams & Wilkins; 2006:432–437.
Namm JP, Li Q, Lao X, et al. B lymphocytes as effector cells in the immunotherapy of cancer. *J Surg Oncol.* 2012;105(4):431–435.
Ribas A, Butterfield LH, Glaspy JA, Economou JS. Current developments in cancer vaccines and cellular immunotherapy. *J Clin Oncol.* 2003;21(12):2415–2432.

Question 8 *Adenovirus varieties are used not only as a viral vector for gene therapy but also can function as an oncolytic virus. How does adenoviral protein E1b contribute to virus propagation in infected human cells expressing wild-type p53?*

Answer 8

Viral protein E1b interacts with and inactivates a normal p53 protein, blocking p53-induced apoptosis. The delayed apoptosis allows the virus to replicate, package its genome, lyse the cells, and spread to neighboring cells.

Ridgway PJ, Hall AR, Myers CJ, Braithwaite AW. P53/E1b58kDa complex regulates adenovirus replication. *Virology.* 1997;237:404–413.
Yew PR, Berk AJ. Inhibition of p53 transactivation required for transformation by adenovirus early 1B protein. *Nature.* 1992;357(6373):82–85.

Question 9
Adenovirus with *E1b* gene deleted or inactivated is used to target only cancer cells. How would you explain the mechanism by which it kills only cancer cells and spares normal cells?

Question 10
Adenoviral protein E1a targets a tumor suppressor protein Rb. What is the role of E1a in virus propagation?

Question 11
Adenovirus with *E1a* gene deleted is used to target only cancer cells. What is the mechanism by which it kills cancer cells and spares normal cells?

Question 12
What are cancer vaccines?

Question 9 *Adenovirus with* E1b *gene deleted or inactivated is used to target only cancer cells. How would you explain the mechanism by which it kills only cancer cells and spares normal cells?*

Answer 9

When *E1b*-deleted adenovirus infects normal cells with wild-type p53, it is prevented from replicating by the action of p53. On the other hand, this engineered virus can replicate in the absence of functional p53. Because most cancer cells are defective in p53 function, the *E1b*-deficient adenovirus can replicate in most cancer cells expressing no or mutant p53, leading to cell lysis. Cancer cells expressing wild-type p53 is not targeted by the *E1b*-deleted virus.

Barker DD, Berk AJ. Adenovirus proteins from both E1B reading frames are required for transformation of rodent cells by viral infection and DNA transfection. *Virology*. 1987;156(1):107–121.

Hall EJ, Giaccia AJ. Gene therapy. In: Hall EJ, Giaccia AJ, eds. *Radiobiology for the Radiologist*. 6th ed. Philadelphia, PA: Lippincott Williams & Wilkins; 2006:432–437.

Hann B, Balmain A. Replication of an E1B 5-kilodalton protein-deficient adenovirus (ONYX-015) is restored by gain-of-function rather than loss-of-function p53 mutation. *J Virol*. 2003;11588–11595.

Harada N, Maniwa Y, Yoshimura M, et al. E1B-deleted adenovirus replicates in p53-deficient lung cancer cells due to the absence of apoptosis. *Oncol Rep*. 2005;14(5):1155–1163.

Question 10 *Adenoviral protein* E1a *targets a tumor suppressor protein Rb. What is the role of* E1a *in virus propagation?*

Answer 10

The E1a protein is the first viral protein synthesized after adenoviral infection and is required for viral replication. One of the targets of E1a protein is Rb, which modulates the cell cycle. Binding of E1a to Rb protein results in the release of E2F transcription factor from preexisting E2F-Rb complexes. The free E2F then activates the E2 promoter of the adenoviral gene as well as several human genes related to cell cycle regulation. The E2F-induced cellular proteins help synthesis of viral DNA, resulting in multiple virus particles.

Dyson N, Harlow E. Adenovirus E1A targets key regulators of cell proliferation. *Cancer Surv*. 1992;12:161–195.

Question 11 *Adenovirus with* E1a *gene deleted is used to target only cancer cells. What is the mechanism by which it kills cancer cells and spares normal cells?*

Answer 11

Adenovirus with a deletion in the Rb-binding domain of the E1a protein can be used for gene therapy. When normal cells are infected with E1a-deficient adenovirus, host cells cannot enter S phase because of the action of active Rb protein. Therefore, E1a-deleted virus can replicate only in cells with inactive Rb. As Rb is already inactivated in most cancer cells, leading to uncontrolled proliferation, the E1a-deficient virus can replicate only in cancer cells.

Fueyo J, Gomez-Manzano C, Alemany R, et al. A mutant oncolytic adenovirus targeting the Rb pathway produces anti-glioma effect in vivo. *Oncogene*. 2000;19(1):2–12.

Hall EJ, Giaccia AJ. Gene therapy. In: Hall EJ, Giaccia AJ, eds. *Radiobiology for the Radiologist*. 6th ed. Philadelphia, PA: Lippincott Williams & Wilkins; 2006:432–437.

Ulasov IV, Tyler MA, Rivera AA, Nettelbeck DM, Douglas JT, Lesniak MS. Evaluation of E1A double mutant oncolytic adenovectors in anti-glioma gene therapy. *J Med Virol*. 2008;80(9):1595–1603.

Question 12 *What are cancer vaccines?*

Answer 12

Cancer vaccines stimulate immune responses to cancer. They are effective against metastatic lesions. They are intended to delay or stop cancer growth, prevent cancer recurrence, or eliminate cancer cells by stimulating immune responses.

Hall EJ, Giaccia AJ. Gene therapy. In: Hall EJ, Giaccia AJ, eds. *Radiobiology for the Radiologist*. 6th ed. Philadelphia, PA: Lippincott Williams & Wilkins; 2006:432–437.

Question 13
There are several ways to stimulate immune responses using gene therapy technologies. How is gene therapy used to induce cytokines that activate immune cells?

Question 14
Tumor antigens stimulate B cells that produce tumor-specific antibodies and cytotoxic T cells that directly attack cancer cells. What are several realistic ways to introduce tumor antigens into the body to enhance immune responses?

Question 15
p53 is an important transcription factor involved in cell cycle checkpoint, DNA repair, apoptosis, and angiogenesis. Most cancer cells are deficient in the function of p53 through its mutation or deletion. What types of gene therapy can be applied to correct the deficiency of p53?

Question 16
The ideal strategy for gene therapy is to replace a gene whose mutation initiates or maintains the malignant phenotype. What are limitations of this strategy?

Question 13 *There are several ways to stimulate immune responses using gene therapy technologies. How is gene therapy used to induce cytokines that activate immune cells?*

Answer 13

DNA encoding cytokines can be injected directly into a tumor. Cytokines are naturally produced by immune cells and regulate immune responses. Some cytokines, such as IL-2, GM-CSF, IFNγ, and IFNα, increase the activity of cytotoxic T cells, which act against cancer cells. Tumor cells can be injected with DNA encoding these cytokines.

Hall EJ, Giaccia AJ. Gene therapy. In: Hall EJ, Giaccia AJ, eds. *Radiobiology for the Radiologist*. 6th ed. Philadelphia, PA: Lippincott Williams & Wilkins; 2006:432–437.

Berzofsky JA, Terabe M, Wood LV. Strategies to use immune modulators in therapeutic vaccines against cancer. *Semin Oncol*. 2012;39(3):348–357.

Question 14 *Tumor antigens stimulate B cells that produce tumor-specific antibodies and cytotoxic T cells that directly attack cancer cells. What are several realistic ways to introduce tumor antigens into the body to enhance immune responses?*

Answer 14

1. Synthetic peptide of tumor antigen can be injected systemically. The synthetic peptide is often modified to stimulate immune responses that are stronger than those caused by the original antigens.
2. DNA encoding tumor antigens can be injected into a patient as a "naked nucleic acid" vaccine or packaged in viruses. The introduced DNA is incorporated into a cellular genome and produces large quantities of antigens to stimulate a strong immune response.
3. Cancer cells lysed by oncolytic virus release tumor antigens.

Berzofsky JA, Wood LV, Terabe M. Cancer vaccines: 21st century approaches to harnessing an ancient modality to fight cancer. *Expert Rev Vaccines*. 2013;12(10):1115–1118.

Hall EJ, Giaccia AJ. Gene therapy. In: Hall EJ, Giaccia AJ, eds. *Radiobiology for the Radiologist*. 6th ed. Philadelphia, PA: Lippincott Williams & Wilkins; 2006:432–437.

Question 15 *p53 is an important transcription factor involved in cell cycle checkpoint, DNA repair, apoptosis, and angiogenesis. Most cancer cells are deficient in the function of p53 through its mutation or deletion. What types of gene therapy can be applied to correct the deficiency of p53?*

Answer 15

Transduction of cells with wild-type p53 can inhibit growth and angiogenesis or initiate apoptosis. Clinical trials have been conducted combining *p53* gene therapy with radiation therapy (RT) in patients. Clinical trials reveal that this treatment is safe and far less harmful to normal cells than chemotherapy. Combination *p53* gene therapy and RT is significantly more effective than radiation treatment alone in lung cancer.

Hall EJ, Giaccia AJ. Gene therapy. In: Hall EJ, Giaccia AJ, eds. *Radiobiology for the Radiologist*. 6th ed. Philadelphia, PA: Lippincott Williams & Wilkins; 2006:432–437.

Wang Z, Sun Y. Targeting p53 for novel anticancer therapy. *Transl Oncol*. 2010;3(1):1–12.

Question 16 *The ideal strategy for gene therapy is to replace a gene whose mutation initiates or maintains the malignant phenotype. What are limitations of this strategy?*

Answer 16

1. Many genetic changes are needed for malignant transformation.
2. The genes causing or maintaining the malignant phenotype have not been fully identified.
3. Gene replacement affects only a minority of tumor cells.

Brower V. Cancer gene therapy steadily advances. *J Natl Cancer*. 2008;Inst100(18):1276–1278.

Hall EJ, Giaccia AJ. Gene therapy. In: Hall EJ, Giaccia AJ, eds. *Radiobiology for the Radiologist*. 6th ed. Philadelphia, PA: Lippincott Williams & Wilkins; 2006:432–437

Question 17

How can we manipulate a therapeutic gene to be induced only in response to radiation?

Question 18

What is the advantage of radiation-inducible gene therapy (radiogenetic therapy)?

Question 19

A hallmark of the cancer is dysregulation of growth and signal transduction pathways that often results in resistance to radiation therapy. What are some pathways that are commonly deregulated in cancer and targets of biological agents?

Question 20

Many therapeutic approaches are aimed at epidermal growth factor receptor (EGFR), whose expression is higher in cancer cells. How can we inhibit EGFR pathway activation?

Question 21

In some cancer patients, epidermal growth factor receptor (EGFR) is consistently activated due to mutation in its cytoplasmic domain. What is the most practical way to target EGFR mutant tumors?

Question 17 *How can we manipulate a therapeutic gene to be induced only in response to radiation?*

Answer 17

Cancer cells are transduced with a chimeric gene that can be activated by radiation. The chimeric gene includes a cytotoxic gene, such as tumor necrosis factor (TNF)-α, under a promoter/enhancer that is activated by radiation, such as early growth response gene (*Egr-1*). TNFα is expressed only in the radiation field by activated *Egr-1* promoter, causing vascular destruction as well as apoptosis of tumor cells.

Hall EJ, Giaccia AJ. Gene therapy. In: Hall EJ, Giaccia AJ, eds. *Radiobiology for the Radiologist*. 6th ed. Philadelphia, PA: Lippincott Williams & Wilkins; 2006:432–437.

Question 18 *What is the advantage of radiation-inducible gene therapy (radiogenetic therapy)?*

Answer 18

Total body toxicity can be avoided in this therapy since the gene is expressed only in the radiation field.

Hall EJ, Giaccia AJ. Gene therapy. In: Hall EJ, Giaccia AJ, eds. *Radiobiology for the Radiologist*. 6th ed. Philadelphia, PA: Lippincott Williams & Wilkins; 2006:432–437.

Question 19 *A hallmark of the cancer is dysregulation of growth and signal transduction pathways that often results in resistance to radiation therapy. What are some pathways that are commonly deregulated in cancer and targets of biological agents?*

Answer 19

Because epidermal growth factor receptor (EGFR), Raf-1, and NFκB pathway are disrupted in a wide spectrum of human cancers, they have been targeted for cancer therapy. Their activities can be regulated using monoclonal antibodies and low-molecular weight chemical inhibitors.

Hall EJ, Giaccia AJ. Gene therapy. In: Hall EJ, Giaccia AJ, eds. *Radiobiology for the Radiologist*. 6th ed. Philadelphia, PA: Lippincott Williams & Wilkins; 2006:432–437.

Question 20 *Many therapeutic approaches are aimed at epidermal growth factor receptor (EGFR), whose expression is higher in cancer cells. How can we inhibit EGFR pathway activation?*

Answer 20

Monoclonal antibody inhibitors are used to block the epidermal growth factor (EFG) binding site on the extracellular domain of EGFR. Since EGF cannot attach to EGFR, the downstream signaling cascade from EGFR is not activated. We can also use small-molecule inhibitors that target the tyrosine kinase activity of the cytoplasmic domain of EGFR.

Sgambato A, Casaluce F, Maione P, et al. The role of EGFR tyrosine kinase inhibitors in the first-line treatment of advanced non-small cell lung cancer patients harboring EGFR mutation. *Curr Med Chem*. 2012;19(20):3337–3352.

Yan L, Hsu K, Beckman RA. Antibody-based therapy for solid tumors. *Cancer J*. 2008;14(3):178–183.

Question 21 *In some cancer patients, epidermal growth factor receptor (EGFR) is consistently activated due to mutation in its cytoplasmic domain. What is the most practical way to target EGFR mutant tumors?*

Answer 21

Some specific mutations in the cytoplasmic domain of EGFR cause the constitutive tyrosine kinase activation of EGFR. Because it is a downstream event of ligand binding, blocking EGFR with monoclonal antibodies cannot block this constitutive activation. Only tyrosine kinase inhibitors specific for mutated EGFR are effective in blocking EGFR signaling.

Sgambato A, Casaluce F, Maione P, et al. The role of EGFR tyrosine kinase inhibitors in the first-line treatment of advanced non small cell lung cancer patients harboring EGFR mutation. *Curr Med Chem*. 2012; 19(20):3337–3352.

Question 22

More than 30 mutations in the *BRAF* gene are identified to be associated with human cancer. The most common mutation is V600E. What is a practical approach to target cancers with the BRAF-V600E mutation?

Question 23

Although therapeutic gene constructs are often injected into a tumor, they cannot completely avoid normal tissue toxicity. To increase tumor specificity, what promoters can be used in gene therapy constructs?

Question 24

Recently developed nuclease-based genomic editing technologies, including zinc finger nucleases (ZENs) or clustered regularly interspaced short palindromic repeats (CRISPR)-Cas9, have the potential to be powerful tools for gene therapy. What are the advantages of these technologies over other gene therapy tools?

Question 22 *More than 30 mutations in the* BRAF *gene are identified to be associated with human cancer. The most common mutation is V600E. What is a practical approach to target cancers with the BRAF-V600E mutation?*

Answer 22

BRAF inhibitors, which disable BRAF kinase activity, are used alone or in combination with MEK inhibitors. MEK is a downstream kinase of BRAF. Several RAF inhibitors have been developed to combat cancers with BRAF-V600E.

Long GV, Stroyakovskiy D, Gogas H, et al. Combined BRAF and MEK inhibition versus BRAF inhibition alone in melanoma. *N Engl J Med.* 2014;371(20):1877–1888.

Maurer G, Tarkowski B, Baccarini M. Raf kinases in cancer-roles and therapeutic opportunities. *Oncogene.* 2011; 30(32):3477–3488.

Question 23 *Although therapeutic gene constructs are often injected into a tumor, they cannot completely avoid normal tissue toxicity. To increase tumor specificity, what promoters can be used in gene therapy constructs?*

Answer 23

1. A hypoxia-sensitive element can be added to the gene therapy construct. The hypoxia-inducible factor will bind to the hypoxia-sensitive element and activate transcription of therapeutic cytotoxic genes in hypoxic conditions. This strategy kills cancer cells dwelling in regions of hypoxia, where chemotherapy and radiation therapy are not particularly effective.
2. Tumor-specific promoters can be added to the gene therapy construct. Tumor-specific promoters are active in specific tumor cells, such as breast cancer or prostate cancer. Some tumor-specific promoters are constitutively activated at high levels in malignant cells but not in normal tissues.

Hall EJ, Giaccia AJ. Gene therapy. In: Hall EJ, Giaccia AJ, eds. *Radiobiology for the Radiologist.* 6th ed. Philadelphia, PA: Lippincott Williams & Wilkins; 2006:432–437.

Question 24 *Recently developed nuclease-based genomic editing technologies, including zinc finger nucleases (ZENs) or clustered regularly interspaced short palindromic repeats (CRISPR)-Cas9, have the potential to be powerful tools for gene therapy. What are the advantages of these technologies over other gene therapy tools?*

Answer 24

These technologies use nucleases to make site-specific double-stranded breaks in the genome. They can inactivate genes, correct mutated sequences, or insert intact genes by a wide range of genome alterations, including localized mutagenesis, local and dispersed sequence replacement, large and small insertions and deletions, and even chromosomal translocations.

Corrigan-Curay J, O'Reilly M, Kohn DB, et al. Genome editing technologies: defining a path to clinic. *Mol Ther.* 2015;23(5):796–806.

Question 25

What is the advantage of the clustered regularly interspaced short palindromic repeats (CRISPR)-Cas9 system over other nuclease-based gene editing technologies?

Question 25 *What is the advantage of the clustered regularly interspaced short palindromic repeats (CRISPR)-Cas9 system over other nuclease-based gene editing technologies?*

Answer 25

To target specific gene sequences, other gene editing nucleases use a protein domain that recognizes and binds to the target DNA sequence. The CRISPR-Cas9 system uses an RNA-guided system to recognize the target sequence. Due to the relative ease of engineering the RNA-based targeting component, various regions of the genome can be targeted. When multiple guide RNAs (gRNA) are used, multiple targets can be edited. The gRNA recognizes 20 bp target sites on the genome and engages the Cas9 nuclease to cleave the target complementary DNA sequence (Figure 24.1).

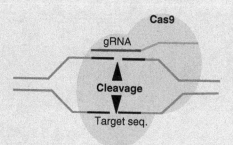

Figure 24.1 RNA-guided endonuclease CRISPR-Cas9.

Corrigan-Curay J, O'Reilly M, Kohn DB, et al. Genome editing technologies: defining a path to clinic. *Mol Ther*. 2015;23(5):796–806.

25

CHEMOTHERAPY AND TARGETED AGENTS

NIKHIL JOSHI AND NEIL WOODY

Question 1
What are the broad classifications of chemotherapy agents?

Question 2
How is emetogenecity of chemotherapy classified (chemotherapy-induced nausea and vomiting [CINV])?

Question 3
What is the mechanism of action of cisplatin? What are some of its toxicities?

Turn page to see the answers.

Question 1 *What are the broad classifications of chemotherapy agents?*

Answer 1

Alkylating agents—these drugs substitute hydrogen atoms for alkyl groups (methyl-, ethyl-, etc.) on the DNA. Alkylating agents are subdivided into nitrogen mustards, ethylenimine derivatives, alkyl sulfonates, triazine derivatives, and nitrosoureas.

Antibiotics—these directly bind or intercalate (insert between layers) into DNA, preventing replication or RNA synthesis.

Antimetabolites—chemicals that mimic normal molecules in cells. These can act in several ways such as substituting for a normal drug (cytarabine substituting for cytosine in DNA synthesis), competing with a normal enzyme substrate (5-fluorouracil competing with uracil for binding to thymidylate synthetase), or by inhibiting a key enzyme related to the manufacture of nucleotides (methotrexate).

Mitotic inhibitors—these inhibit construction or deconstruction of the mitotic spindle (Vinca alkaloids and taxanes).

Topoisomerase inhibitors—these inhibit enzymes responsible for twisting and coiling of DNA (e.g., Etoposide).

Hall EJ, Giaccia AJ. Chemotherapeutic agents from the perspective of the radiation biologist. In: Hall EJ, Giaccia AJ, eds. *Radiobiology for the Radiologist*. 7th ed. Philadelphia, PA: Lippincott Williams & Wilkins; 2012:448–489.

Question 2 *How is emetogenecity of chemotherapy classified (chemotherapy-induced nausea and vomiting [CINV])?*

Answer 2

It is categorized as high (>90% chance of CINV without prophylaxis), moderately high (60%–90% chance of CINV without prophylaxis), moderate (30%–60% chance of CINV without prophylaxis), low (10%–30% chance of CINV without prophylaxis), and minimal (<10% chance of CINV without prophylaxis).

Lindley CM, Bernard S, Fields SM. Incidence and duration of chemotherapy-induced nausea and vomiting in the outpatient oncology population. *J Clin Oncol*. 1989;7:1142–1149.

Question 3 *What is the mechanism of action of cisplatin? What are some of its toxicities?*

Answer 3

Cisplatin undergoes an aquation reaction and then binds to DNA, causing interstrand and intrastrand DNA adducts. This DNA crosslinking damages the DNA structure, causing problems with mitosis, and initiates apoptosis that eventually leads to cell death. Cisplatin can cause neutropenia, thrombocytopenia, ototoxicity, nephrotoxicity, nausea, and vomiting.

Hall EJ, Giaccia AJ. Chemotherapeutic agents from the perspective of the radiation biologist. In: Hall EJ, Giaccia AJ, eds. *Radiobiology for the Radiologist*. 7th ed. Philadelphia, PA: Lippincott Williams & Wilkins; 2012:448–489.

Question 4
What is the mechanism of action of paclitaxel? What are some of its toxicities?

Question 5
What are the principal side effects of taxanes? What are some major indications for the use of taxanes?

Question 6
What is the mechanism of action for 5-fluorouracil (5-FU)? What are some indications for its usage?

Question 7
How does methotrexate act? What are some of its toxicities?

Question 4 *What is the mechanism of action of paclitaxel? What are some of its toxicities?*

Answer 4

Paclitaxel binds to the beta subunit of tubulin in the mitotic spindle and stabilizes the microtubule assembly, thus preventing disassembly and blocking mitosis. This causes a premitosis cell cycle block and activation of apoptosis. Paclitaxel can cause neutropenia, alopecia, and neuropathy. Ixabepilone is an epothilone B analogue that has more potent antitumor activity in vitro than paclitaxel. It preferentially inhibits the beta III-tubulin isotype of the microtubules.

Dumontet C, Jordan MA, Lee FY. Ixabepilone: targeting βIII-tubulin expression in taxane-resistant malignancies. *Mol Cancer Ther*. 2009;8(1):17–25.

Question 5 *What are the principal side effects of taxanes? What are some major indications for the use of taxanes?*

Answer 5

Peripheral neuropathy, alopecia, nausea, and vomiting are seen with paclitaxel. Docetaxel also causes fluid retention and epiphora (excessive watering of the eye) as well. Both agents cause neutropenia. Some major indications include lung cancer, breast cancer, pancreatic cancer, and head and neck cancer.

Guastalla JP III, Diéras V. The taxanes: toxicity and quality of life considerations in advanced ovarian cancer. *Br J Cancer*. 2003;89:S16–S22.

Question 6 *What is the mechanism of action for 5-fluorouracil (5-FU)? What are some indications for its usage?*

Answer 6

5-FU inhibits the enzyme thymidylate synthetase. This prevents the formation of thymidine and thus cancers die due to a lack of thymidine. Folinic acid or leucovorin enhances the stability of 5-FU—thymidylate synthetase interaction and hence enhances its cytotoxicity. 5-FU is used in the treatment of head and neck cancer, colon cancer, rectal cancer, pancreatic cancer, and breast cancer.

Longley DB, Harkin DP, Johnston PG. 5-fluorouracil: mechanisms of action and clinical strategies. *Nat Rev Cancer*. 2003;3:330–338.

Question 7 *How does methotrexate act? What are some of its toxicities?*

Answer 7

Methotrexate inhibits the enzyme dihydrofolate reductase, thus blocking the conversion of dihydrofolate to tetrahydrofolate that is required for the synthesis of DNA, RNA, and proteins. Toxicities include mucositis, myelosuppression, fatigue, nausea, and vomiting.

Tian H, Cronstein BN. Understanding the mechanisms of action of methotrexate: implications for the treatment of rheumatoid arthritis. *Bull NYU Hosp Jt Dis*. 2007;65:168–173.

Question 8

What is the use and mechanism of action for leucovorin rescue with high-dose methotrexate? What is one indication for high-dose methotrexate use?

Question 9

What is the mechanism of temozolomide? What enzyme repairs its damage? What drug is used with it for preventing pneumocystis pneumonia?

Question 8 *What is the use and mechanism of action for leucovorin rescue with high-dose methotrexate? What is one indication for high-dose methotrexate use?*

Answer 8

Leucovorin is a 5-formyl derivative of tetrahydrofolic acid, which gets converted to tetrahydrofolate, thus bypassing the enzyme dihydrofolate reductase that is blocked by methotrexate. Thus, it can be used to rescue normal cells after high-dose methotrexate. Doses of methotrexate above 3 g/m^2 are usually considered high dose.

High-dose methotrexate is used in the treatment of primary central nervous system (CNS) lymphoma. Precautions must be taken to ensure high-volume urine flow and alkaline urine. This prevents the precipitation of methotrexate in urine, thereby preventing nephrotoxicity.

Treon SP, Chabner BA. Concepts in use of high-dose methotrexate therapy. *Clin Chem.* 1996;42:1322–1329.

Question 9 *What is the mechanism of temozolomide? What enzyme repairs its damage? What drug is used with it for preventing pneumocystis pneumonia?*

Answer 9

Temozolomide is an alkylating agent which alkylates (methylates) tumor cell DNA at the *N*-7 or *O*-6 position of guanine. This DNA damage then triggers cell death pathways, leading to cell kill. This damage is repaired by the enzyme O6-methylguanine DNA methyltransferase (MGMT). Methylation of the MGMT promoter and reduced activity of the *MGMT* gene has been associated with improved responses to temozolomide. Trimethoprim/sulfamethoxazole or pentamidine are used for prophylaxis against pneumocystis pneumonia, which is caused by *Pneumocystis jirovecii*.

Bobola MS, Tseng SH, Blank A, Berger MS, Silber JR. Role of O6-methylguanine-DNA methyltransferase in resistance of human brain tumor cell lines to the clinically relevant methylating agents temozolomide and streptozotocin. *Clin Cancer Res.* 1996;2:735–741.

Hegi ME, Liu L, Herman JG, et al. Correlation of O6-methylguanine methyltransferase (MGMT) promoter methylation with clinical outcomes in glioblastoma and clinical strategies to modulate MGMT activity. *J Clin Oncol.* 2008;26:4189–4199.

Stupp R, Hegi ME, Mason WP, et al. Effects of radiotherapy with concomitant and adjuvant temozolomide versus radiotherapy alone on survival in glioblastoma in a randomised phase III study: 5-year analysis of the EORTC-NCIC trial. *Lancet Oncol.* 2009;10:459–466.

Question 10
What is the mechanism of pemetrexed? What are some of its main indications?

Question 11
Why is pemetrexed not used for squamous cell lung cancer?

Question 12
How does Mesna prevent the cystitis associated with ifosfamide?

Question 13
What is the mechanism of action of actinomycin D? What are some of its toxicities? What are some of its indications in oncology?

Question 10 *What is the mechanism of pemetrexed? What are some of its main indications?*

Answer 10

Pemetrexed is an antifolate chemotherapy agent, which inhibits thymidylate synthase, dihydrofolate reductase, and glycinamide ribonucleotide formyltransferase, thereby preventing DNA and RNA synthesis, leading to cell death. Folic acid and vitamin B_{12} supplementation are recommended on treatment with pemetrexed. It is mainly used for nonsquamous lung cancer and mesothelioma.

Scagliotti G, Hanna N, Fossella F, et al. The differential efficacy of pemetrexed according to NSCLC histology: a review of two phase III studies. *Oncologist.* 2009;14:253–263.

Question 11 *Why is pemetrexed not used for squamous cell lung cancer?*

Answer 11

The main target for pemetrexed is the enzyme thymidylate synthase. This is amplified in squamous cell carcinoma versus adenocarcinoma lung. Thus, pemetrexed is more efficacious in adenocarcinoma lung.

Scagliotti G, Hanna N, Fossella F, et al. The differential efficacy of pemetrexed according to NSCLC histology: a review of two phase III studies. *Oncologist.* 2009;14:253–263.

Question 12 *How does Mesna prevent the cystitis associated with ifosfamide?*

Answer 12

Ifosfamide usage was initially limited by hemorrhagic cystitis, which was dose limiting. This is prevented by the concurrent administration of Mesna (mercaptoethane sulfonate sodium). This is a thiol compound, which detoxifies the acrolein metabolite of ifosfamide in the urinary bladder, only without affecting its antitumor efficacy.

Tascilar M, Loos WJ, Seynaeve C, Verweij J, Sleijfer S. The pharmacologic basis of ifosfamide use in adult patients with advanced soft tissue sarcomas. *Oncologist.* 2007;12:1351–1360.

Question 13 *What is the mechanism of action of actinomycin D? What are some of its toxicities? What are some of its indications in oncology?*

Answer 13

The two major mechanisms are DNA intercalation and the stabilization of cleavable complexes of topoisomerases I and II with DNA. However, there are several other possible mechanisms of action reported. Toxicities include bone marrow suppression, alopecia, fatigue, and diarrhea. Actinomycin D is used in various cancers like gestational trophoblastic neoplasia, Wilms' tumor, Rhabdomyosarcoma, and Ewing's sarcoma.

Sobell HM. Actinomycin and DNA transcription. *Proc Natl Acad Sci USA.* 1985;82:5328–5331.

Question 14

What is the mechanism of action of gemcitabine? What is the most common toxicity?

Question 15

What is the mechanism of action of mitomycin C? What are some of its toxicities?

Question 16

What is the mechanism of action of vincristine and its principal dose-limiting toxicity?

Question 17

What is the mechanism of doxorubicin? What are some common indications?

Question 14 *What is the mechanism of action of gemcitabine? What is the most common toxicity?*

Answer 14

Gemcitabine is a cytidine analog. It gets converted intracellularly to false nucleotides, which lead to inhibition of DNA polymerase and ribonucleotide reductase. The incorporation of false nucleotides into DNA also causes strand termination. Myelosuppression, especially thrombocytopenia, is the most common toxicity.

Mini E, Nobili S, Caciagli B, Landini I, Mazzei T. Cellular pharmacology of gemcitabine. *Ann Oncol.* 2006;17(suppl 5):v7–v12.

Question 15 *What is the mechanism of action of mitomycin C? What are some of its toxicities?*

Answer 15

Mitomycin C is an antitumor antibiotic, which is most active under anaerobic conditions. Once reduced, it is converted into a highly reactive bis-electrophilic intermediate that alkylates the DNA (major mechanism of action). Other actions include inhibition of rRNA as well. Toxicities include delayed myelosuppression, stomatitis, and fatigue.

Paz MM, Zhang X, Lu J, Holmgren A. A new mechanism of action for the anticancer drug mitomycin C: mechanism-based inhibition of thioredoxin reductase. *Chem Res Toxicol.* 2012;25:1502–1511.

Question 16 *What is the mechanism of action of vincristine and its principal dose-limiting toxicity?*

Answer 16

Vincristine inhibits microtubule polymerization and blocks mitosis, thus inducing a cell cycle arrest and eventually cell death. As a vesicant, vincristine should be administered with precautions against extravasation. The principal toxicity is peripheral neuropathy, which is most commonly manifested in the hands and feet.

Hall EJ, Giaccia AJ. Chemotherapeutic agents from the perspective of the radiation biologist. In: Hall EJ, Giaccia AJ, eds. *Radiobiology for the Radiologist.* 7th ed. Philadelphia, PA: Lippincott Williams & Wilkins; 2012:448–489.
Jordan MA. Mechanism of action of antitumor drugs that interact with microtubules and tubulin. *Curr Med Chem Anticancer Agents.* 2002;2:1–17.

Question 17 *What is the mechanism of doxorubicin? What are some common indications?*

Answer 17

There are two proposed mechanisms by which doxorubicin acts in the cancer cell, namely intercalation into DNA and disruption of topoisomerase-II-mediated DNA repair and generation of free radicals and their damage to cellular membranes, DNA, and proteins. Common indications include breast cancer, Hodgkin's lymphoma, and soft tissue sarcomas.

Thorn CF, Oshiro C, Marsh S, et al. Doxorubicin pathways: pharmacodynamics and adverse effects. *Pharmacogenet Genomics.* 2011;21:440–446.

Question 18

How does doxorubicin cause cardiotoxicity? What agent is known to prevent it?

Question 19

How does the cardiotoxicity of doxorubicin differ from that of trastuzumab? What are some indications for its use?

Question 20

What is the mechanism of action of etoposide? What are some of the toxicities?

Question 21

What is the mechanism of action of capecitabine? What are some of its indications?

Question 18 *How does doxorubicin cause cardiotoxicity? What agent is known to prevent it?*

Answer 18

It is postulated that doxorubicin causes cardiotoxicity by inducing iron-related free radicals and formation of doxorubicinol metabolite along with mitochondrial disruption. Dexrazoxane can prevent this cardiotoxicity by sequestering the intracellular iron, preventing free radical generation.

Thorn CF, Oshiro C, Marsh S, et al. Doxorubicin pathways: pharmacodynamics and adverse effects. *Pharmacogenet Genomics.* 2011;21:440–446.

Question 19 *How does the cardiotoxicity of doxorubicin differ from that of trastuzumab? What are some indications for its use?*

Answer 19

The cardiotoxicity of doxorubicin is characterized at least to some degree by the loss of myocytes (a cumulative toxic dose is seen and the toxicity is more likely to be irreversible) while the cardiotoxicity of trastuzumab is associated with a loss of cardiac myocyte contractility and is more likely to be reversible without a cumulative dose or association with myocyte death.

Trastuzumab is used for breast cancer and HERr2 expressing gastric cancer in the metastatic setting.

Telli ML, Hunt SA, Carlson RW, Guardino AE. Trastuzumab-related cardiotoxicity: calling into question the concept of reversibility. *J Clin Oncol.* 2007; 25:3525–3533.

Question 20 *What is the mechanism of action of etoposide? What are some of the toxicities?*

Answer 20

Etoposide interferes with the scission–reunion reaction of mammalian topoisomerase II by stabilizing a cleavable complex. This induces DNA damage and eventually cell death. Toxicities include myelosuppression, alopecia, menopause in women, and infertility.

van Maanen JM, Retel J, de Vries J, Pinedo HM. Mechanism of action of antitumor drug etoposide: a review. *J Natl Cancer Inst.* 1988;80:1526–1533.

Question 21 *What is the mechanism of action of capecitabine? What are some of its indications?*

Answer 21

Capecitabine is a prodrug of 5-fluorouracil (5-FU), which is converted to 5 FU by thymidine phosphorylase inside the cell. Higher levels of this enzyme are found in tumor cells versus normal cells. The cytotoxicity then follows that of 5-FU. Capecitabine is associated with an elevated risk of hand foot syndrome relative to 5-FU.

Indications include breast cancer, colon cancer, rectal cancer, and pancreatic cancer.

Petrelli F, Cabiddu M, Barni S. 5-fluorouracil or capecitabine in the treatment of advanced colorectal cancer: a pooled-analysis of randomized trials. *Med Oncol.* 2012;29:1020–1029.

Question 22
What are the common suffixes to differentiate types of targeted therapies?

Question 23
What is the mechanism of action of cetuximab? What is its dose in head and neck cancer? What are two important side effects?

Question 24
What is the mechanism of action of trastuzumab?

Question 25
What is the mechanism of action of rituximab?

Question 22 *What are the common suffixes to differentiate types of targeted therapies?*

Answer 22

mab—**M**onoclonal **antib**ody-based drug (e.g., cetuximab)
Ib—Small molecule inh**ib**itor (erlotinib)
Ximab—Ch**i**meric monoclonal antibody (e.g., rituximab)
Zumab—H**u**manized monoclonal antibody (e.g., trastuzumab)

American Medical Association. Naming biologics: monoclonal antibodies. http://www.ama-assn.org/ama/pub/
physician-resources/medical-science/united-states-adopted-names-council/naming-guidelines/naming-biologics/
monoclonal-antibodies.page? Accessed August 2, 2016.

Question 23 *What is the mechanism of action of cetuximab? What is its dose in head and neck cancer? What are two important side effects?*

Answer 23

Cetuximab is an IgG1 chimeric monoclonal antibody against the external domain of the epidermal growth factor receptor (EGFR). It prevents the binding of endogenous ligands with the EGFR that leads to shutting down of the receptor-dependent transduction pathway, eventually leading to cell death.

The loading dose with radiation is 400 mg/m^2 week 1 (1 week before the start of radiation) followed by 250 mg/m^2 every week. Skin rash and infusion reactions are two common side effects.

Lenz H. Cetuximab in the management of colorectal cancer. *Biologics*. 2007;1:77–91.

Question 24 *What is the mechanism of action of trastuzumab?*

Answer 24

Trastuzumab is a humanized IgG1 monoclonal antibody against the external domain of the Her2 protein located on the tumor cell surface. This blocks intracellular signaling, leading to cell death. Another mechanism is the induction of antibody-dependent cellular cytotoxicity by the Fc portion of the antibody.

Pohlmann PR, Mayer IA, Mernaugh R. Resistance to trastuzumab in breast cancer. *Clin Cancer Res*. 2009;15:
7479–7491.

Question 25 *What is the mechanism of action of rituximab?*

Answer 25

Rituximab is a chimeric monoclonal antibody directed against the pan-B cell marker CD20. Mechanisms of cell destruction that have been demonstrated to be activated by rituximab binding to CD20 include direct signaling of apoptosis, complement activation, and cell-mediated cytotoxicity.

Smith MR. Rituximab (monoclonal anti-CD20 antibody): mechanisms of action and resistance. *Oncogene*.
2003;22:7359–7368.

Question 26
What is T-DM1? How does it act?

Question 27
How does erlotinib work?

Question 28
What is afatinib and what important differences does it exhibit from erlotinib?

Question 29
What is the mechanism of crizotinib?

Question 26 *What is T-DM1? How does it act?*

Answer 26

T-DM1 or trastuzumab emtansine is an antibody-drug conjugate. Several mechanisms of action include those of trastuzumab and those of DM1, a cytotoxic antimicrotubule agent released within the target cells upon degradation of the human epidermal growth factor receptor-2 (HER2)-T-DM1 complex in lysosomes.

Barok M, Joensuu H, Isola J. Trastuzumab emtansine: mechanisms of action and drug resistance. *Breast Cancer Res.* 2014;16:209.

Question 27 *How does erlotinib work?*

Answer 27

Erlotinib is a small molecule tyrosine kinase reversible inhibitor of the intracellular domain of the epidermal growth factor receptor (EGFR). This prevents downstream signaling, leading to tumor cell death. About 90% of *EGFR* gene mutations affect a small region of the gene within exons 18–24, which code for the tyrosine kinase domain.

Gridelli C, Bareschino MA, Schettino C, Rossi A, Maione P, Ciardiello F. Erlotinib in non-small cell lung cancer treatment: current status and future development. *Oncologist.* 2007;12:840–849.
Schettino C, Bareschino MA, Ricci V, Ciardiello F. Erlotinib: an EGF receptor tyrosine kinase inhibitor in non-small-cell lung cancer treatment. *Expert Rev Respir Med.* 2008;2:167–178.

Question 28 *What is afatinib and what important differences does it exhibit from erlotinib?*

Answer 28

Afatinib is an irreversible inhibitor of the epidermal growth factor receptor (EGFR) and HERr2 tyrosine kinase domain. While most tyrosine kinase inhibitors such as erlotinib bind to the kinase domain, irreversible inhibitors may bind on the edge of the ATP binding cleft. As a result, afatinib exhibits significant anticancer activity in patients harboring T790M mutations, which are resistant to erlotinib and gefitinib.

Karachaliou N, Rosell R. Systemic treatment in EGFR-ALK NSCLC patients: second line therapy and beyond. *Cancer Biol Med.* 2014;11:173–181.

Question 29 *What is the mechanism of crizotinib?*

Answer 29

Crizotinib binds competitively to the tyrosine kinase domain of the EML4-anaplastic lymphoma kinase (ALK) fusion gene product. It also inhibits c-met and hepatocyte growth factor that contributes to oncogenesis. It is a targeted agent against non-small cell lung cancer (NSCLC) with ALK rearrangement (about 4% of all NSCLCs harbor this rearrangement). Ceritinib is a second generation tyrosine kinase inhibitor (TKI) against the same target.

Sahu A, Prabhash K, Noronha V, Joshi A, Desai S. Crizotinib: a comprehensive review. *SAJC.* 2013;2:91–97.

Question 30

What is the mechanism of action of imatinib? What are some of its uses?

Question 31

What is brentuximab vedotin and what is its mechanism of cytotoxicity and cellular target?

Question 32

What are some targeted therapies for thyroid cancer? What are their mechanisms of action?

Question 30 *What is the mechanism of action of imatinib? What are some of its uses?*

Answer 30

Imatinib inhibits multiple tyrosine kinases. It has specific activity against the TK domain in ABL (the Abelson proto-oncogene), c-kit, and PDGF-R (platelet-derived growth factor receptor). It is commonly used for chronic myeloid leukemia where it targets the *BCR-ABL* gene product tyrosine kinase domain.

Imatinib is used for chronic myeloid leukemia, certain c-kit mutated melanomas, and for progressive or recurrent aggressive fibromatosis.

Marcucci G, Perrotti D, Caligiuri MA. Understanding the molecular basis of imatinib mesylate therapy in chronic myelogenous leukemia and the related mechanisms of resistance. Commentary re: A. N. Mohamed et al., the effect of imatinib mesylate on patients with Philadelphia chromosome-positive chronic myeloid leukemia with secondary chromosomal aberrations. *Clin Cancer Res.* 9: 1333–1337, 2003. *Clin Cancer Res.* 2003;9:1248–1252.

Question 31 *What is brentuximab vedotin and what is its mechanism of cytotoxicity and cellular target?*

Answer 31

Brentuximab is a chimeric monoclonal antibody-drug conjugate against CD30. The antitumor effect is due to the vedotin component (monomethyl auristatin E) that blocks polymerization of tubulin. The CD30 antigen is expressed predominantly on the Reed-Sternberg cell in Hodgkin's lymphoma, and studies have shown high response rates even in the setting of progression after autologous stem cell transplant.

Ansell SM. Hodgkin lymphoma: diagnosis and treatment. *Mayo Clin Proc.* 2015;90:1574–1583.
Younes A, Bartlett NL, Leonard JP, et al. Brentuximab vedotin (SGN-35) for relapsed CD30-positive lymphomas. *N Engl J Med.* 2010;363:1812–1821.

Question 32 *What are some targeted therapies for thyroid cancer? What are their mechanisms of action?*

Answer 32

Vandetanib—multiple tyrosine kinase inhibitor targeting RET kinases, vascular endothelial growth factor (VEGFR), and epidermal growth factor receptor (EGFR).
Cabozantinib—multiple tyrosine kinase inhibitor targeting MET, VEGFR2, and RET kinases.
Lenvatinib—multikinase inhibitor targeting VEGFR1-3, FGFR1-4, PDGFRβ, RET, and c-KIT.

Carneiro RM, Carneiro BA, Agulnik M, Kopp PA, Giles FJ. Targeted therapies in advanced differentiated thyroid cancer. *Cancer Treat Rev.* 2015;41:690–698.

Question 33

What are some targeted therapies used for metastatic renal cell carcinoma? What are their mechanisms of action?

Question 34

What is aprepitant? What is its mechanism of action?

Question 33 *What are some targeted therapies used for metastatic renal cell carcinoma? What are their mechanisms of action?*

Answer 33

Bevacizumab—antibody against vascular endothelial growth factor (VEGF).

Sunitinib—small molecule multikinase including inhibition of platelet derived growth factor receptor (PDGFR), vascular endothelial growth factor receptor (VEGFR), and FMS-like tyrosine kinase-3 (FLT3).

Sorafenib—small molecule inhibitor of kinases inhibiting VEGFR, PDGFRβ, and FLT3, as well as intracellular Raf kinases (e.g., BRAF).

Pazopanib—multi tyrosine kinase inhibitor including inhibition of VEGFR, PDGFRβ, fibroblast growth factor receptors (FGFR), and others.

Axitinib—second generation selective inhibitor of VEGFR receptors 1, 2, and 3.

Everolimus—inhibitor of mTOR (mammalian target of Rapamycin).

Minguet J, Smith KH, Bramlage CP, Bramlage P. Targeted therapies for treatment of renal cell carcinoma: recent advances and future perspectives. *Cancer Chemother Pharmacol.* 2015;76:219–233.

Question 34 *What is aprepitant? What is its mechanism of action?*

Answer 34

Aprepitant is an oral neurokinin-1 (NK-1) inhibitor used for emesis prophylaxis when administering highly emetogenic drugs like cisplatin. NK-1 inhibitors block the binding of substance P to the NK-1 receptor and thus have a mechanism independent of other antiemetic drugs such as corticosteroids or 5-hydroxytryptamine ($5HT_3$) inhibitors. A prodrug IV fosaprepitant is also available.

Aapro M, Carides A, Rapoport BL, et al. Aprepitant and fosaprepitant: a 10-year review of efficacy and safety. *Oncologist.* 2015;20:450–458.

26

HYPERTHERMIA

SHARVARI DHARMAIAH, VINAY RAO, AND JENNIFER S. YU

Question 1
What is hyperthermia?

Question 2
What are the different methods of local hyperthermia?

Question 3
What are the different methods of regional hyperthermia?

Turn page to see the answers.

Question 1 *What is hyperthermia?*

Answer 1

Hyperthermia is a form of cancer treatment wherein body tissues are exposed to ablative (50°C–60°C) or fever range (39°C–43°C) temperatures. Hyperthermia improves cancer control through multiple mechanisms including directly damaging or killing cancer cells, increasing perfusion to improve radiation sensitivity and drug delivery, and improving the antitumor immune response. It is most often used alongside other forms of cancer therapy, such as radiation and chemotherapy.

Chu K, Dupuy D. Thermal ablation of tumors: biological mechanisms and advances in therapy. *Nat Rev Cancer.* 2014;14(3):199–208.

Hall EJ, Giaccia AJ. Hyperthermia. In: Hall EJ, Giaccia AJ, eds. *Radiobiology for the Radiologist.* 7th ed. Philadelphia, PA: Lippincott Williams & Wilkins; 2006:490–511.

Question 2 *What are the different methods of local hyperthermia?*

Answer 2

In local hyperthermia, heat is applied to a small area. Based on the location of the tumor, hyperthermia can be administered by external, intraluminal, or interstitial approaches. The external method is used to treat superficial tumors and utilizes external applicators that focus energy on the tumor. Intraluminal or endocavitary methods are typically used within body cavities, for example, for treatment of advanced cervical cancer. Probes are inserted through the cavity into the tumor to deliver direct heat energy. Interstitial applications are used to treat deep tumors. Under anesthesia, a catheter is inserted into the tumor and the heat source is then inserted into the catheter to heat the tumor.

Hall EJ, Giaccia AJ. Hyperthermia. In: Hall EJ, Giaccia AJ, eds. *Radiobiology for the Radiologist.* 7th ed. Philadelphia, PA: Lippincott Williams & Wilkins; 2006:490–511.

van der Zee J. Heating the patient: a promising approach? *Ann Oncol.* 2002;13(8):1173–1184.

Question 3 *What are the different methods of regional hyperthermia?*

Answer 3

In regional hyperthermia, various methods are used to heat large areas of the body such as a limb, body cavity, or an organ. The different approaches utilized are deep tissue, regional perfusion, or continuous hyperthermic peritoneal perfusion (CHPP) techniques. Deep tissue methods are used to treat tumors within the body where external applicators are positioned around the target organ or cavity and radiofrequency or microwave energy is administered. Regional perfusion is used to treat tumors in the arms and legs or cancers in some internal organs. In this method, which is often combined with chemotherapy, a portion of the patient's blood is removed, heated, and then perfused through the limb or organ. CHPP is used to treat cancers within the peritoneal cavity. During surgery, the treatment is administered through the use of heated anticancer drugs that flow from a warming device through the peritoneal cavity.

Hall EJ, Giaccia AJ. Hyperthermia. In: Hall EJ, Giaccia AJ, eds. *Radiobiology for the Radiologist.* 7th ed. Philadelphia, PA: Lippincott Williams & Wilkins; 2006:490–511.

van der Zee J. Heating the patient: a promising approach? *Ann Oncol.* 2002;13(8):1173–1184.

Question 4
In in vitro models, what is the relationship between temperature and cell death?

Question 5
What are some major factors that differentiate hyperthermia from irradiation treatment?

Question 6
How is the Arrhenius plot useful in assessing the effects of thermal damage in tissues?

Question 4 *In in vitro models, what is the relationship between temperature and cell death?*

Answer 4

In in vitro models, cell death occurs in an exponential pattern that can be modeled with the rate of killing increasing as the temperature increases.

Hall EJ, Giaccia AJ. Hyperthermia. In: Hall EJ, Giaccia AJ, eds. *Radiobiology for the Radiologist*. 7th ed. Philadelphia, PA: Lippincott Williams & Wilkins; 2006:490–511.

Question 5 *What are some major factors that differentiate hyperthermia from irradiation treatment?*

Answer 5

- Following radiation treatment, cells frequently die when attempting to undergo mitosis (mitotic cell death). In hyperthermia, heat-induced damage can facilitate necrosis or apoptosis of cells throughout the cell cycle.
- Hyperthermia can impair DNA repair.
- Hyperthermia affects both differentiating and dividing cells.
- Tissue damage is expressed immediately if the temperature is high enough.
- Tissue hypoxia can reduce the sensitivity of cells to radiation but can increase heat-induced damage in hyperthermia.

Hall EJ, Giaccia AJ. Hyperthermia. In: Hall EJ, Giaccia AJ, eds. *Radiobiology for the Radiologist*. 7th ed. Philadelphia, PA: Lippincott Williams & Wilkins; 2006:490–511.

Question 6 *How is the Arrhenius plot useful in assessing the effects of thermal damage in tissues?*

Answer 6

The Arrhenius plot serves as a basis for understanding the thermal doses necessary in clinical hyperthermia applications. In an Arrhenius plot, the slope designates the activation energy (E_a) of the chemical process involved in killing cancer cells. Above the "breakpoint," a temperature point (about 43°C) in which there is a significant change in the slope of the plot, a change in 1°C signifies a doubling of the rate of cell killing. Below this value, the rate of cell death can drop by a factor between 2 and 4 for each degree Celsius drop. Differences in activation energy both below and above this breakpoint may demonstrate different means of cell killing or the development of thermotolerance in some cells. The Arrhenius equation is described by $\ln k = \ln A - E_a/RT$, where k is the rate constant, T is the temperature in Kelvin, A is a preexponential factor, E_a is the activation energy, and R is the universal gas constant. The y-intercept $= \ln A$ and slope $= -E_a/R$.

Arrhenius Plot

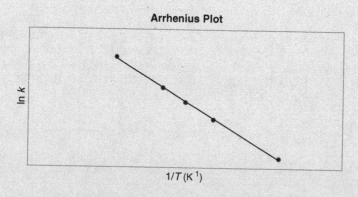

Hall EJ, Giaccia AJ. Hyperthermia. In: Hall EJ, Giaccia AJ, eds. *Radiobiology for the Radiologist*. 7th ed. Philadelphia, PA: Lippincott Williams & Wilkins; 2006:490–511.

Question 7

What is a thermal enhancement ratio (TER)?

Question 8

What are the factors that affect the sensitivity of direct cellular damage due to hyperthermia?

Question 9

What is the therapeutic gain factor?

Question 10

What is the importance of indirect effects of hyperthermia on heat and the tumor microenvironment?

Question 7 *What is a thermal enhancement ratio (TER)?*

Answer 7

TER is the ratio of radiation doses with and without the administration of heat necessary to produce a specific level of biological damage. The TER increases with increasing temperature and can be used to predict effective treatment doses. TER from clinical data ranges from 1.15 to 1.5.

Hall EJ, Giaccia AJ. Hyperthermia. In: Hall EJ, Giaccia AJ, eds. *Radiobiology for the Radiologist.* 7th ed. Philadelphia, PA: Lippincott Williams & Wilkins; 2006:490–511.

Question 8 *What are the factors that affect the sensitivity of direct cellular damage due to hyperthermia?*

Answer 8

Factors that improve the sensitivity of cells to direct damage by hyperthermia include:

- An acidic environment
- A hypoxic environment
- A state of nutritional deprivation
- Poor vascularization or an increased distance from capillaries
- Destabilization of cell membrane structure through the use of agents, such as alcohols, that may modify the lipid content within cells
- Dysregulation of the normal cell growth cycle

Hall EJ, Giaccia AJ. Hyperthermia. In: Hall EJ, Giaccia AJ, eds. *Radiobiology for the Radiologist.* 7th ed. Philadelphia, PA: Lippincott Williams & Wilkins; 2006:490–511.

Question 9 *What is the therapeutic gain factor?*

Answer 9

The therapeutic gain factor is defined as the ratio of the thermal enhancement ratio (TER) in the tumor to the TER in normal tissues.

Hall EJ, Giaccia AJ. Hyperthermia. In: Hall EJ, Giaccia AJ, eds. *Radiobiology for the Radiologist.* 7th ed. Philadelphia, PA: Lippincott Williams & Wilkins; 2006:490–511.

Question 10 *What is the importance of indirect effects of hyperthermia on heat and the tumor microenvironment?*

Answer 10

Mild hyperthermia has the potential to promote large-scale changes in the tumor microenvironment that can improve the efficacy of radiation therapy. Hyperthermia can facilitate reoxygenation of hypoxic tissues following radiotherapy that can improve response rates. Hyperthermia can also change pH, cell metabolism, and protein and gene expressions.

Hall EJ, Giaccia AJ. Hyperthermia. In: Hall EJ, Giaccia AJ, eds. *Radiobiology for the Radiologist.* 7th ed. Philadelphia, PA: Lippincott Williams & Wilkins; 2006:490–511.

Question 11
What is thermotolerance?

Question 12
What role do heat shock proteins (HSPs) play in hyperthermia?

Question 13
Why is thermotolerance not a likely issue during normal heating conditions used in the clinic?

Question 14
What are some possible immunologic effects of hyperthermia?

Question 11 *What is thermotolerance?*

Answer 11

Thermotolerance, also known as induced thermal resistance, is an acquired resistance to the effects of hyperthermia following an initial heat treatment. The clinical significance of thermotolerance is controversial. In vitro studies have shown that cancer cells are initially sensitive to hyperthermia but become more resistant in subsequent treatments due to the induction of heat shock proteins (HSPs). Thermotolerance can occur in under as little as a few hours posttreatment and can take significant time, up to a week, for cells to become sensitive to hyperthermia again.

Hall EJ, Giaccia AJ. Hyperthermia. In: Hall EJ, Giaccia AJ, eds. *Radiobiology for the Radiologist.* 7th ed. Philadelphia, PA: Lippincott Williams & Wilkins; 2006:490–511.

Question 12 *What role do heat shock proteins (HSPs) play in hyperthermia?*

Answer 12

HSPs are activated after cells are exposed to hyperthermia. HSPs possess the ability to protect against the potentially lethal heat exposures brought about by hyperthermia. HSPs stabilize proteins to protect against cell death. Current research is investigating the role of HSPs in mediating T lymphocyte activity and antitumor immune mechanisms.

Hall EJ, Giaccia AJ. Hyperthermia. In: Hall EJ, Giaccia AJ, eds. *Radiobiology for the Radiologist.* 7th ed. Philadelphia, PA: Lippincott Williams & Wilkins; 2006:490–511.

Question 13 *Why is thermotolerance not a likely issue during normal heating conditions used in the clinic?*

Answer 13

Hyperthermia improves perfusion and therefore oxygenation of the tumor. When hyperthermia is used in conjunction with radiation, the increased oxygenation and inhibition of DNA repair processes more than counter the effects of thermotolerance.

Hall EJ, Giaccia AJ. Hyperthermia. In: Hall EJ, Giaccia AJ, eds. *Radiobiology for the Radiologist.* 7th ed. Philadelphia, PA: Lippincott Williams & Wilkins; 2006:490–511.

Question 14 *What are some possible immunologic effects of hyperthermia?*

Answer 14

Hyperthermia can increase immunogenicity by facilitating exposure or spillage of tumor antigens, activation of immune effector cells, and improvement in perfusion that increases effector immune cell recruitment into the tumors.

Hall EJ, Giaccia AJ. Hyperthermia. In: Hall EJ, Giaccia AJ, eds. *Radiobiology for the Radiologist.* 7th ed. Philadelphia, PA: Lippincott Williams & Wilkins; 2006:490–511.

Question 15
How does the cumulative equivalent minutes (CEM) concept affect thermal dose?

Question 16
What is the importance of the thermal isoeffect dose formulation?

Question 17
In what cancers has adjuvant hyperthermia shown to improve local control?

Question 18
What is the benefit of administering hyperthermia in combination with chemotherapeutic treatment?

Question 15 *How does the cumulative equivalent minutes (CEM) concept affect thermal dose?*

Answer 15

Developed by Sapareto and Dewey, CEM is used to calculate the thermal isodose effect to allow for comparisons in thermal dose among patients. According to the Arrhenius plot, there is a predictable relationship between the rate of cell death and temperature. CEM allows physicians to normalize the time and temperature data across patients.

CEM 43°C T_{90} is the measure of thermal dose that refers to the number of CEM at 43°C exceeded by 90% of the time points. CEM 43°C is calculated for the entire hyperthermia treatment as follows:

$$CEM\ 43°C = \Sigma\ t_i R^{(43 - T_i)}$$

where CEM 43°C is the cumulative number of equivalent minutes at 43°C, t is the i-th time interval, R is the constant of proportionality ($R = 0.25$ if $T < 43°C$, $R = 0.5$ if $T > 43°C$), and T_i is the average temperature during time interval t_i. The temperature of 43°C was chosen because the Arrhenius plot indicates that it is the breakpoint temperature for most cells in the body.

Hall EJ, Giaccia AJ. Hyperthermia. In: Hall EJ, Giaccia AJ, eds. *Radiobiology for the Radiologist*. 7th ed. Philadelphia, PA: Lippincott Williams & Wilkins, 2006:490–511.

Question 16 *What is the importance of the thermal isoeffect dose formulation?*

Answer 16

The thermal isoeffect dose formulation is defined as cumulative equivalent minutes (CEM) of 43°C and is used to compare thermal dosing across patients as tumors vary in their ability to be heated. CEM 43°C is used to evaluate the quality of hyperthermia treatment.

Hall EJ, Giaccia AJ. Hyperthermia. In: Hall EJ, Giaccia AJ, eds. *Radiobiology for the Radiologist*. 7th ed. Philadelphia, PA: Lippincott Williams & Wilkins; 2006:490–511.

Question 17 *In what cancers has adjuvant hyperthermia shown to improve local control?*

Answer 17

Many clinical trials have shown the direct and significant benefit of combination therapy with hyperthermia. Local control has improved in the following types of cancer: cervical cancer, superficial localized breast cancer, malignant melanoma, nodal metastases from head and neck cancer, glioma, esophageal cancer, and high-risk sarcoma.

Hall EJ, Giaccia AJ. Hyperthermia. In: Hall EJ, Giaccia AJ, eds. *Radiobiology for the Radiologist*. 7th ed. Philadelphia, PA: Lippincott Williams & Wilkins; 2006:490–511.

Question 18 *What is the benefit of administering hyperthermia in combination with chemotherapeutic treatment?*

Answer 18

The goal of combined therapy is to improve the therapeutic ratio. Hyperthermia synergizes with chemotherapy including melphalan, cisplatin, anthracyclines, bleomycin, mitomycin C, nitrosoureas, and nitrogen mustards. Additionally, increased temperature (even as little as 1°C–2°C) enhances sensitization for various chemotherapeutic agents.

Hall EJ, Giaccia AJ. Hyperthermia. In: Hall EJ, Giaccia AJ, eds. *Radiobiology for the Radiologist*. 7th ed. Philadelphia, PA: Lippincott Williams & Wilkins; 2006:490–511.
Kowel CD, Bertino JR. Possible benefits of hyperthermia to chemotherapy. *Cancer Res*. 1979;39:2285–2289.

Question 19
What are mechanisms by which hyperthermia improves the efficacy of chemotherapy in vivo?

Question 20
What are the effects of hypoxia in hyperthermia?

Question 21
How does the enhanced permeability and retention (EPR) effect improve tumor targeting of chemotherapy?

Question 22
What are the surgical modalities that can benefit from chemotherapy and hyperthermia treatment?

Question 19 *What are mechanisms by which hyperthermia improves the efficacy of chemotherapy in vivo?*

Answer 19

- Increase in drug uptake and/or retention.
- Inhibit DNA repair.
- Increase reactive oxygen species that cause further damage to the cell.
- Increase perfusion to improve delivery of chemotherapy to the tumor.

Hall EJ, Giaccia AJ. Hyperthermia. In: Hall EJ, Giaccia AJ, eds. *Radiobiology for the Radiologist*. 7th ed. Philadelphia, PA: Lippincott Williams & Wilkins; 2006:490–511.

Question 20 *What are the effects of hypoxia in hyperthermia?*

Answer 20

While hypoxia protects cells from x-rays, it does not protect cells from heat. Regions of mild to severe hypoxia in tumors are likely due to aberrant vascular function and metabolic abnormalities that result from rapid tumor proliferation. Hyperthermia can improve oxygenation by increasing blood flow in hypoxic areas.

Dewhirst MW, Cao Y, Moeller B. Cycling hypoxia and free radicals regulate angiogenesis and radiotherapy response. *Nat Rev Cancer*. 2008;8(6):425–437.
Hall EJ, Giaccia AJ. Hyperthermia. In: Hall EJ, Giaccia AJ, eds. *Radiobiology for the Radiologist*. 7th ed. Philadelphia, PA: Lippincott Williams & Wilkins; 2006:490–511.

Question 21 *How does the enhanced permeability and retention (EPR) effect improve tumor targeting of chemotherapy?*

Answer 21

EPR effect is defined as the tendency of molecules of certain sizes, usually liposomes or macromolecular drugs, to preferably aggregate in tumor tissue compared to normal tissue. Endothelial cell membrane pores can lead to drug accumulation in tumors. Hyperthermia can enhance drug delivery by directly increasing the size of these pores. Thus, the EPR effect in hyperthermia treatment can yield a four- to five-fold improvement in drug delivery in patients experiencing concurrent hyperthermia and chemotherapy.

Thermosensitive liposomes loaded with chemotherapy show promising results. These liposomes preferentially accumulate in tumor cells. When heated, the liposomes release the chemotherapy to deliver high local concentrations of drug into the tumor.

Hall EJ, Giaccia AJ. Hyperthermia. In: Hall EJ, Giaccia AJ, eds. *Radiobiology for the Radiologist*. 7th ed. Philadelphia, PA: Lippincott Williams & Wilkins; 2006:490–511.

Question 22 *What are the surgical modalities that can benefit from chemotherapy and hyperthermia treatment?*

Answer 22

Three surgical modalities benefit from adjuvant therapy: isolated limb perfusion (ILP), isolated limb infusion (ILI), and intraperitoneal chemotherapy. ILP and ILI are used for the treatment of melanoma (in transit metastases) and extremity sarcomas. The goal of ILP is to administer the highest possible regional drug concentrations into the affected limb and reduce systemic side effects. A tourniquet is placed on the affected limb to reduce systemic delivery of the drug. ILI is similar to ILP, but it does not involve the surgical insertion of arterial and venous catheters, significantly lowering morbidity in patients. Intraperitoneal chemotherapy is used in patients at high risk for peritoneal seeding, such as patients with ovarian cancer, and is used in combination with hyperthermia. The chemotherapy solution is heated before it is administered to the abdominal cavity and exposed to the affected organs.

Hall EJ, Giaccia AJ. Hyperthermia. In: Hall EJ, Giaccia AJ, eds. *Radiobiology for the Radiologist*. 7th ed. Philadelphia, PA: Lippincott Williams & Wilkins; 2006:490–511.

Question 23
What are some technical problems associated with localized hyperthermia?

Question 24
What are the three basic kinds of invasive thermometers?

Question 25
What techniques have been implemented to improve patient evaluation and their respective thermal dose estimates?

Question 26
What are the benefits of proton resonance frequency shift-based magnetic resonance thermal imaging (PFRS-based MRTI)?

Question 23 *What are some technical problems associated with localized hyperthermia?*

Answer 23

There are technical problems involved in cases of localized hyperthermia treatment of tumors via microwaves, radiofrequency (RF)-induced currents, or ultrasound. Microwaves are typically limited to treatment of superficial lesions. RF-induced currents lack efficient sensitizers that selectively target cancer cells. The use of RF-induced currents therefore may lead to acute and/or chronic side effects in patients. Ultrasound can be distorted by bone or air cavities.

Hall EJ, Giaccia AJ. Hyperthermia. In: Hall EJ, Giaccia AJ, eds. *Radiobiology for the Radiologist*. 7th ed. Philadelphia, PA: Lippincott Williams & Wilkins; 2006:490–511.

Question 24 *What are the three basic kinds of invasive thermometers?*

Answer 24

The three basic kinds of invasive thermometers are: electrically conducting, minimally conducting, and optical sensors. Examples of electrically conducting thermometers are thermistors and thermocouple sensors with metallic leads. These are not suitable for electromagnetic (EM) hyperthermia. High-resistivity thermistors with carbon-impregnated plastic leads are commonly used as minimally conducting thermometers. These thermometers provide accurate measurements in strong EM environments due to the high-resistivity material. Nonconducting optical sensors, which are also used in EM hyperthermia, use an optical fiber with optical properties that are a known function of temperature. Direct heating of either the sensor or catheter (in which the sensor is placed) can lead to incorrect temperature measurements. The use of minimally conducting and optical sensors has eliminated this error in EM hyperthermia.

Hall EJ, Giaccia AJ. Hyperthermia. In: Hall EJ, Giaccia AJ, eds. *Radiobiology for the Radiologist*. 7th ed. Philadelphia, PA: Lippincott Williams & Wilkins; 2006:490–511.

Question 25 *What techniques have been implemented to improve patient evaluation and their respective thermal dose estimates?*

Answer 25

Real-time temperature monitoring is needed to deliver high-quality hyperthermia. Noninvasive techniques include infrared thermography, thermal monitoring sheet fiber-optic arrays, electrical impedance tomography, microwave tomography, ultrasonic temperature estimation techniques, and magnetic resonance thermal imaging (MRTI).

Hall EJ, Giaccia AJ. Hyperthermia. In: Hall EJ, Giaccia AJ, eds. *Radiobiology for the Radiologist*. 7th ed. Philadelphia, PA: Lippincott Williams & Wilkins; 2006:490–511.

Question 26 *What are the benefits of proton resonance frequency shift-based magnetic resonance thermal imaging (PFRS-based MRTI)?*

Answer 26

PRFS-based MRTI is the most promising method to monitor three-dimensional temperature distributions during thermal therapy. It has been a successful approach in both EM and ultrasound heating therapy. PRFS-based MRTI has an accuracy of 1°C per 1 cm^3 of tissue in multiple slices obtained once per minute, at the least. It provides a precise measurement of volumetric temperature distribution to help gauge the heat focus in the tumor. This technique also shares data for treatment planning and feedback control of treatment delivery. Additionally, it provides a simultaneous real-time and posttreatment assessment of tissue damage that helps predict the clinical response of the patient. These benefits of PRFS-based MRTI greatly enhance the efficacy of clinical trials of hyperthermia.

Hall EJ, Giaccia AJ. Hyperthermia. In: Hall EJ, Giaccia AJ, eds. *Radiobiology for the Radiologist*. 7th ed. Philadelphia, PA: Lippincott Williams & Wilkins; 2006:490–511.

Question 27

What is thermal tumor ablation?

Question 28

How is thermal tumor ablation administered?

Question 29

Why is it important to identify the biomarkers of heating efficacy in hyperthermia?

Question 27 *What is thermal tumor ablation?*

Answer 27

Thermal tumor ablation is defined as the destruction of tissue by extreme hyperthermia. It is used primarily in the treatment of tumors of the liver, kidney, lung, bone, adrenal gland, or prostate. Tumors are heated at high temperatures (between 50°C and 100°C) at short intervals to ablate tumors. The heat is focused on the tumor and 5 to 10 mm of the surrounding tissue.

Brace C. Thermal tumor ablation in clinical use. *IEEE Pulse*. 2011;2(5): 28–38.

Hall EJ, Giaccia AJ. Hyperthermia. In: Hall EJ, Giaccia AJ, eds. *Radiobiology for the Radiologist*. 7th ed. Philadelphia, PA: Lippincott Williams & Wilkins; 2006:490–511.

Question 28 *How is thermal tumor ablation administered?*

Answer 28

The location and size of the tumor is identified and the applicator is inserted with the assistance of imaging. Next, the zone of ablation is determined; using follow-up imaging, the entire tumor with margins is included in the ablation zone. While surgical removal involves physical excision of the tumor, thermal ablation kills cancer tissue in situ and the dead tissue is then absorbed by the body. Thermal tumor ablation can be performed using open, laparoscopic, or endoscopic or percutaneous approaches.

Hall EJ, Giaccia AJ. Hyperthermia. In: Hall EJ, Giaccia AJ, eds. *Radiobiology for the Radiologist*. 7th ed. Philadelphia, PA: Lippincott Williams & Wilkins; 2006:490–511.

Brace C. Thermal tumor ablation in clinical use. *IEEE Pulse*. 2011;2(5):28–38.

Question 29 *Why is it important to identify the biomarkers of heating efficacy in hyperthermia?*

Answer 29

The efficacy of hyperthermia depends on whether or not the tumor is heatable. If the tumor does not receive sufficient heat, hyperthermia treatment may be ineffective. Therefore, identification of biomarkers is crucial in determining whether the patient will benefit from hyperthermia.

Hall EJ, Giaccia AJ. Hyperthermia. In: Hall EJ, Giaccia AJ, eds. *Radiobiology for the Radiologist*. 7th ed. Philadelphia, PA: Lippincott Williams & Wilkins; 2006:490–511.

27

STEM CELLS

HAIDONG HUANG AND JENNIFER S. YU

Question 1
What are stem cells and what are their roles in the body?

Question 2
What are totipotent, pluripotent, multipotent, and unipotent stem cells?

Question 3
What are embryonic stem (ES) cells?

Question 4
What are the main approaches for researchers to obtain mouse and human embryonic stem (ES) cells?

Turn page to see the answers.

Question 1 *What are stem cells and what are their roles in the body?*

Answer 1

Stem cells are specific cells in the body that have the potential to develop into many different cell types. Stem cells have two major important characteristics: self-renewal and differentiation. As stem cells divide, the daughter cells can either retain stem cell features or differentiate. Under certain physiological or experimental conditions, stem cells can differentiate into tissue- or organ-specific cells with special functions. Stem cells in the body produce cells to support tissue formation and function and replace aging or dead cells. Stem cells can also be stimulated after tissue injury to produce differentiated cells to repair or replace the damaged tissue.

Goodell MA, Nguyen H, Shroyer N. Somatic stem cell heterogeneity: diversity in the blood, skin and intestinal stem cell compartments. *Nat Rev Mol Cell Biol*. 2015;16:299–309.
Martello G, Smith A. The nature of embryonic stem cells. *Annu Rev Cell Dev Biol*. 2014;30:647–675.

Question 2 *What are totipotent, pluripotent, multipotent, and unipotent stem cells?*

Answer 2

These are all stem cells with the ability of self-renewal and differentiation, but they vary in their differentiation potential. Totipotent stem cells can differentiate into any cell type or give rise to an entire organism. The fertilized egg and cells produced by the first few divisions are totipotent. Pluripotent stem cells can differentiate into nearly all cells, but not an entire organism. Embryonic stem (ES) cells are a subtype of pluripotent stem cells. Multipotent stem cells are limited to differentiating into closely related families of cells, often from the same germ layer from which the stem cell was derived. Unipotent stem cells can differentiate into only one specific cell type.

Hans RS. The potential of stem cells: an inventory. In: Knoepffler N, Schipanski D, Sorgner SL, eds. *Human Biotechnology as Social Challenge*. Burlington, PA: Ashgate Publishing; 2007:chap 3; 28.

Question 3 *What are embryonic stem (ES) cells?*

Answer 3

ES cells are obtained from the inner cell mass in the mid-blastocyst stage (in the mouse, it is embryonic day 3.5 and in the human, it is 3 to 5 days after an egg cell is fertilized by a sperm). In normal development, the cells inside the inner cell mass are pluripotent and will produce all kinds of differentiated cells of tissues and organs in the entire body. These cells can be extracted and grown in vitro under specific conditions to retain the properties of ES cells.

Goodell MA, Nguyen H, Shroyer N. Somatic stem cell heterogeneity: diversity in the blood, skin and intestinal stem cell compartments. *Nat Rev Mol Cell Biol*. 2015;16:299–309.
Martello G, Smith A. The nature of embryonic stem cells. *Annu Rev Cell Dev Biol*. 2014;30:647–675.

Question 4 *What are the main approaches for researchers to obtain mouse and human embryonic stem (ES) cells?*

Answer 4

Mouse ES cells can be obtained by directly isolating the inner cell mass from mouse blastocyst (usually 10–20 cells per embryo). These cells can grow in the laboratory with the proper nutrients to keep their pluripotent ability. Human ES cells are also obtained from blastocyst stage embryos, which are created by in vitro fertilization in a petri dish.

Goodell MA, Nguyen H, Shroyer N. Somatic stem cell heterogeneity: diversity in the blood, skin and intestinal stem cell compartments. *Nat Rev Mol Cell Biol*. 2015;16:299–309.
Martello G, Smith A. The nature of embryonic stem cells. *Annu Rev Cell Dev Biol*. 2014;30:647–675.

Question 5
What are adult stem cells?

Question 6
How are adult stem cells identified?

Question 7
What are the main approaches for researchers to obtain adult stem cells?

Question 5 *What are adult stem cells?*

Answer 5

Adult stem cells are undifferentiated cells in adult animals that can self-renew and also give rise to differentiated cells. Adult stem cells have been identified in the brain, blood vessels, muscle, skin, teeth, and liver and therefore have their own names corresponding to their tissue origins (e.g., neural stem cells, muscle stem cells). Adult stem cells are thought to live in a specific niche in each tissue, where they either divide continuously to produce new cells to replace dead cells, or remain dormant for years, dividing and creating new cells as needed.

Goodell MA, Nguyen H, Shroyer N. Somatic stem cell heterogeneity: diversity in the blood, skin and intestinal stem cell compartments. *Nat Rev Mol Cell Biol*. 2015;16:299–309.

Martello G, Smith A. The nature of embryonic stem cells. *Annu Rev Cell Dev Biol*. 2014;30:647–675.

Question 6 *How are adult stem cells identified?*

Answer 6

To identify some cells as adult stem cells, scientists use both in vivo and in vitro methods. In vivo, through lineage tracing, these cells are labeled with molecular markers and the specialized cell types that they generate are determined. These cells can also be isolated and then transplanted into other normal animals, to determine whether the cells replace their tissue of origin, or into other animals without these stem cells, to determine whether the transplanted cells can form their tissue of origin.

In vitro, stem cell properties can be enriched using methods such as clonogenic assays, side population assays, and Aldefluor assay. Stem cells can also be enriched in vivo and in vitro by the expression of a distinctive set of markers including cell surface antigens and transcription factors. However, in vitro culture conditions can alter the phenotype. Some stem cell markers may not be expressed only in stem cells and so using a combination of several markers is needed to help identify stem cells. Functional validation should be performed with serial extreme limiting dilution in vivo. All these methods have their advantages and limitations and are often combined to identify stem cells.

Goodell MA, Nguyen H, Shroyer N. Somatic stem cell heterogeneity: diversity in the blood, skin and intestinal stem cell compartments. *Nat Rev Mol Cell Biol*. 2015;16:299–309.

Martello G, Smith A. The nature of embryonic stem cells. *Annu Rev Cell Dev Biol*. 2014;30:647–675.

Question 7 *What are the main approaches for researchers to obtain adult stem cells?*

Answer 7

Adult stem cells exist in special locations of many tissues and organs and can be obtained by many different methods. (a) Some stem cells can be isolated from the body directly. For example, blood stem cells can be taken from a donor's bone marrow, from blood in the umbilical cord, or from a person's circulating blood. Neural stem cells have been isolated from the brain and spinal cord. (b) Amniotic fluid contains a mixture of stem cells that have the ability to develop into skin, cartilage, cardiac tissue, nerves, muscle, and bone. (c) Some types of adult stem cells can be produced through inducing embryonic stem (ES) cells with particular chemical and mechanical factors. (d) Other adult stem cells can transform or differentiate into apparently unrelated cell types (e.g., brain stem cells that differentiate into blood cells). Although this transdifferentiation has been reported in animals, its mechanism is not clear and its application is very limited.

Cananzi M, Atala A, De Coppi P. Stem cells derived from amniotic fluid: new potentials in regenerative medicine. *Reprod Biomed Online*. 2009;18:17–27.

Question 8
What is asymmetric division of stem cells?

Question 9
What is a stem cell niche?

Question 10
What is the quiescent state of stem cells?

Question 8 *What is asymmetric division of stem cells?*

Answer 8

Stem cells can perform symmetric and asymmetric division when needed. In symmetric division, a stem cell produces two identical daughter cells, two stem cells, or two differentiated cells. An asymmetric stem cell division gives rise to two daughter cells with different fates, which may show differences in size, morphology, gene expression pattern, or the number of subsequent cell divisions. Some specific RNAs, proteins, metabolites, or cytoskeletons are asymmetrically distributed during or after asymmetric division, which instruct different cell fates. One of the daughter cells keeps the stem cell characteristics and the other forms a differentiated cell.

Knoblich JA. Mechanisms of asymmetric stem cell division. *Cell.* 2008;132:583–597.
Yamashita YM, Yuan H, Cheng J, Hunt AJ. Polarity in stem cell division: asymmetric stem cell division in tissue homeostasis. *Cold Spring Harb Perspect Biol.* 2010;2:a001313.

Question 9 *What is a stem cell niche?*

Answer 9

Stem cell populations in the tissue or organ are localized in specific anatomical areas called "niches." A stem cell niche is the local microenvironment that the stem cell directly contacts or indirectly interacts with, including adhesion molecules, extracellular matrix components, and other signaling factors from neighboring stem cells or differentiated cells (including differentiated tumor cells, blood vessels, immune infiltrates, and other stromal cells) that directly contact the stem cell surface to transduce signals into the stem cells. In addition, secreted factors from neighboring or distant cells diffuse around stem cells, enter stem cells, or bind to specific receptors on the stem cell. Other factors including oxygen tension and pH, ionic strength (e.g., Ca^{2+} concentration), and metabolites around stem cells are also important niche signals.

Morrison SJ, Spradling AC. Stem cells and niches: mechanisms that promote stem cell maintenance throughout life. *Cell.* 2008;132:598–611.
O'Brien LE, Bilder D. Beyond the niche: tissue-level coordination of stem cell dynamics. *Annu Rev Cell Dev Biol.* 2013;29:107–136.

Question 10 *What is the quiescent state of stem cells?*

Answer 10

Stem cells are undifferentiated, long-lived cells that support tissue integrity throughout the life of the organism, but they do not keep dividing and proliferating. Many adult stem cells are predominantly in a quiescent state, in which stem cells remain in the G_0 state until they are stimulated to divide. Quiescent stem cells are able to respond to stimuli that originate from their niche by activating and entering the cell cycle to resume proliferation and contribute to tissue regeneration or repair. The quiescent state is important for long-term maintenance of stem cells through many mechanisms that help to maintain the DNA integrity, such as the following: (a) Quiescent stem cells stay at the G_0 stage and avoid telomere shortening that occurs with each round of replication. (b) Cell proliferation may increase the level of reactive oxygen species (ROS); quiescent stem cells are metabolically inactive with lower generations of ROS, thereby reducing cell aging and damage. (c) Reduced DNA replication, which has low levels of error, contributes to DNA damage. Stem cell quiescence reduces DNA replication and damage and preserves genetic integrity.

Cheung TH, Rando TA. Molecular regulation of stem cell quiescence. *Nat Rev Mol Cell Biol.* 2013;14:329–340.

Question 11

What is stem cell aging? What factors cause or affect stem cell aging?

Question 12

What is stem cell therapy? What is the main procedure of stem cell therapy?

Question 13

What are the obstacles and risk factors associated with stem cell therapy?

Question 11 *What is stem cell aging? What factors cause or affect stem cell aging?*

Answer 11

Although stem cells are usually in a quiescent state, their life-long persistence in the body makes them particularly susceptible to the accumulation of cellular damage, which may change their stem cell state, affect stem cell capability, and ultimately lead to stem cell death, senescence, loss of regenerative function, or malignant transformation. Thus, stem cells in many tissues have been found to undergo profound changes with age, including a decline in their capability to renew themselves and produce differentiated cells, blunted response to tissue injury, and genetic/epigenetic changes that can be passed down to daughter cells, which could result in reduced cell replacement and tissue regeneration. Factors having effects on stem cell aging include: (a) random somatic mutations that accumulate in the long life of the stem cell, (b) loss of some of their histone and DNA methylation state during organism aging, and (c) alteration of stem cell niche factors (e.g., cytokine CCL11; inflammatory cytokine, Rantes; and other immune system-associated molecules, C1q, β2-microglobulin) during aging that affect stem cells' function.

Goodell MA, Rando TA. Stem cells and healthy aging. *Science*. 2015;350:1199–1204.
Oh J, Lee YD, Wagers AJ. Stem cell aging: mechanisms, regulators and therapeutic opportunities. *Nat Med*. 2014;20:870–880.

Question 12 *What is stem cell therapy? What is the main procedure of stem cell therapy?*

Answer 12

Stem cell therapy is the technology to use stem cells (adult or embryonic) or cells derived from stem cells to create living and functional tissues in vivo and in vitro to regenerate and repair tissue damage due to age, disease, and congenital defects. Embryonic stem (ES) cells or adult stem cells derived from either peripheral blood, cord blood, bone marrow, or any adult tissue are isolated, dissociated, and then cultured in specific media in the laboratory. These stem cells can be injected directly into patients or forced to differentiate into the required cell types before injection into the patient. These cells in the body can reach the site of injury/tissues in response to homing signals from the injured tissue.

Avior Y, Sagi I, Benvenisty N. Pluripotent stem cells in disease modelling and drug discovery. *Nat Rev Mol Cell Biol*. 2016;17:170–182.
Nadig RR. Stem cell therapy—Hype or hope? A review. *J Conserv Dent*. 2009;12:131–138.

Question 13 *What are the obstacles and risk factors associated with stem cell therapy?*

Answer 13

Some obstacles and risk factors should be considered during the stem cell therapy: (a) Ethical controversy: obtaining embryonic stem (ES) cells for therapy usually involves destruction of an embryo that could potentially become a viable organism. (b) Immune rejection: a donor's ES cells may be rejected by the patient's immune system. (c) Risk of teratoma: despite best efforts to differentiate stem cells prior to transplantation, a small fraction of stem cells may remain undifferentiated. These cells have the potential to transform into teratomas. (d) In vitro expansion and culture of stem cells can change the stem cell properties and cause unpredictable results after transplantation into the patient.

Avior Y, Sagi I, Benvenisty N. Pluripotent stem cells in disease modelling and drug discovery. *Nat Rev Mol Cell Biol*. 2016;17:170–182.
Nadig RR. Stem cell therapy—Hype or hope? A review. *J Conserv Dent*. 2009;12:131–138.

Question 14

What are induced pluripotent stem cells (iPSCs)?

Question 15

What are the major approaches to create induced pluripotent stem cells (iPSCs)?

Question 14 *What are induced pluripotent stem cells (iPSCs)?*

Answer 14

iPSCs are cells that have been reprogrammed in the lab from tissue-specific cells into an embryonic stem (ES) cell-like state by ectopic expression of specific combinations of transcription factors or treating with chemicals. Like pluripotent stem cells, iPSCs also express stem cell markers and can generate cells with characteristics of all three germ layers. Mouse iPSCs have been proven to be able to develop into many different tissue types when injected into mouse embryos at a very early stage.

Takahashi K, Yamanaka S. A decade of transcription factor-mediated reprogramming to pluripotency. *Nat Rev Mol Cell Biol*. 2016;17:183–193.

Yamanaka S. Induced pluripotent stem cells: past, present, and future. *Cell Stem Cell*. 2012;10:678–684.

Question 15 *What are the major approaches to create induced pluripotent stem cells (iPSCs)?*

Answer 15

iPSC technology has evolved rapidly since it was first developed in 2006. Approaches to generating iPSCs include use of viral vectors and chemical inducers. (a) Retroviral vectors are used to deliver reprogramming factors. The first generation of iPSCs used retroviral vectors to deliver reprogramming factors OCT3/4, SOX2, KLF4, and MYC (collectively referred to as OSKM). Retroviruses randomly integrate into the host genome and can alter the regulation of the reprogramming factors themselves or genes near the integration site. (b) Transient expression of reprogramming factors can be achieved with adenoviruses, plasmids, transposons, Sendai viruses, synthetic mRNAs, and recombinant proteins. (c) Chemical compounds can induce iPSCs when used alone or in combination with transcription factors to enhance the efficiency of generating iPSCs. These chemicals (RG108, 5-azacytidine; RG108, 5-azacytidine; MEK inhibitor PD035901; TGF-beta receptor inhibitor SB431542) affect chromatin modifications or influence signal transduction. (d) Defined media and matrix proteins can be used to generate and maintain human iPSCs.

Takahashi K, Yamanaka S. A decade of transcription factor-mediated reprogramming to pluripotency. *Nat Rev Mol Cell Biol*. 2016;17:183–193.

Yamanaka S. Induced pluripotent stem cells: past, present, and future. *Cell Stem Cell*. 2012;10:678–684.

Question 16

How can induced pluripotent stem cells (iPSCs) be used in medicine? What are some concerns about their use?

Question 17

What are cancer stem cells (CSCs)? What are the differences between cancer and normal stem cells?

Question 18

Why are cancer stem cells (CSCs) important therapeutic targets?

Question 16 *How can induced pluripotent stem cells (iPSCs) be used in medicine? What are some concerns about their use?*

Answer 16

iPSCs reprogrammed from normal individuals or patients carrying specific molecular defect(s) can be used broadly in medicine. (a) Organ synthesis and tissue repair: like normal stem cells, iPSCs can be induced to any type of cell in vivo or in vitro to replace or repair dysfunctional or injured tissues. (b) Disease modeling: somatic cells from patients are reprogrammed into iPSCs that are then induced to differentiate into the needed cell types and cultured in vitro. These cells can be used to discover mechanisms underlying the disease including genetic and epigenetic changes and dysregulation of signaling pathways. (c) Drug testing and drug discovery: iPSC-derived disease-specific cells or tissues can be used as models of that disease for drug screening. Because these cells are derived from humans, they can better represent physiological and phenotypic attributes than cells or tissues derived from animals, so they can be used to predict toxicology and therapeutic response to drugs.

There are some limitations and disadvantages associated with the use of iPSCs. (a) Generation of iPSCs often uses retroviral or lentiviral systems that may cause additional and unpredictable effects on the host genome. The use of small molecules to create iPSCs may reduce this risk. (b) Altered expression of reprogramming transcription factors used to create the iPSCs may cause disease. (c) iPSCs have the potential to form tumors. (d) Although iPSCs have the same genetic background as the diseased cells from which they are derived, they still have limitations in mimicking the in vivo physiological conditions for efficient drug testing and therapeutic target discovery.

Avior Y, Sagi I, Benvenisty N. Pluripotent stem cells in disease modelling and drug discovery. *Nat Rev Mol Cell Biol.* 2016;17:170–182.

Hirschi KK, Li S, Roy K. Induced pluripotent stem cells for regenerative medicine. *Annu Rev Biomed Eng.* 2014;16:277–294.

Singh VK, Kalsan M, Kumar N, Saini A, Chandra R. Induced pluripotent stem cells: applications in regenerative medicine, disease modeling, and drug discovery. *Front Cell Dev Biol.* 2015;3:1–18.

Question 17 *What are cancer stem cells (CSCs)? What are the differences between cancer and normal stem cells?*

Answer 17

CSCs, also known as cancer stem-like cells, tumor-initiating cells, or tumor-propagating cells, are a small subset of cells within the tumor that have a large capacity for self-renewal and give rise to more differentiated tumor cells. Both normal cells and CSCs may use common self-renewal pathways to maintain themselves and may share expression of some common markers. CSCs have tumorigenic activity and can form tumors when serially transplanted into animals. CSCs often carry genetic and epigenetic mutations that promote their survival.

Beck B, Blanpain C. Unravelling cancer stem cell potential. *Nat Rev Cancer.* 2013;13:727–738.

Nguyen LL, Vanner R, Dirks, P, Eaves CJ. Cancer stem cells: an evolving concept. *Nat Rev Cancer.* 2012;12:133–143.

Question 18 *Why are cancer stem cells (CSCs) important therapeutic targets?*

Answer 18

CSCs contribute to cancer relapse as they are more resistant to conventional chemotherapy and radiation therapy (RT) compared to differentiated tumor cells. Many CSCs are in a quiescent state and therefore are resistant to cytotoxic therapies that preferentially target highly proliferating tumor cells. CSCs also have high expression of drug efflux channels. CSCs can preferentially activate DNA-damage checkpoints so that they can repair DNA damage more efficiently after ionizing radiation. CSCs have more migratory and invasive potential and therefore facilitate metastasis. Some CSCs also reside within hypoxic niches, where they have reduced exposure to chemotherapy and render RT less efficacious.

Beck B, Blanpain C. Unravelling cancer stem cell potential. *Nat Rev Cancer.* 2013;13:727–738.

Magee JA, Piskounova E, Morrison SJ. Cancer stem cells: impact, heterogeneity, and uncertainty. *Cancer Cell.* 2012;21:283–296.

Question 19
How can cancer stem cells (CSCs) be targeted?

Question 20
What is the cancer stem cell (CSC) niche? How do these niches contribute to CSC properties?

Question 19 *How can cancer stem cells (CSCs) be targeted?*

Answer 19

There are two main strategies to target CSCs: (a) Promote differentiation of CSCs into terminal cancer cells that can more easily be treated with conventional cancer therapy. (b) Target CSC-specific pathways that are needed for their survival or maintenance. Antibodies and small molecules have been designed to target the CSC population.

Beck B, Blanpain C. Unravelling cancer stem cell potential. *Nat Rev Cancer*. 2013;13:727–738.
Magee JA, Piskounova E, Morrison SJ. Cancer stem cells: impact, heterogeneity, and uncertainty. *Cancer Cell*. 2012;21:283–296.

Question 20 *What is the cancer stem cell (CSC) niche? How do these niches contribute to CSC properties?*

Answer 20

CSC niches are anatomically distinct microenvironments surrounding CSCs. There are many kinds of cells in the niches that produce factors that maintain the undifferentiated state of stem cells, stimulate CSC self-renewal and proliferation, and promote tumor cell invasion and metastasis. (a) Cancer-associated fibroblasts (CAFs): CSCs and endothelial cells can produce factors that transform normal fibroblast cells into CAFs, which in turn activate stem cell programs including WNT and NOTCH pathways. (b) Mesenchymal stem cells (MSCs): MSCs are stromal cells that can secrete many factors including CXCL12, interleukin (IL) 6, and IL8, Gremlin 1 to promote cancer stemness. (c) Inflammatory cells: Several immunosuppressive cells, including tumor-associated macrophages (TAMs), tumor-associated neutrophils (TANs), and myeloid-derived suppressor cells (MDSCs), secrete cytokines to enhance CSC proliferation, migration, and invasion. (d) Hypoxia and angiogenesis: Hypoxia helps maintain CSCs through inhibition of immunosurveillance, enhancing resistance to chemotherapy and radiation therapy (RT), and may facilitate epithelial to mesenchymal transition (EMT) through reactive oxygen species. Endothelial cells can promote self-renewal of CSCs by direct cell–cell contact or by nitric oxide (NO) production via the NOTCH pathway.

Beck B, Blanpain C. Unravelling cancer stem cell potential. *Nat Rev Cancer*. 2013;13:727–738.
Plaks V, Kong N, Werb Z. The cancer stem cell niche: how essential is the niche in regulating stemness of tumor cells? *Cell Stem Cell*. 2015;16:225–238.

28

IMMUNOTHERAPY

NIKHIL JOSHI AND NEIL WOODY

Question 1

What are the components of the human immune system?

Question 2

What cell surface markers identify T cell, B cell, and natural killer (NK) cell components of the immune system?

Question 3

What are the names of some immune activating and immune inhibitory receptors on the T cell?

Question 4

What are the nonspecific host defense mechanisms included under innate immunity?

Question 1 *What are the components of the human immune system?*

Answer 1

The immune system broadly consists of the innate immune system and the adaptive immune system. The innate immune system includes a host of immune-related cells including macrophages, dendritic cells, mast cells, neutrophils, basophils, eosinophils, natural killer (NK) cells, T cells, and nonspecific host defenses. The adaptive immune system includes T cells, B cells, and antibodies against specific antigens. While the innate immune system works quickly, it lacks memory. The adaptive immune system is delayed in its initial response but is associated with memory. The response is quicker with repeated exposure to the same stimulus.

Warrington R, Watson W, Kim HL, Antonetti FR. An introduction to immunology and immunopathology. *Allergy Asthma Clin Immunol.* 2011;7(suppl 1):S1,1492-7-S1-S1.

Question 2 *What cell surface markers identify T cell, B cell, and natural killer (NK) cell components of the immune system?*

Answer 2

All Leukocytes: CD45
T Cell: T cell antigen receptor (TcR), which includes the signaling component CD3, CD5
Cytotoxic T Cell: CD8
Helper T Cell: CD4
B Cell: CD19, CD20, CD22, CD24, CD38
NK cell: CD16, CD30, CD31, CD38, CD56

Haynes BF, Soderberg KA, Fauci AS. Introduction to the immune system. In: Kasper D, Fauci A, Hauser S, et al., eds. *Harrison's Principles of Internal Medicine.* 19e. New York, NY: McGraw-Hill Education; 2015.

Question 3 *What are the names of some immune activating and immune inhibitory receptors on the T cell?*

Answer 3

Activating receptors include CD28, OX40, GITR, CD137, CD27, HVEM.
Inhibitory receptors include cytotoxic T-lymphocyte-associated protein 4 (CTLA-4), PD-1, TIM-3, BTLA, VISTA, LAG-3

Thaventhiran T, Sethu S, Yeang HXA, et al. T cell co-inhibitory receptors—functions and signalling mechanisms. *J Clin Cell Immunol.* 2012;3(suppl12):S12,004, 1–12.

Question 4 *What are the nonspecific host defense mechanisms included under innate immunity?*

Answer 4

Nonspecific host-defense barriers include anatomical barriers like the skin and mucous membrane. Physiological barriers include the body temperature that is regulated tightly, acidic pH of the stomach, bacterial lysozymes, interferons, and complement-mediated microbial lysis. Phagocytic/endocytic barriers include the process of endocytosis, monocytes, macrophages, and neutrophils. The inflammatory barrier involves leakage of vascular fluid containing serum proteins that have antibacterial activity.

Warrington R, Watson W, Kim HL, Antonetti FR. An introduction to immunology and immunopathology. *Allergy Asthma Clin Immunol.* 2011;7(suppl1):S1,1492-7-S1-S1.

Question 5
How do natural killer (NK) cells detect abnormal cells?

Question 6
What is one mechanism by which tumors evade natural killer (NK) cell detection?

Question 7
What is the basis for T cell adoptive immunotherapy? Name one example for its use.

Question 8
What is the role of local radiation in generating antitumor T cells?

Question 5 *How do natural killer (NK) cells detect abnormal cells?*

Answer 5

NK cells identify surface proteins on cells, specifically human leukocyte antigen (HLA) class I antigens, which are anti-activating antigens. In the absence of cell surface markers, NK cells do not induce cell death. In cases where HLA class I antigens are absent and activating antigens are present, NK cells attack the target cell. In cases where both HLA class I antigens and activating antigens are present, the balance of signals determines if the NK cell will attack. NK cells are both cytotoxic and capable of activating other components of the immune system. Tumors have been shown to secrete soluble NKG2D ligands, which are an activating antigen for NK cells. These soluble ligands make it difficult for NK cells to detect the abnormal tumor cells.

Lanier LL. NK cell recognition. *Annu Rev Immunol.* 2005;23:225–274.
Vivier E, Raulet DH, Moretta A, et al. Innate or adaptive immunity? The example of natural killer cells. *Science.* 2011;331:44–49.

Question 6 *What is one mechanism by which tumors evade natural killer (NK) cell detection?*

Answer 6

Tumors have been shown to secrete soluble NKG2D ligands, which are an activating antigen for NK cells. These soluble ligands make it difficult for NK cells to detect the abnormal tumor cells.

Vivier E, Raulet DH, Moretta A, et al. Innate or adaptive immunity? The example of natural killer cells. *Science.* 2011;331:44–49.

Question 7 *What is the basis for T cell adoptive immunotherapy? Name one example for its use.*

Answer 7

T cell adoptive immunotherapy is a technique in which T cells are cultured in laboratory to elicit an immune response to antigens. Either naturally occurring T cells or genetically engineered cells expressing chimeric antigen receptors (CARs) may be employed. When the cells are transferred to the patient the patient "adopts" the immune response to the antigen. An example is a CAR expressing T cell against CD19, a cell surface molecule found in almost all cases of B cell acute lymphoblastic leukemia (ALL). The CAR activates a signaling cascade in the immune effector T cell against the selected antigen.
A fundamental principle for T cell adoptive immunotherapy is that T cells activated via the T cell receptor alone are prone to anergy. Modern CARs involve costimulatory molecules. Some examples include CD28, OX40, and DAP10. Thus, a variety of targets can be selected to engineer CARs and use them for adoptive immunotherapy.

Fry TJ, Mackall CL. T-cell adoptive immunotherapy for acute lymphoblastic leukemia. Hematology. *Am Soc Hematol Educ Program.* 2013;2013:348–353.

Question 8 *What is the role of local radiation in generating antitumor T cells?*

Answer 8

Local radiation causes immunogenic cell death of cancer cells. This process promotes uptake and cross-presentation of tumor antigens by dendritic cells to T cells in the draining nodes. The tumor-derived DNA induces interferon beta production by the dendritic cell. These proimmunogenic signals result in increased immunogenic action against the tumor cells. Local radiation is also thought to improve T cell recruitment and infiltration into the tumor by reprogramming macrophages to secrete nitric oxide, leading to normalization of the vasculature and also via enhanced tumor secretion of chemokines like CXCL10 and CXCL16 that recruit CD 8+ T cells and VCAM-1 expression on the endothelium, which permits extravasation.

Demaria S, Golden EB, Formenti SC. Role of local radiation therapy in cancer immunotherapy. *JAMA Oncol.* 2015;1:1325–1332.

Question 9

What is ipilimumab? What is its mechanism of action?

Question 10

What is pembrolizumab? What is its mechanism of action?

Question 11

What role do dendritic cells play in suppression of immune response to tumors?

Question 12

How does Bacillus Calmette–Guerin (BCG) work as immunotherapy?

Question 9 *What is ipilimumab? What is its mechanism of action?*

Answer 9

Ipilimumab is a fully human IgG1, monoclonal antibody against cytotoxic T-lymphocyte-associated protein 4 (CTLA-4). CTLA-4 is an immune checkpoint protein receptor, which downregulates the action of cytotoxic T lymphocytes (CTL). By binding to the CTLA-4 receptor, ipilimumab prevents CTLA-4 from competing with CD28 for binding CD80/CD86. The resulting increased signaling through CD28 increases the cytotoxic T-lymphocytes response. This agent is used in metastatic melanoma.

Hodi FS, O'Day SJ, McDermott DF, et al. Improved survival with ipilimumab in patients with metastatic melanoma. *N Engl J Med.* 2010;363:711–723.

Question 10 *What is pembrolizumab? What is its mechanism of action?*

Answer 10

Pembrolizumab is a therapeutic antibody against PD-1. Programmed death 1 (PD-1) protein is an immune checkpoint receptor expressed by activated T cells that binds PD-1 ligands PD1-L1 (B7-H1) and PD1-L2 (B7-DC) expressed on tumor cells, thereby evading the immune system. Pembrolizumab blocks this interaction, thereby activating the immune system against the tumor cells. Another example is nivolumab.

Topalian SL, Hodi FS, Brahmer JR, et al. Safety, activity, and immune correlates of anti-PD-1 antibody in cancer. *N Engl J Med.* 2012;366:2443–2454.

Question 11 *What role do dendritic cells play in suppression of immune response to tumors?*

Answer 11

Dendritic cells can become tolerant to surrounding tumor cells within the microenvironment and may suppress an inflammatory response. Radiation therapy (RT) alone may be insufficient to reverse the tolerogenic effect of these dendritic cells. Toll-like receptor agonists may help to reverse this dendritic cell tolerance and allow RT to stimulate an immune response.

Adams S. Toll-like receptor agonists in cancer therapy. *Immunotherapy.* 2009;1:949–964.

Question 12 *How does Bacillus Calmette–Guerin (BCG) work as immunotherapy?*

Answer 12

BCG is a live attenuated preparation of *Mycobacterium bovis* (Calmette–Guerin strain). It acts by stimulating the Toll-like receptor 2 (TLR2) and Toll-like receptor 4 (TLR4) through its cell wall and peptidoglycans. The bacterial DNA also stimulates the Toll-like receptor 9 (TLR9) receptor. BCG is approved for Tis, T1, and Ta bladder cancer as adjuvant therapy after transurethral bladder resection.

Adams S. Toll-like receptor agonists in cancer therapy. *Immunotherapy.* 2009;1:949–964.
Lamm DL, Blumenstein BA, Crawford ED, et al. A randomized trial of intravesical doxorubicin and immunotherapy with Bacille Calmette-Guerin for transitional-cell carcinoma of the bladder. *N Engl J Med.* 1991;325:1205–1209.

Question 13

What is imiquimod? What is its mechanism of action, side-effect profile, and indication for usage?

Question 14

What is tasquinimod? What is its mechanism of action, side-effect profile, and indication for usage?

Question 15

What is talimogene laherparepvec (T-VEC) and what is its mechanism of action in melanoma cells?

Question 16

What is sipuleucel-T and what is its mechanism of action?

Question 13 *What is imiquimod? What is its mechanism of action, side-effect profile, and indication for usage?*

Answer 13

Imiquimod is a Toll-like receptor 7 (TLR7)-agonist often used as a topical cream. It results in upregulation of major histocompatibility complex (MHC) class I on tumor cells, recruitment of T cells into the tumor, enhancement of their effector function and mobilization of Langerhans cells and inflammatory DCs, as well as interleukin (IL)-17 production by dermal T cells. The side effects are mostly local (skin redness, burning sensation, dry skin, itching, skin breakdown, skin crusting or scabbing, skin drainage, skin flaking, etc.). It is used for superficial basal cell carcinomas (BCCs) and actinic keratosis.

Walter A, Schafer M, Cecconi V, et al. Aldara activates TLR7-independent immune defence. *Nat Commun*. 2013;4:1560–1572.

Question 14 *What is tasquinimod? What is its mechanism of action, side-effect profile, and indication for usage?*

Answer 14

Tasquinimod is an orally active quinoline-3-carboxamide. While the detailed mechanism of action remains unknown, it is believed that the drug acts via inhibition of angiogenesis by modulating the expression of thrombospondin-1 and downregulation of hypoxia inducible factor 1 alpha. It is used in metastatic castrate-resistant prostate cancer. The dose-limiting toxicity is amylase elevation without pancreatitis and sinus tachycardia.

Jennbacken K, Welen K, Olsson A, et al. Inhibition of metastasis in a castration resistant prostate cancer model by the quinoline-3-carboxamide tasquinimod (ABR-215050). *Prostate*. 2012;72:913–924.

Question 15 *What is talimogene laherparepvec (T-VEC) and what is its mechanism of action in melanoma cells?*

Answer 15

T-VEC is a genetically modified herpes simplex virus, type 1. This oncolytic virus preferentially replicates in cancer cells, resulting in lysis, release of new viral particles, tumor-associated antigens, and danger-associated molecular factors. The release of new viral particles causes continued infection of tumor cells. The local efflux of tumor antigens and danger signals can help promote an immune response, which is enhanced by viral expression of granulocyte macrophage colony-stimulating factor (GM-CSF).

Kohlhapp FJ, Kaufman HL. Molecular pathways: mechanism of action for talimogene laherparepvec, a new oncolytic virus immunotherapy. *Clin Cancer Res*. 2016;22(5):1048–1054.

Question 16 *What is sipuleucel-T and what is its mechanism of action?*

Answer 16

Sipuleucel-T is an active cellular immunotherapy agent used in the treatment of metastatic castration-resistant prostate cancer. It is a therapeutic cancer vaccine consisting of autologous peripheral-blood mononuclear cells, including antigen-presenting cells that have been activated ex vivo with a recombinant fusion protein (PA2024). PA2024 consists of a prostate antigen, prostatic acid phosphatase that is fused to granulocyte macrophage colony-stimulating factor, which acts as an immune-cell activator.

Kantoff PW, Higano CS, Shore ND, et al. Sipuleucel-T immunotherapy for castration-resistant prostate cancer. *N Engl J Med*. 2010;363:411–422.

Question 17

What is the abscopal effect? What are some examples of cancers that show the effect? What are the suggested mechanisms responsible for this effect?

Question 18

What is the pseudoabscopal effect?

Question 19

What are some mechanisms of immune suppression in the tumor microenvironment?

Question 20

What are the side effects of nivolumab/pembrolizumab and ipilimumab?

Question 17 *What is the abscopal effect? What are some examples of cancers that show the effect? What are the suggested mechanisms responsible for this effect?*

Answer 17

The abscopal effect is a rare clinical response to radiation therapy (RT) where tumor regression is noted at sites distant to the irradiated volume. This phenomenon is seen in renal cell carcinoma, melanoma, and hepatocellular carcinoma but can also be seen with other cancers, including neuroblastoma. Possible mechanisms include cytokine release, immune activation, enhanced immune recognition, and mounting an adaptive immune response. Three molecular signals are primarily responsible: the promotion of uptake of dying cells by dendritic cells, the cross-presentation of tumor-derived antigens to T cells, and the activation of antitumor T cells.

Siva S, MacManus MP, Martin RF, et al. Abscopal effects of radiation therapy: a clinical review for the radiobiologist. *Cancer Lett.* 2015;356:82–90.

Question 18 *What is the pseudoabscopal effect?*

Answer 18

The pseudoabscopal effect is an explanation offered for the abscopal effect noted in certain hematological malignancies. An example would be the abscopal effect seen in systemic bone marrow and peripheral blood as a result of cytotoxic effects on these circulating neoplastic cells passing through the irradiated spleen.

Siva S, MacManus MP, Martin RF, et al. Abscopal effects of radiation therapy: a clinical review for the radiobiologist. *Cancer Lett.* 2015;356:82–90.

Question 19 *What are some mechanisms of immune suppression in the tumor microenvironment?*

Answer 19

These include downregulation of major histocompatibility complex (MHC)-1, thus preventing cytotoxic T lymphocyte (CTL)-mediated killing; inhibition of CTL function through expression of PD-L1 and PD-L2, which interacts with PD-1 receptors on CTLs; secretion of HIF-1 alpha and IL-10, which in turn inhibits CTLs; and secretion of TGF beta, reactive oxygen species (ROS), reactive nitrogen intermediates (RNI), arginase, and nitric oxide synthase (NOS), which are enzymes that deplete l-arginine, an important metabolite for CTL function.

Vatner RE, Cooper BT, Vanpouille-Box C, Demaria S, Formenti SC. Combinations of immunotherapy and radiation in cancer therapy. *Front Oncol.* 2014;325:1–15.

Question 20 *What are the side effects of nivolumab/pembrolizumab and ipilimumab?*

Answer 20

These include autoimmune-like syndromes (colitis, optic neuritis, and endocrinopathies), fatigue, pruritus, and rash. The side effects seen with ipilimumab appear to be dose related while those associated with nivolumab/pembrolizumab are more or less the same regardless of the dose. Toxicities of PD-1 antibodies may vary with disease treated. Symptomatic pneumonitis is rare with ipilimumab, but PD-1 antibodies may cause more severe pneumonitis. Drug-related hepatitis is yet another rare but important complication.

Weber JS, Yang JC, Atkins MB, Disis ML. Toxicities of immunotherapy for the practitioner. *J Clin Oncol.* 2015;33:2092–2099.

Question 21

What is the mechanism of action of interferon alpha 2b for melanoma? What are the side effects?

Question 22

What is the mechanism of interleukin (IL)-2 for melanoma? What are the side effects?

Question 23

What are some glioblastoma multiforme (GBM) vaccine strategies that are currently being studied?

Question 21 *What is the mechanism of action of interferon alpha 2b for melanoma? What are the side effects?*

Answer 21

Interferon has diverse immunomodulatory effects on tumor cells, like direct antiproliferative effect, enhancement of natural killer (NK) cell activity, and the upregulation of tumor antigens and/or human leukocyte antigen (HLA) class I and class II antigens. Constitutional symptoms and neuropsychiatric manifestations including depression, myelosuppression, and hepatotoxicity are the major side effects. In the adjuvant Eastern Cooperative Oncology Group (ECOG) trial for interferon alpha 2b, two thirds of the patients had a grade 3 toxicity, 9% had life-threatening toxicity, and two patients died of hepatic failure.

Sabel MS, Sondak VK. Pros and cons of adjuvant interferon in the treatment of melanoma. *Oncologist*. 2003;8:451–458.

Question 22 *What is the mechanism of interleukin (IL)-2 for melanoma? What are the side effects?*

Answer 22

IL-2 antitumor activity is thought to be mediated by activation of natural killer (NK) cells to lymphokine-activated killing activity (LAK). Side effects include nausea, vomiting, anorexia, diarrhea, transaminitis, cholestasis, fever, chills, fatigue, increased vascular permeability, fluid retention, pulmonary edema, hypotension, and prerenal azotemia. Thrombocytopenia, anemia, coagulopathy, increased risk of catheter site infections, autoimmunity, neurotoxicity, and myocarditis are also known. High-dose IL-2 should be administered in an inpatient setting with close monitoring.

Jen EY, Poindexter NJ, Farnsworth ES, Grimm EA. IL-2 regulates the expression of the tumor suppressor IL-24 in melanoma cells. *Melanoma Res*. 2012;22:19–29.

Question 23 *What are some glioblastoma multiforme (GBM) vaccine strategies that are currently being studied?*

Answer 23

These include whole tumor cell vaccines (autologous, allogenic, and gene modified), dendritic cell vaccines (tumor pulsed, peptide/protein pulsed, or gene modified), protein vaccines, peptide vaccines, heat shock protein vaccine, and viral/bacterial vectors or plasmid DNA vaccines. A popular example of a peptide vaccine is the EGFRvIII vaccine directed against a single GBM-specific antigen.

Xu LW, Chow KK, Lim M, Li G. Current vaccine trials in glioblastoma: a review. *J Immunol Res*. 2014;796856 1–10.

Question 24

What is the role for adjuvant interferon alpha 2b for locally advanced cutaneous melanoma?

Question 25

What is the role of combination ipilimumab and nivolumab versus monotherapy alone for metastatic melanoma patients?

Question 24 *What is the role for adjuvant interferon alpha 2b for locally advanced cutaneous melanoma?*

Answer 24

The Eastern Cooperative Oncology Group (ECOG) EST 1684 trial showed a relapse-free and overall survival benefit with 52 weeks of subcutaneous interferon alpha 2b versus observation after surgery for stage IIB and stage III cutaneous melanoma patients after initial surgery. This included regionally recurrent melanoma patients at any interval provided they had surgery for their recurrence. A later update of this study, however, did not show a survival benefit.

Kirkwood JM, Strawderman MH, Ernstoff MS, Smith TJ, Borden EC, Blum RH. Interferon alfa-2b adjuvant therapy of high-risk resected cutaneous melanoma: the Eastern Cooperative Oncology Group trial EST 1684. *J Clin Oncol.* 1996;14:7–17.

Question 25 *What is the role of combination ipilimumab and nivolumab versus monotherapy alone for metastatic melanoma patients?*

Answer 25

The CheckMate 067 trial explored this question for unresectable stage III/IV melanoma and found that for PD-1 positive tumors, progression-free survival (PFS) was the same (14 months) for combination or nivolumab alone while for PD-1 negative tumors, PFS was longer for the combination versus nivolumab alone (11.2 months versus 5.3 months). Treatment-related adverse events were more likely in the combination group. PD-1 positivity was defined as at least 5% of tumor cells showing PD-L1 staining of any intensity on the cell surface in a section containing at least 100 tumor cells that could be evaluated.

Larkin J, Chiarion-Sileni V, Gonzalez R, et al. Combined nivolumab and ipilimumab or monotherapy in untreated melanoma. *N Engl J Med.* 2015;373:23–34.

29

RADIOGENOMICS

MOHAMED E. ABAZEED

Question 1
What is radiogenomics?

Question 2
What is precision medicine?

Question 3
What is the rationale for the genetic basis for the variation in normal tissue and tumor radiosensitivity?

Turn page to see the answers. **489**

Question 1 *What is radiogenomics?*

Answer 1

Radiogenomics refers to the study of genetic variation associated with normal tissue toxicity and tumor response after radiation therapy (RT). The goal is to measure associations between the genetic content of patients' germline and tumor DNA and normal tissue toxicity and tumor response, respectively. This could permit the prediction of radiation-related toxicity and/or the likelihood of tumor response prior to treatment delivery.

Andreassen CN, Schack LM, Laursen LV, Alsner J. Radiogenomics - current status, challenges and future directions. *Cancer Lett*, (2016). doi: 10.1016/j.canlet.2016.01.035.

Yard BD, Adams DJ, Chie EK, et al. A genetic basis for the variation in the vulnerability of cancer to DNA damage. *Nat Commun*. 2016;7:11428.

Question 2 *What is precision medicine?*

Answer 2

Precision medicine is a paradigm that medical decisions, practices, and/or products can be tailored to the individual patient. In radiation therapy (RT), the ability to predict normal tissue toxicity and/or tumor response using radiogenomics could result in greater precision of care or more personalized treatment regimens.

Yard B, Chie EK, Adams DJ, Peacock C, Abazeed ME. Radiotherapy in the era of precision medicine. *Semin Radiat Oncol*. 2015;25(4):227–236.

Question 3 *What is the rationale for the genetic basis for the variation in normal tissue and tumor radiosensitivity?*

Answer 3

There are significant differences in sequence alterations in the genome of patients and their tumors. The observation that there is significant heterogeneity in normal tissue and tumor radiosensitivity and this variation appears to be characterized by a continuous variable rather than falling into distinct bins of response strongly suggests a polygenetic basis for variation in normal tissue and tumor radiosensitivity. Moreover, there has been direct evidence that tumors can respond predictably to ionizing radiation based on their genetic content.

Andreassen CN. Can risk of radiotherapy-induced normal tissue complications be predicted from genetic profiles?. *Acta oncologica*. 2005;44(8):801–815.

Yard BD, *et al*. A genetic basis for the variation in the vulnerability of cancer to DNA damage. *Nat Commun* 7, 11428 (2016).

Question 4
What are the tools for measuring the genetic contents of patients and their tumors?

Question 5
Are there any definitive links between normal tissue toxicity and genetic changes?

Question 6.
What is a genome-wide association study (GWAS)?

Question 4 *What are the tools for measuring the genetic contents of patients and their tumors?*

Answer 4

A. Single nucleotide polymorphism (SNP): A single base substitution in which the least common allele has an abundance of 1% or more in the general population. SNPs account for approximately 90% of the interindividual sequence variation within human populations.

B. Transcriptomic profiling: The measurement of the full range of messenger RNA (mRNA) expressed in the cell.

C. Whole genome sequencing: The determination of the complete DNA sequence of a sample's genome.

D. Whole exome sequencing: The determination of the DNA sequence of the expressed genes of a sample's genome.

E. Epigenomics: The study of the functionally relevant changes to the genome that do not involve a change in the sequence of the DNA (e.g., DNA methylation or histone modification).

Garraway LA. Genomics-driven oncology: framework for an emerging paradigm. *J Clin Oncol.* 2013;31(15):1806–1814.

Question 5 *Are there any definitive links between normal tissue toxicity and genetic changes?*

Answer 5

Not to date. Almost all previously published associations between candidate single nucleotide polymorphisms (SNPs) in genes presumed to be related to the manifestation of acute and late radiation toxicity in healthy tissues appear to be false-positive associations. This underlies the high risk of overfitting and false-positive results.

Andreassen CN. A simulated SNP experiment indicates a high risk of over-fitting and false positive results when a predictive multiple SNP model is established and tested within the same dataset. *Radiother Oncol.* 2015;114(3):310–313.

Question 6 *What is a genome-wide association study (GWAS)?*

Answer 6

The GWAS measures the association between single nucleotide polymorphisms (SNPs) and an acute or delayed toxicity of interest. It is not a directed search informed by prior knowledge. Instead, it is an agnostic search for associations across the genome without any need for a prior understanding of the biology of toxicity. Although this method is thought to be more sensitive for identifying associations, there remains a substantial risk of overfitting and false discovery. These limitations can be partially addressed by adjusting the significance threshold.

Andreassen CN, Schack LM, Laursen LV, Alsner J. Radiogenomics - current status, challenges and future directions. *Cancer Lett,* (2016). doi: 10.1016/j.canlet.2016.01.035.

Question 7

What are the distributions of response after irradiation in cancer cell lines within most cancer types?

Question 8

Are there cancer type specific determinants of cancer's resistance or vulnerability to ionizing radiation?

Question 7 *What are the distributions of response after irradiation in cancer cell lines within most cancer types?*

Answer 7

Gaussian or normal distributions. This indicates that there is significant underlying biological diversity in the response of cancer cells to ionizing radiation and this diversity has been shown to be mediated mainly by the genetic content of these cells.

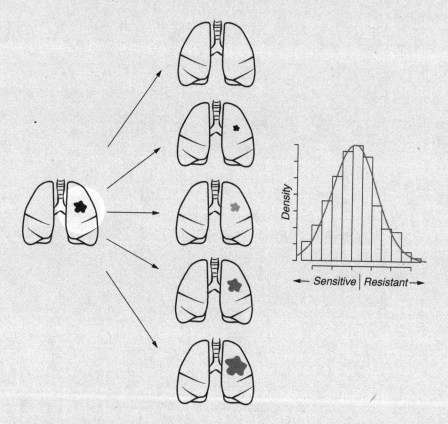

Source: Figure from Yard BD, *et al.* A genetic basis for the variation in the vulnerability of cancer to DNA damage. *Nat Commun* 7, 11428 (2016). With permission from Nature Publishing Group.

Question 8 *Are there cancer type specific determinants of cancer's resistance or vulnerability to ionizing radiation?*

Answer 8

Yes. For example, the androgen receptor confers resistance to radiation in prostate *and* breast cancer. The androgen receptor's messenger RNA (mRNA) is frequently elevated in both of these cancer types. Also, the antioxidant regulating transcription factor, Nrf2, confers resistance to radiation in cancers of the upper aerodigestive tract (head and neck, lung, and esophagus) and in liver cancer. The gene encoding Nrf2, *NFE2L2*, and the adaptor responsible for its degradation, encoded by *KEAP1*, are frequently genetically altered in these cancer types. Therefore, although heteregeneous, cancer genomes may have redundant genetic events that confer resistance to radiation therapy (RT). This may translate to the personalization of care based on stratification into genetically similar subpopulations rather than individual patients.

Abazeed ME, Adams DJ, Hurov KE, et al. Integrative radiogenomic profiling of squamous cell lung cancer. *Cancer Res.* 2013;73(20):6289–6298.

Yard BD, *et al.* A genetic basis for the variation in the vulnerability of cancer to DNA damage. *Nat Commun* 7, 11428 (2016).